T0362282

Chiari I Malformation

Editors

DAVID D. LIMBRICK, Jr
JEFFREY R. LEONARD

NEUROSURGERY
CLINICS OF NORTH AMERICA

www.neurosurgery.theclinics.com

Consulting Editors
RUSSELL R. LONSER
DANIEL K. RESNICK

January 2023 • Volume 34 • Number 1

ELSEVIER

1600 John F. Kennedy Boulevard • Suite 1800 • Philadelphia, Pennsylvania, 19103-2899

http://www.theclinics.com

NEUROSURGERY CLINICS OF NORTH AMERICA Volume 34, Number 1
January 2023 ISSN 1042-3680, ISBN-13: 978-0-323-93855-6

Editor: Stacy Eastman
Developmental Editor: Ann Gielou Posedio

© **2023 Elsevier Inc. All rights reserved.**

This periodical and the individual contributions contained in it are protected under copyright by Elsevier, and the following terms and conditions apply to their use:

Photocopying

Single photocopies of single articles may be made for personal use as allowed by national copyright laws. Permission of the Publisher and payment of a fee is required for all other photocopying, including multiple or systematic copying, copying for advertising or promotional purposes, resale, and all forms of document delivery. Special rates are available for educational institutions that wish to make photocopies for non-profit educational classroom use. For information on how to seek permission visit www.elsevier.com/permissions or call: (+44) 1865 843830 (UK)/(+1) 215 239 3804 (USA).

Derivative Works

Subscribers may reproduce tables of contents or prepare lists of articles including abstracts for internal circulation within their institutions. Permission of the Publisher is required for resale or distribution outside the institution. Permission of the Publisher is required for all other derivative works, including compilations and translations (please consult www.elsevier.com/permissions).

Electronic Storage or Usage

Permission of the Publisher is required to store or use electronically any material contained in this periodical, including any article or part of an article (please consult www.elsevier.com/permissions). Except as outlined above, no part of this publication may be reproduced, stored in a retrieval system or transmitted in any form or by any means, electronic, mechanical, photocopying, recording or otherwise, without prior written permission of the Publisher.

Notice

No responsibility is assumed by the Publisher for any injury and/or damage to persons or property as a matter of products liability, negligence or otherwise, or from any use or operation of any methods, products, instructions or ideas contained in the material herein. Because of rapid advances in the medical sciences, in particular, independent verification of diagnoses and drug dosages should be made.

Although all advertising material is expected to conform to ethical (medical) standards, inclusion in this publication does not constitute a guarantee or endorsement of the quality or value of such product or of the claims made of it by its manufacturer.

Neurosurgery Clinics of North America (ISSN 1042-3680) is published quarterly by Elsevier Inc., 360 Park Avenue South, New York, NY 10010-1710. Months of issue are January, April, July, and October. Business and Editorial Offices: 1600 John F. Kennedy Blvd., Suite 1800, Philadelphia, PA 19103-2899. Customer Service Office: 11830 Westline Industrial Drive, St. Louis, MO 63146. Periodicals postage paid at New York, NY, and additional mailing offices. Subscription prices are $451.00 per year (US individuals), $821.00 per year (US institutions), $484.00 per year (Canadian individuals), $1,019.00 per year (Canadian institutions), $562.00 per year (international individuals), $1,019.00 per year (international institutions), $100.00 per year (US students), $255.00 per year (international students), and $100.00 per year (Canadian students). International air speed delivery is included in all *Clinics* subscription prices. All prices are subject to change without notice. **POSTMASTER:** Send address changes to *Neurosurgery Clinics of North America*, Elsevier Periodicals Customer Service, 11830 Westline Industrial Drive, St. Louis, MO 63146. **Customer Service: 1-800-654-2452 (US and Canada). From outside the US and Canada, call: 1-314-453-7041. Fax: 1-314-453-5170. E-mail: JournalsCustomerService-usa@elsevier.com (for print support) and journalsonlinesupport-usa@elsevier.com (for online support).**

Reprints. For copies of 100 or more, of articles in this publication, please contact the Commercial Reprints Department, Elsevier Inc., 360 Park Avenue South, New York, NY 10010-1710. Tel. 212-633-3874; Fax: 212-633-3820; E-mail: reprints@elsevier.com.

Neurosurgery Clinics of North America is covered in *MEDLINE/PubMed (Index Medicus), EMBASE/Excerpta Medica, and Current Contents/Clinical Medicine (CC/CM).*

Contributors

CONSULTING EDITORS

RUSSELL R. LONSER, MD
Professor and Chair, Department of
Neurological Surgery, The Ohio State
University Wexner Medical Center, Columbus,
Ohio, USA

DANIEL K. RESNICK, MD, MS
Professor and Vice Chairman, Program
Director, Department of Neurosurgery,
University of Wisconsin-Madison School of
Medicine and Public Health, Madison,
Wisconsin, USA

EDITORS

DAVID D. LIMBRICK, Jr, MD, PhD
T.S. Park Chair and Chief of Pediatric
Neurosurgery, Executive Vice Chair of
Neurological Surgery, Washington University
School of Medicine, Neurosurgeon-in-Chief,
St. Louis Children's Hospital, St Louis,
Missouri, USA

JEFFREY R. LEONARD, MD
Chief, Neurosurgery, Division of Neurological
Surgery, Fellowship Director, The Robert F.
and Edgar T. Wolfe Foundation Endowed Chair
in Neurosurgery, Nationwide Children's
Hospital, Professor, Department of
Neurological Surgery, The Ohio State
University College of Medicine, The Ohio State
University Wexner Medical Center, Columbus,
Ohio, USA

AUTHORS

RICHARD C. E. ANDERSON, MD
Department of Neurological Surgery,
Hassenfeld Children's Hospital, NYU Langone
Health, New York, New York, USA

SYED HASSAN ABBAS AKBARI, MD, MSCI
Johns Hopkins School of Medicine, Johns
Hopkins All Children's Hospital, St Petersburg,
Florida, USA

KENAN I. ARNAUTOVIĆ, MD, PhD
Department of Neurosurgery, Semmes
Murphey Neurologic and Spine Institute,
The University of Tennessee Health
Science Center, Memphis, Tennessee,
USA

ALISA ARNAUTOVIĆ, BS
George Washington University School of
Medicine, Washington, DC, USA

DIANE J. AUM, MD
Resident Physician, Department of
Neurosurgery, Washington University,
Washington University School of Medicine, St
Louis, Missouri, USA

ULRICH BATZDORF, MD
Professor of Neurosurgery, Department of
Neurosurgery, David Geffen School of
Medicine at UCLA, Los Angeles, California,
USA

AKSHAY BHAMIDIPATI, MS
School of Medicine, Vanderbilt University,
Nashville, Tennessee, USA

WALEED BRINJIKJI, MD
Departments of Neurosurgery and Radiology,
Mayo Clinic, Rochester, Minnesota,
USA

DOUGLAS L. BROCKMEYER, MD
Department of Neurosurgery, University of Utah, Division of Pediatric Neurosurgery, Intermountain Primary Children's Hospital, Salt Lake City, Utah, USA

ARINDAM R. CHATTERJEE, MD
Department of Neurological Surgery, Mallinckrodt Institute of Radiology, Department of Neurology, Washington University School of Medicine, St Louis, Missouri, USA

SARAH N. CHIANG, BS
Department of Neurological Surgery, Washington University School of Medicine, St Louis, Missouri, USA

SILKY CHOTAI, MD
Resident Physician, Department of Neurosurgery, Vanderbilt University Medical Center, Nashville, Tennessee, USA

MICHAEL J. COOLS, MD
Monroe Carell Jr. Children's Hospital at Vanderbilt University Medical Center, Nashville, Tennessee, USA

JEREMY K. CUTSFORTH-GREGORY, MD
Department of Neurology, Mayo Clinic, Rochester, Minnesota, USA

SOMNATH DAS, MD
Neurological Surgery; University of Alabama, Birmingham, Alabama, USA

YOSEF M. DASTAGIRZADA, MD
Department of Neurological Surgery, Hassenfeld Children's Hospital, NYU Langone Health, New York, New York, USA

BRIAN J. DLOUHY, MD
Associate Professor of Neurosurgery and Pediatrics, University of Iowa Hospitals & Clinics, University of Iowa Stead Family Children's Hospital, Iowa City, Iowa, USA

MEGHAN ELLINGTON
Department of Medical and Molecular Genetics, Indiana University School of Medicine, Indianapolis, Indiana, USA

FARAZ FARZAD, BA
University of Virginia School of Medicine, Charlottesville, Virginia, USA

CLAIR A. FRANCOMANO, MD
Professor, Department of Medical and Molecular Genetics, Indiana University School of Medicine, Indianapolis, Indiana, USA

JAKUB GODZIK, MD
Department of Neurological Surgery, The University of Alabama, Birmingham, Alabama, USA

GABE HALLER, PhD
Assistant Professor of Neurosurgery, Department of Neurosurgery, Washington University, St Louis, Missouri, USA

TODD C. HANKINSON, MD
Department of Neurological Surgery, University of Colorado School of Medicine, Aurora, Colorado, USA

JOHN D. HEISS, MD
Head, Clinical Unit, Surgical Neurology Branch, National Institute of Neurological Diseases and Stroke, National Institutes of Health, Bethesda, Maryland, USA

KATHERINE G. HOLSTE, MD
Department of Neurosurgery, University of Michigan, Ann Arbor, Michigan, USA

BERMANS J. ISKANDAR, MD
Department of Neurological Surgery, University of Wisconsin-Madison, University of Wisconsin Hospital and Clinics, Madison, Wisconsin, USA

JOHN A. JANE Jr, MD
Department of Neurological Surgery, University of Virginia Health System, Charlottesville, Virginia, USA

JEREMY Y. JONES, MD
Assistant Professor, Pediatric Radiology, Department of Radiology, Nationwide Children's Hospital, Columbus, Ohio, USA

MICHAEL KELLY, MD
Department of Orthopedic Surgery, Rady Children's Hospital, San Diego, California, USA

RAHUL KUMAR, MD, PhD
Department of Neurosurgery, Mayo Clinic, Rochester, Minnesota, USA

DAVID B. KURLAND, MD, PhD
Department of Neurological Surgery, Hassenfeld Children's Hospital, NYU Langone Health, New York, New York, USA

DAVID C. LAUZIER, BS
Department of Neurological Surgery,
Washington University School of Medicine,
St Louis, Missouri, USA

JEFFREY R. LEONARD, MD
Chief, Neurosurgery, Division of Neurological
Surgery, Fellowship Director, The Robert F.
and Edgar T. Wolfe Foundation Endowed Chair
in Neurosurgery, Nationwide Children's
Hospital, Professor, Department of
Neurological Surgery, The Ohio State
University College of Medicine, The Ohio State
University Wexner Medical Center, Columbus,
Ohio, USA

DAVID D. LIMBRICK, Jr, MD, PhD
T.S. Park Chair and Chief of Pediatric
Neurosurgery, Executive Vice Chair of
Neurological Surgery, Washington University
School of Medicine, Neurosurgeon-in-Chief,
St. Louis Children's Hospital, St Louis,
Missouri, USA

CORMAC O. MAHER, MD
Department of Neurosurgery, University of
Michigan, Ann Arbor, Michigan,
USA

ZIYAD MAKOSHI, MBBS, MSC, FRCSC
Division of Neurological Surgery, Nationwide
Children's Hospital, Columbus, Ohio,
USA; Division of Neurosurgery, The Ottawa
Hospital, 1053 Carling Avenue, Ottawa,
Ontario, Canada

ALEXANDRIA C. MARINO, MD, PhD
Department of Neurological Surgery, University
of Virginia Health System, University of Virginia
Health Sciences Center, Charlottesville,
Virginia, USA

AARON S. MCALLISTER, MS, MD
Assistant Professor, Pediatric Radiology,
Department of Radiology, Nationwide
Children's Hospital, Columbus, Ohio,
USA

ARNOLD H. MENEZES, MD
Professor of Neurosurgery and
Pediatrics, University of Iowa Hospitals &
Clinics, University of Iowa Stead Family
Children's Hospital, Iowa City, Iowa,
USA

NISHIT MUMMAREDDY, MD
Department of Neurological Surgery,
Vanderbilt University Medical Center,
Nashville, Tennessee, USA

KARIN M. MURASZKO, MD
Department of Neurosurgery, University of
Michigan, Ann Arbor, Michigan,
USA

JOSHUA W. OSBUN, MD
Department of Neurological Surgery,
Mallinckrodt Institute of Radiology,
Department of Neurology, Washington
University School of Medicine, St Louis,
Missouri, USA

LINDSAY S. PETRACEK, BSC
Research Assistant, Department of Pediatrics,
Division of Adolescent and Young Adult
medicine, The Johns Hopkins University
School of Medicine, Baltimore Maryland, USA

JONATHAN PINDRIK, MD
Associate Professor of Neurological Surgery,
The Ohio State Department of Neurological
Surgery, Division of Pediatric Neurosurgery,
Nationwide Children's Hospital, Columbus,
Ohio, USA

MIRZA POJSKIĆ, MD
Department of Neurosurgery, University of
Marburg, Marburg, Germany; Faculty of
Medicine, Josip Juraj Strossmayer University,
Osijek, Croatia

VIJAY M. RAVINDRA, MD, MSPH
Department of Neurosurgery, Naval Medical
Readiness Training Command, Department of
Neurosurgery, University of California San
Diego, San Diego, California, USA; Department
of Neurosurgery, University of Utah, Salt Lake
City, Utah, USA

PETER C. ROWE, MD
Professor, Department of Pediatrics, Division
of Adolescent and Young Adult medicine, The
Johns Hopkins University School of Medicine,
Baltimore Maryland, USA

BROOKE SADLER, PhD
Assistant Professor of Pediatrics, Department
of Pediatrics, Washington University, St Louis,
Missouri, USA

CHEVIS N. SHANNON, DrPH, MBA, MPH, MERC
Department of Neurosurgery, The University of Alabama at Birmingham, Birmingham, Alabama, USA

LAUREN STONE, MD
Department of Orthopedic Surgery, University of California, San Diego, San Diego, California, USA

JENNIFER M. STRAHLE, MD
Associate Professor of Neurological Surgery, Orthopedic Surgery, and Pediatrics, Director, Pediatric Neuro-Spine Program, Associate Professor, Department of Neurosurgery, Washington University, Washington University School of Medicine, Saint Louis Children's Hospital, St Louis, Missouri, USA

JOHN C. WELLONS III, MD, MSPH
Monroe Carell Jr. Children's Hospital at Vanderbilt University Medical Center, Nashville, Tennessee, USA

ALEXANDER T. YAHANDA, MD, MPHS
Department of Neurological Surgery, Washington University School of Medicine, St Louis, Missouri USA

Contents

The current nomenclature of Chiari malformations includes the standard designations, Chiari 1–4, which were described by Hans Chiari in the late nineteenth century, and more recent additions, Chiari 0, 0.5, and 1.5, which emerged when the standard nomenclature failed to include important anatomical variations. The authors describe these entities and propose that to best optimize clinical care and research, it would be wise to place less focus on the eponyms and more effort on developing a descriptive or pathophysiological nomenclature.

Chiari I malformation is a common condition seen by adult and pediatric neurosurgeons. With increased utilization of MRI over time, incidental findings of Chiari I malformation are occurring more frequently. The prevalence of symptomatic Chiari I malformation is much smaller than that of asymptomatic Chiari I malformation. The prevalence of Chiari I malformation-associated syringomyelia is likely overestimated in the literature. The epidemiology of Chiari I malformation and associated syringomyelia differs based on age, sex, ethnicity, race, and socioeconomic status. The natural history of Chiari I malformation and associated syringomyelia appears to be quite benign as few patients who are managed nonsurgically later require surgical intervention.

Socioeconomic and demographic factors affect the care of patients with Chiari I malformations. This article describes the current cost of surgical treatment of Chiari I malformations and highlights how careful patient selection, treatment selection, postoperative protocols, and varying payment models may serve as cost-reducing measures. In addition, the article highlights racial disparities resulting in delayed diagnosis and greater disease progression in non-white patients, as well as the relative parity in the workup and treatment of Chiari I malformation based on insurance status. These findings illustrate the need for greater access to neurosurgical care and greater outreach to community physicians by the neurosurgical community.

Chiari 1 malformation (CM1) includes a spectrum of clinical manifestations. These signs and symptoms result from compression at the cervicomedullary junction and alteration in cerebrospinal fluid dynamics thus affecting several structures above, at, and below the cervicomedullary junction. Differences in presentation exist among different age groups and high clinical suspicion should be present in younger children. Additionally, CM1 can be associated with other diagnoses and can have unusual acute presentations that should be recognized to ensure excellent outcomes.

Sleep-disordered breathing (SDB) is a frequent symptomatic feature of pediatric Chiari I, reported in at least 24% of patients presenting to neurosurgeons. Here the epidemiology, natural history, pathophysiology, and diagnosis of SDB in Chiari I is reviewed. Diagnosis requires polysomnography, which should be pursued in young or symptomatic patients or those with prominent imaging findings. Review of case series of surgical decompression suggest that surgical decompression can improve SDB in selected patients.

Individuals with Chiari malformation can present with symptoms of fatigue, light-headedness, and syncope—the cardinal features of orthostatic intolerance. Similar orthostatic symptoms can complicate the clinical course following Chiari decompression. The presence of orthostatic intolerance in patients with Chiari malformation is not surprising given the location of the major circulatory control centers and their pathways in the brainstem. This article reviews the normal physiologic response to upright posture and the common forms of orthostatic intolerance encountered in clinical practice. The authors describe the relationship between orthostatic intolerance and Chiari malformation and provide suggestions regarding the evaluation and management of these disorders.

Several studies have been performed to elucidate the genetic basis of Chiari I malformation (CM1). The heritability of CM1 is clear from twin studies, familial clustering, and the prevalence of CM1 among certain classes of Mendelian disorders, namely connective tissue disorders, brain overgrowth disorders, disorders of CSF homeostasis, certain tumors, disorders of skull development and vascular conditions. A comprehensive understanding of the causes of CM1 will require large cohorts of patients for genetic studies and in-depth phenotyping of cases to better understand the biological mechanisms underlying disease.

The heritable disorders of connective tissue (HDCTs) are a heterogeneous group of inherited disorders caused by pathogenic variants in genes encoding a wide range of molecules involved in the structure and function of the extracellular matrix. Currently, more than 450 HDCTs are recognized. These include the Ehlers-Danlos syndrome (EDS), Marfan syndrome, Loeys-Dietz syndrome (LDS), Stickler syndrome, and a wide range of skeletal dysplasias. Recent evidence suggests that people with the HDCTs are at an increased risk of Chiari I malformation (CM1).

Imaging in Chiari I Malformation   67

Jonathan Pindrik, Aaron S. McAllister, and Jeremy Y. Jones

Chiari I Malformation represents a hindbrain anomaly best demonstrated radiographically with MRI. Brain and spine MRI provide optimal anatomic detail of cerebellar tonsillar descent below the foramen magnum and may reveal additional imaging features including ventriculomegaly (potentially leading to the diagnosis of hydrocephalus), characteristics of intracranial hypertension or hypotension, spinal cord syrinx, scoliosis, and/or tethered spinal cord. Specialized imaging sequences provide enhanced visualization of ventral and dorsal cervicomedullary cisterns and cerebrospinal fluid flow. Although these studies contribute critical information for evaluation, their impact on surgical decision-making remains uncertain. Additional radiographic measures (pBC2 and clival-axial angle) may impact surgical planning and risk assessment.

Cerebrospinal Fluid Hydrodynamics in Chiari I Malformation and Syringomyelia: Modeling Pathophysiology   81

John D. Heiss

Anatomic MRI, MRI flow studies, and intraoperative ultrasonography demonstrate that the Chiari I malformation obstructs CSF pathways at the foramen magnum and prevents normal CSF movement through the foramen magnum. Impaired CSF displacement across the foramen magnum during the cardiac cycle increases pulsatile hindbrain motion, pressure transmission to the spinal subarachnoid space, and the amplitude of CSF subarachnoid pressure waves driving CSF into the spinal cord. Central canal septations in adults prevent syrinx formation by CSF directly transmitting its pressure wave from the fourth ventricle to the central canal

Adult Chiari Malformation Type I: Surgical Anatomy, Microsurgical Technique, and Patient Outcomes   91

Alisa Arnautovic, Mirza Pojskić, and Kenan I. Arnautović

 Video content accompanies this article at http://www.neurosurgery.theclinics.com.

In this study, the authors summarize the current knowledge on epidemiology, demographics, risk factors, and prognostic factors that influence outcomes in patients with adult Chiari malformation type I (CM-I) who underwent posterior fossa decompression surgery with duraplasty. Furthermore, they describe the contribution of their research group to the field of adult CM-I treatment, including the association of increased body mass index with severity of CM-I and syringomyelia, relevant surgical anatomy, and surgical technique of 270° microsurgical decompression of foramen magnum. The authors also report on common complications in the literature and describe techniques for prevention of complications.

Posterior fossa decompression (PFD) with/without duraplasty is the standard surgical treatment for symptomatic CM-1. Posterior fossa decompression without duraplasty (PFD) may be associated with shorter operative times and hospital stays, fewer complications, and may yield improvements in symptoms and syrinx sizes. Posterior fossa decompression with duraplasty (PFDD) may be associated with superior long-term symptomatic improvements, larger syrinx reductions, and a lower need for revision decompression. Various dural graft materials may be used for PFDD, though the ideal type of graft has not been definitively established. Other adjunct surgical procedures may be added to PFD/PFDD given certain symptomatic or anatomical considerations.

Surgery is the treatment of choice for symptomatic patients with Chiari anomalies Although the surgical treatment of Chiari anomalies in adults is a straightforward procedure, complications and less than satisfactory outcomes do occur. Understanding these complications is important for correcting the problem as well as preventing the recurrence of similar problems. In this article, the author review the short-term and long-term complications associated with posterior fossa decompression for Chiari malformation.

Craniovertebral junction (CVJ) abnormalities are associated with the Chiari malformation type I. These abnormalities may lead to ventral brainstem compression which can be reduced with traction and posterior reduction using instrumentation. In other cases, the irreducible CVJ pathology with persistent ventral brainstem compression requires ventral decompression. In all cases, a posterior extradural or extra-intradural decompression is required along with an occipitocervical fusion to maintain the reduced and realigned CVJ or stabilize the CVJ after a ventral decompression.

Studies have documented that 1% to 4% of patients undergoing MRI of the brain or cervical spine will be diagnosed with Chiari Malformation I. More recently, CM have been described as a spectrum of disease (Chiari 0, 1.5, complex). Craniocervical junction instability may be more prevalent in certain Chiari phenotypes. Despite the very low incidence of CVJ instability in the CMI population at large, clinicians must be aware of the important radiographic and clinical factors that are associated with various versions of Chiari malformations so the best clinical management decisions can be made.

The term "complex Chiari malformation" (CCM) refers to a subset of clinical and radiographic findings that describe a subpopulation of Chiari patients with craniocervical kyphosis and secondary brainstem compression. These patients are at a greater risk for unsuccessful surgical treatment with standard Chiari surgical decompressive procedures and may require craniocervical fusion and/or odontoid resection. This article reviews concepts related to the diagnosis, management, and treatment of CCM and discusses possible directions for future research.

The management of scoliosis in patients with Chiari I malformation and syringomyelia is a complex decision-making process, which is changing due to evolving evidence. Headache and scoliosis are common presenting symptoms of an underlying Chiari. History, physical examination, and screening with MRI are cornerstones of diagnosis. Posterior fossa decompression provides curve stabilization or regression in about half of patients. In those who require spinal fusion, careful attention must be paid to intraoperative neurological monitoring data to minimize risk of neurologic injury.

CM-I-associated syringomyelia is a risk factor for scoliosis where a larger syrinx size is more likely to be associated with scoliosis. Therefore, the effect of syrinx on scoliosis progression may be alleviated by PFD. There is no difference in the need for fusion surgery between patients undergoing PFD with duraplasty vs. those undergoing extradural decompression; however, PFD with duraplasty is associated with an improvement in curve magnitude compared to extradural decompression alone. Further study on the comparison of PFD techniques for this cohort of patients is needed. PFD is a durable surgical option for patients with CM-I, syrinx, and scoliosis. Early decompression of CM-I in younger patients and those with smaller curve magnitude at presentation is recommended as there is a higher likelihood of halting curve progression.

The purpose of this article was to consider, evaluate, and compare the clinical outcomes measurement tools that are used to assess patients with Chiari I malformation. This article highlights the variety of general and disease-specific outcome measures used in both the pediatric and adult Chiari I malformation patient populations. Although general measures can be associated with clinical outcomes and quality of life, that association is not often found to be statistically significant, and they do not often have the capabilities to assess and measure factors that directly impact the Chiari patient population. However, limitations exist when considering the disease-specific outcome measures, as these tools most often have not been rigorously evaluated externally from the initial validation or have been externally validated but results cannot be replicated. Identifying an outcomes measurement tool for both adults and patients will contribute to the clinical tools available to providers for decision-making and management.

Mounting evidence has suggested a relationship between Chiari I malformation and idiopathic intracranial hypertension, with some studies implicating anomalies of the cerebral venous system in the development of these conditions. However, precise mechanisms explaining these associations are not well described. There is a clear need to clarify the interplay between these conditions to guide further study in this area. In tandem with these efforts, it is necessary to review proper diagnosis and management to improve outcomes in patients suffering from these diseases.

Spontaneous intracranial hypotension (SIH) occurs secondary to cerebrospinal fluid (CSF) hypovolemia in the setting of noniatrogenic spinal CSF leak. Although orthostatic headache is characteristic, atypical presentations can occur. Cranial imaging can disclose characteristic imaging features of SIH but spinal imaging is needed for leak localization. Although advanced diagnostic workup and treatment depend on the type of CSF leak, differentiation of SIH from other headache pathologic conditions, such as Chiari I malformation, is crucial to prevent misdiagnosis and ineffective treatment.

NEUROSURGERY CLINICS OF NORTH AMERICA

SERIES OF RELATED INTEREST

Neurologic Clinics
https://www.neurologic.theclinics.com/
Neuroimaging Clinics
https://www.neuroimaging.theclinics.com/

THE CLINICS ARE AVAILABLE ONLINE!
Access your subscription at:
www.theclinics.com

NEUROSURGERY CLINICS OF NORTH AMERICA

FORTHCOMING ISSUES

April 2023
Ablative Therapies in Neurosurgery
Peter Nakaji and Oliver Bozinov, editors

July 2023
Meningioma
Randy L. Jensen and Gabriel Zada, editors

October 2023
Spinal Deformity Update
Sigurd Berven and Praveen V. Mummaneni,
editors

RECENT ISSUES

October 2022
Update on Open Vascular Surgery
Michael T. Lawton, Editor

July 2022
Pain Management
Joshua M. Rosenow and Julie G. Pilitsis, Editors

April 2022
Recent Advances in Endovascular
Neurosurgery
Elad I. Levy, Adnan H. Siddiqui, and Justin M.
Cappuzzo, Editors

SERIES OF RELATED INTEREST

Neurologic Clinics
https://www.neurologic.theclinics.com/

Neuroimaging Clinics
https://www.neuroimaging.theclinics.com/

THE CLINICS ARE AVAILABLE ONLINE!
Access your subscription at:
www.theclinics.com

Preface
Advances in the Field of Chiari I Malformation and Integrating Them into Clinical Practice

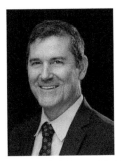 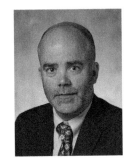

David D. Limbrick, Jr, MD, PhD   Jeffrey R. Leonard, MD
Editors

The field of Chiari type 1 malformation (CM-1) presents an interesting contrast between the past and the future. The diagnosis itself is steeped in history and irrevocably tied to the initial classification schema described by Hans Chiari in 1891. Meanwhile, leading-edge work in genetics, dynamic imaging, patient-oriented research, and other advances is driving the future of the field. This issue of *Neurosurgery Clinics of North America*, entitled "Chiari I Malformation," reconciles the vast chasm between past and future of this commonly encountered disorder.

Far more than simply an update of the previous issue on this topic in 2015, "Chiari I Malformation" addresses head-on the nosology of CM-1 and the intersection of epidemiology and disparities in care among disadvantaged groups. In addition to expert reviews of clinical features and current and emerging radiologic tools, the articles contained herein consider next-level complexity in the management of CM-1, including ventral brainstem compression, craniovertebral junction instability, and spinal deformity. Emerging strategies to evaluate and treat comorbid idiopathic intracranial hypertension and cerebrospinal fluid (CSF) leaks are also discussed.

This issue of *Neurosurgery Clinics of North America* also provides a state-of-the-field analysis of the pathophysiology of CM-1, from the genetic basis of CM-1 and its relationship to various comorbidities to CSF hydrodynamics and pulsatility. Notably, controversies regarding the management of dysautonomia and postural intolerance and the putative role of heritable disorders of connective tissue are discussed in detail by true content experts.

We would like to conclude by thanking each of the contributing authors for sharing their accumulated knowledge, experience, and wisdom. This work is built on the shoulders of giants, such as Ed Oldfield, and we hope that you find this collection valuable as you build expertise in this complex disease and its contemporary management.

Sincerely,

David D. Limbrick Jr, MD, PhD
Washington University School of Medicine
St. Louis Children's Hospital

Jeffrey R. Leonard, MD
Neurosurgery
Nationwide Children's Hospital
Neurological Surgery
The Ohio State University School of Medicine
Columbus, OH 43205, USA

E-mail addresses:
limbrickd@wustl.edu (D.D. Limbrick)
jeffrey.leonard@nationwidechildrens.org
(J.R. Leonard)

Neurosurg Clin N Am 34 (2023) xv
https://doi.org/10.1016/j.nec.2022.10.001
1042-3680/23/© 2022 Published by Elsevier Inc.

The Nomenclature of Chiari Malformations

Michael J. Cools, MD[a],*, John C. Wellons III, MD, MSPH[a], Bermans J. Iskandar, MD[b,c]

KEYWORDS

• Chiari malformation • Nomenclature • Category • Naming • Cerebellar tonsils

KEY POINTS

• The standard nomenclature of Chiari malformations comprises 4 types: Chiari 1–4, originally described by Hans Chiari, and which consist of congenital abnormalities of posterior fossa structures.
• Chiari 1 is the most common type, which consists of a tonsil position >5 mm below the foramen magnum and can cause syringomyelia.
• Chiari 2 represents herniation of all posterior fossa structures (brainstem, vermis, and fourth ventricle) in spina bifida patients.
• Chiari 3 and 4 are rare posterior fossa abnormalities that are distinct from Chiari 1 and 2 and are probably multifactorial.
• Recently, variations on Chiari I have emerged, including Chiari 0, 0.5, and 1.5, implying that tonsillar descent may not be the only defining pathology.
• Since these are vastly disparate entities with no common pathophysiology, shifting from the Chiari eponym to a more descriptive nomenclature may help guide clinical management and research efforts.

INTRODUCTION

Hans Chiari first described the malformation that bears his name in 1891, starting with a report of a 17-year-old girl with hydrocephalus and a "cone-shaped projection" of the cerebellar tonsil with descent into the cervical spinal canal.[1–3] In the subsequent articles, he characterized the malformation into three types. The type 1 malformation consisted of "elongation of the cerebellar tonsils and medial parts of the inferior lobes of the cerebellum into cone-like projections, which accompany the medulla oblongata into the spinal canal."[2,4] The type 2 malformation comprised displacement of parts of the cerebellum and elongated fourth ventricle into a widened cervical spinal canal. Chiari later amended his description to include displacement of the cerebellar vermis, pons, and medulla, in addition to elongation of the fourth ventricle.[4] The type 3 malformation, represented by only one example, consisted of herniation of cerebellar tissue through the foramen magnum and into a hydromyelocele in the upper cervical spine.[4] Lastly, the type 4 malformation comprised a parietal encephalocele, hydrocephalus, and hypoplasia of the cerebellum.[5,6]

There was disagreement about nomenclature even in Chiari's time. Students of Julius Arnold noted that Arnold had described a Chiari 2 malformation before Chiari's description, and thus dubbed this malformation an Arnold-Chiari malformation.[7,8] In addition, the Chiari 4 malformation has been used to describe several different malformations, from cerebellar hypoplasia without the

[a] Monroe Carell Jr. Children's Hospital at Vanderbilt University Medical Center, 2220 Children's Way, Suite 9226, Nashville, TN 37232, USA; [b] Department of Neurological Surgery, University of Wisconsin at Madison, Madison, WI, USA; [c] University of Wisconsin Hospital and Clinics, 600 Highland Avenue, K4/832, Madison, WI 53792, USA
* Corresponding author.
E-mail address: michaeljcools@gmail.com
Twitter: @michaeljcools (M.J.C.)

Neurosurg Clin N Am 34 (2023) 1–7
https://doi.org/10.1016/j.nec.2022.08.003
1042-3680/23/© 2022 Elsevier Inc. All rights reserved.

Table 1 Current definitions of Chiari malformations		
Chiari 1		**Caudal Descent of the Cerebellar Tonsils by 5 mm or 3-5 mm Below McRae's Line**
	Chiari 0	Syrinx without other identifiable cause that responds to posterior fossa decompression; no tonsillar descent
	Chiari 0.5	Ventrolateral herniation of cerebellar tonsils anterior to a horizontal line drawn through the middle of the caudal medulla at the level of the foramen magnum
	Chiari 1.5	Caudal descent of the cerebellar tonsils with associated descent of the brainstem with obex at or below McRae's Line
Chiari 2		Descent of the cerebellar vermis and brainstem into the upper cervical canal Must be associated with myelomeningocele
Chiari 3		Caudal descent of the medulla and cerebellar herniation into a posterior defect of bifid upper cervical spine with resultant encephalocele
Chiari 4		Cerebellar hypoplasia in association with an occipital encephalocele

parietal encephalocele to the Dandy–Walker malformation.[6] More recently, newer "subtypes" of the Chiari malformations have been proposed, including Chiari 0,[9] Chiari 0.5,[10] Chiari 1.5,[11] and Chiari 3.5 (**Table 1**).[12] The proliferation of these subtypes and questions about their clinical importance has led to calls for a consistent and descriptive nomenclature.[6,13] In this review, we discuss the nomenclature and its implications on management.

CHIARI 1

The Chiari 1 malformation is defined as descent of the cerebellar tonsils by more than 5 mm below McRae's line, which stretches from basion to opisthion (**Fig. 1**).[6,14,15] The cutoff of 5 mm was first proposed by Aboulezz, and colleagues,[16] who conducted an MRI study of patients with Chiari 1 malformations and normal controls in 1985. The authors found that, although in normal subjects the tonsils extended as low as 3 mm below the foramen magnum, they reached at least 5 mm in most patients with symptomatic Chiari 1.[16] In a subsequent study, the MRIs of 25 patients with symptomatic Chiari 1 malformation were compared with 200 patients undergoing MRI for unrelated symptoms.[17] Nearly all patients with a symptomatic Chiari 1 malformation had tonsils that were caudally displaced at least 5 mm, compared with none of the controls, reporting a sensitivity of 92% and specificity of 100% for the 5 mm cutoff in symptomatic Chiari 1

malformations.[17] Although these studies were both limited by small sample sizes and retrospective design, the cutoff of 5 mm became widely used in the radiology literature as the defining criterion for a Chiari 1 malformation.

Over time, neurosurgeons recognized that many asymptomatic individuals had tonsillar herniation exceeding 5 mm. Indeed, MRI studies comprising sample sizes in the thousands later showed that tonsillar descent >5 mm occurred frequently, with a range of 0.7%–0.9% in the general pediatric population, depending on the study.[18,19] Although a 1997–1998 study of 5,248 consecutive pediatric MRI scans at Kaiser Permanente Medical Care Program in northern California in 1997–1998 identified only 58 Chiari 1 malformations,[20] a 2011 study of 14,116 pediatric MRI scans at the University of Michigan revealed a Chiari 1 incidence of 3.6%.[21] Other authors proposed using the appearance of "pegged" tonsils as pathologic,[14,22] but this pegged appearance was also noted in 1% of asymptomatic patients.[23]

Chiari 1 malformations can cause syringomyelia, which is a recognized indication for Chiari decompression surgery.[20,21] In the Kaiser study, 6 of the 58 Chiari 1 patients had syringomyelia (12%),[20] whereas the Michigan study reports syringomyelia in 117 of the 509 Chiari 1 patients (23%).[21] Although the Kaiser study does not report the number of patients with Chari 1 malformation who underwent total spine imaging,[20] the Michigan study notes that only 50% of patients with Chiari 1 patients had spinal MRIs,[21] thus

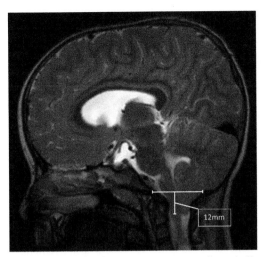

Fig. 1. Chiari 1 malformation. Descent of cerebellar tonsils into the cervical spinal canal without caudal descent of the brainstem.

potentially under-reporting the incidence of syringomyelia in this patient population. Of course, the reported incidence of syringomyelia is much higher in surgical Chiari 1 series ranging between 57% and 65%,[24–26] likely because of a surgical referral bias.

CHIARI 0

Starting with EJ Newton[27] and beyond, multiple theories of pathogenesis of Chiari-related syringomyelia have been advanced, all agreeing that diminution of CSF flow at the foramen magnum seems to be causative.[28] In 1998, Iskandar and colleagues[29] described five patients who presented with syringomyelia without tonsillar herniation who responded to posterior fossa decompression, which came to be known as a Chiari 0 malformation. Their patients all had improvement in clinical symptoms and a decrease in syrinx size.[29] In a subsequent article with 10 additional patients, the authors showed similar findings, showing postoperative syrinx improvement in 9 patients, and stabilization in 1.[9] Kyoshima and colleagues[30] similarly described their experience with four patients with syringomyelia without tonsillar descent that improved after posterior fossa decompression, which they termed "tight cisterna magna."

It later became evident that patients with a Chiari type 0 malformation, whereas they lack tonsillar herniation, seem to have MRI evidence of other more subtle posterior fossa structural abnormalities, including the location of the obex below the level of the foramen magnum, indicating caudal descent of the brainstem,[9,29] an enlarged anterior-posterior brainstem diameter at the level of the foramen magnum on sagittal imaging, and

an increase in the basion to opisthion distance compared with normal controls.[9,29,31] A study of adult patients with Chiari-like symptoms without tonsillar descent revealed a shorter clivus and increased tentorial angle compared with controls.[32] Interestingly, a familial link was reported between Chiari 0 and Chiari 1, identifying five families in which the Chiari 1 proband had a first-degree relative with Chiari 0.[33] Further assessment of affected individuals showed similar clinical and radiological features between Chiari 0 and Chiari 1 individuals, although Chiari 1 patients in general had more severe symptoms and skull base abnormalities than their Chiari 0 relatives. Both groups showed improvement in symptoms and/or syrinx size following craniocervical decompression surgery.[33] Importantly, a minority of patients revealed intraoperatively a veil or adhesions at the foramen magnum as the cause of flow obstruction, and which were not evident on preoperative imaging.

The challenge with the Chiari 0 diagnosis, which keeps it controversial, is our inability to distinguish Chiari 0 from true idiopathic syringomyelia. Although a lower position of the obex and other structural variations noted above, along with crowding of the subarachnoid spaces at the foramen, may be suggestive of Chiari 0[9,30] the only reliable distinguishing feature is the response to posterior fossa decompression (postoperative resolution of the syrinx indicates Chiari 0 pathophysiology). This means that at least for now, Chiari 0 is a postoperative diagnosis, and remains a diagnosis of exclusion, in that all other causes of syringomyelia and symptoms need to be carefully ruled out, including tumor, arachnoiditis, tethered cord, and trauma. It is hoped that further investigations into CSF flow and subtle structural anomalies at the foramen magnum may, in time, provide stronger diagnostic criteria. In addition, further insight into the genetics of this disease process may provide ways to identify Chiari 0 patients early on.

CHIARI 0.5

Recently, Morgenstern and colleagues[10] described a condition in which tonsils are displaced ventrally around the spinal cord, and termed this entity ventral herniation or Chiari 0.5. They retrospectively reviewed all patients presenting to their institution over a 7-year period for Chiari 1 decompression, and found that those who presented with ventral herniation of the tonsils had higher rates of dysphagia, sleep apnea, and behavioral problems compared with the typical Chiari 1 patients.[10] However, most of their patients also met the criteria for a Chiari 1 malformation, with a mean tonsillar descent of 6.5 mm,[10] similar

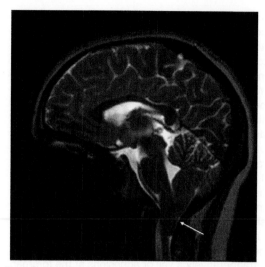

Fig. 2. Chiari 1.5. Note the significant tonsillar descent, as well as the descent of the brainstem and associated position of the obex (*arrow*) below the level of the foramen magnum.

to a case report by Tubbs and colleagues[34] in 2013, describing lateral compression of the brainstem in a patient with Chiari 1 and syringomyelia that improved after posterior fossa decompression.[34] As the Morgenstern and Tubbs articles imply, whereas the concept of ventral herniation of the tonsils is clinically important as an association with tonsillar descent, leading us to consider it a Chiari 1 variant, it is unclear whether any patients have ventral herniation without tonsillar descent, ie, a variant Chiari 0, which could in this case be given the designation of Chiari 0 or Chiari 0.5.

CHIARI 1.5

The Chiari 1.5 malformation was reported in 2004 by Tubbs, and colleagues in patients whose tonsils extended >5 mm below the foramen magnum with accompanying caudal descent of the brainstem (ie, obex located below the foramen magnum) (**Fig. 2**). The terminology of Chiari 1.5 was chosen because descent of both cerebellum and brainstem is reminiscent of Chiari 2 anatomy. Of course, unlike Chiari 2, Chiari 1.5 patients do not have spina bifida and lack common anatomical manifestations of Chiari 2, such as herniation of the vermis and supratentorial anomalies.[6,11,35,36]

The true incidence of Chiari 1.5 malformations is unknown, as large-scale population studies do not differentiate between a Chiari 1 and a 1.5.[23,37] In a description of 150 symptomatic Chiari 1 patients that required surgery, 17% met the criteria for a Chiari 1.5.[25] Despite caudal descent of the brainstem, presenting symptoms appear to be similar to Chiari 1, with no symptoms specifically

attributed to brainstem dysfunction.[6,11] Treatment outcomes, however, may differ between Chiari 1 and 1.5. In a single-center series, Tubbs and colleagues[11,25] reported a 13.6% rate of re-exploration due to persistent syringomyelia in patients with Chiari 1.5, twice the rate of Chiari 1. In addition, Chiari 1.5 may be associated with an increased risk of chronic craniocervical instability requiring occipitocerivcal fusion.[38]

CHIARI 2

In 1894, Julius Arnold described a myelodysplastic patient in whom the fourth ventricle and cerebellum had herniated through the foramen magnum.[7,39] Chiari described a similar case in 1895, and later refined his description to caudal displacement of the vermis, pons, and medulla into the upper cervical spinal canal with elongation of the fourth ventricle.[1,7] Although two of Arnold's students, Schwalbe and Gredig, gave this abnormality the name "Arnold-Chiari malformation,"[8,40] Chiari termed it a Chiari 2 malformation, an eponym preferred by many.[7] The Chiari 2 represents a completely separate entity from Chiari 1, in imaging, clinical findings, indications for surgery, and etiology, and is defined as caudal descent of the cerebellar vermis, brainstem, and fourth ventricle (**Fig. 3**). Importantly, it is seen exclusively in patients with myelomeningocele.[7] Many anatomical MRI findings accompany Chiari 2, including low attachment of the tentorium with steep angle, beaked tectum, large massa intermedia, and enlarged foramen magnum.[41–43] By virtue of the medullary distortion, Chiari 2 patients present with lower brainstem dysfunction including stridor[44–46] impaired airway protection, and generalized hypotonia,[44–46] similar to the youngest Chiari 1 patients, but unlike the majority of older Chiari 1 patients, who present with headaches and other symptoms unrelated to brainstem function.

The cause of Chiari 2 in myelomeningocele remains elusive. Many theories have been proposed,[42,43,47] with the most accepted being the unified hypothesis described by McLone and Knepper, in which *in utero* leakage of CSF results in lack of dilation of the primitive ventricles, resulting in hindbrain herniation.[47] This theory is supported by indirect evidence that prenatal closure of myelomeningocele decreases the occurrence of Chiari 2. In the prospective, randomized Management of Myelomeningocele Study (MOMS), 36% of patients undergoing prenatal repair had no hindbrain herniation, compared with only 4% of patients whose myelomeningoceles were closed postnatally.[48] Grabb and colleagues[49] reported similar results in their retrospective series,

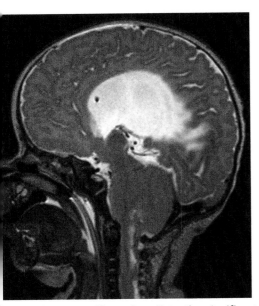

Fig. 3. Chiari 2 malformation. Note the significant tonsillar descent, as well as descent of the pons and medulla. Torcula is low and tectum is beaked.

additionally finding that no patients closed prenatally had significant brainstem dysfunction, compared with 25% of those closed postnatally.[49]

CHIARI 3 AND 3.5

The Chiari 3 malformation is defined as herniation of the posterior fossa contents through a dorsal defect in the lower occipital or upper cervical spine, or a posterior fossa encephalocele.[50–52] This is a rare entity, with only approximately 60 cases reported in the literature.[51,53] The pathophysiology of the lesion remains unclear, with various explanations being proposed, including hydrocephalus with pressure coning, altered CSF dynamics, and failure of induction of endochondral bone leading to an encephalocele physiology.[53,54]

A single variant of the Chiari 3, the so-called Chiari 3.5, was initially described by Giuseppe Muscatello (1866–1951) in 1894.[6,12] This child had multiple congenital abnormalities, including the absence of cervical vertebrae, dura mater that did not extend into the spinal canal, and a fistulous tract between the fourth ventricle and the esophagus. An updated description of this case was presented by Fisahn and colleagues[12] in 2016 and was termed Chiari 3.5. There has only been one documented case of this type of malformation.

CHIARI 4

The Chiari malformation type 4 was described by Hans Chiari in 1895. The main anatomical features included an occipital encephalocele with herniation of the bilateral occipital lobes with hypoplasia of the cerebellum and absence of the tentorium cerebelli.[6] Other types of malformations have since been labeled as Chiari 4 malformations, and many contemporary sources identify a Chiari 4 as simply hypoplasia of the cerebellum.[6,55] It is likely that this malformation is multi-factorial, as both genetic developmental problems and teratogenic insults (eg, phenytoin) can cause cerebellar hypoplasia.

DISCUSSION

The Chiari malformations share only one feature: their location in the posterior fossa. It may be time to remove the eponymic designations and re-configure the nomenclature toward a more descriptive and embryologically relevant terminology.

It seems evident, for example, that Chiari 3 and 4 are anatomical manifestations of varying genetic, teratogenic, or developmental disease processes, and thus may benefit from descriptive or etiological nomenclature. On the contrary, Chiari 2 represents a preventable hindbrain distortion from an open neural tube defect. Of course, although Chiari 1 is the index malformation that occupies a prominent position in a majority of pediatric neurosurgical practices, its pathophysiology remains unresolved. If future study reveals that tonsillar descent is a secondary manifestation of a single genetic or developmental disease process rather than a primary problem with tonsil growth and development, then one would imagine that Chiari 0, 0.5, and 1.5 are but a continuum of the same condition, and which could use re-classification based on severity. Alternatively, if Chiari 1 proves to be a secondary manifestation to multiple congenital and acquired abnormalities (ie, multi-factorial), then the eponymic classification would lose its diagnostic value toward etiological designations. For example, whereas some Chiari 1 malformations are associated with craniocervical abnormalities (platybasia, basilar invagination, etc.), others are not. Notably, although the majority of Chiari 1 malformations are considered developmental, others are acquired, and can be caused by intracranial mass lesions on one end, or prolonged lumbar drainage on the other.[56,57] In addition, Chiari 1 malformations of identical severity on imaging may lead to severe symptoms in some, and no symptoms in others.

Our community's embrace of evidence-based medicine, modern imaging, and basic science in the service of patient care in the past decades positions us to lead the research that would answer these critical questions in the next decade. Thus, although our understanding of these disparate entities has advanced considerably since Professor Chiari first described them, the most exciting era lies ahead. All we need is a commitment to open mind, frank dialogue, and rigorous science.

CLINICS CARE POINTS

- The Chiari malformations are pathophysiological distinct abnormalities of posterior fossa structures.
- The existing nomenclature has been useful for neurosurgeons to define the field and advance clinical care to date, but further advances in diagnosis and treatment would benefit from a more descriptive and pathophysiological re-classification scheme.

DISCLOSURE

The authors have nothing to disclose.

REFERENCES

1. Tubbs RS, Cohen-Gadol AA. Hans Chiari (1851–1916). J Neurol 2010;257(7):1218–20.
2. Chiari H. Ueber Veranderungen des Kleinhirns infolge von Hydrocephalie des Grosshirns. Dt *Deutsche Medizinische Wochenschrift* 1891;17:1172–5.
3. Chiari H. Concerning alterations in the cerebellum resulting from cerebral hydrocephalus. Pediatr Neurosurg 1987;13(1):3–8.
4. Koehler PJ. Chiari's description of cerebellar ectopy (1891): with a summary of Cleland's and Arnold's contributions and some early observations on neural-tube defects. J Neurosurg 1991;75(5):823–6.
5. Tubbs RS, Demerdash A, Vahedi P, et al. Chiari IV malformation: correcting an over one century long historical error. Child's Nerv Syst 2016;32(7):1175–9.
6. Haddad FA, Qaisi I, Joudeh N, et al. The newer classifications of the chiari malformations with clarifications: An anatomical review. Clin Anat 2018;31(3):314–22.
7. Tubbs RS, Oakes WJ. The Chiari Malformations. Published online 2013:5-11. doi:10.1007/978-1-4614-6369-6_2
8. Carmel PW, Markesbery WR. Early descriptions of the Arnold-Chiari malformation: the contribution of John Cleland. J Neurosurg 1972;37(5):543–7.
9. Chern JJ, Gordon AJ, Mortazavi MM, et al. Pediatric Chiari malformation Type 0: a 12-year institutional experience: Clinical article. J Neurosurg Pediatr 2011;8(1):1–5.
10. Morgenstern PF, Tosi U, Uribe-Cardenas R, et al. Ventrolateral tonsillar position defines novel chiari 0.5 classification. World Neurosurg 2020;136:444–53.
11. Tubbs RS, Iskandar BJ, Bartolucci AA, et al. A critical analysis of the Chiari 1.5 malformation. J Neurosurg Pediatr 2004;101(2):179–83.
12. Fisahn C, Shoja MM, Turgut M, et al. The Chiari 3.5 malformation: a review of the only reported case. Child's Nerv Syst 2016;32(12):2317–9.
13. Dellen JR van. Chiari malformation: an unhelpful eponym. World Neurosurg 2021;156:1–3.
14. McClugage SG, Oakes WJ. The Chiari I malformation: JNSPG 75th anniversary invited review article. J Neurosurg Pediatr 2019;24(3):217–26.
15. Headache classification committee of the international headache society (IHS) the international classification of headache disorders, 3rd edition. Cephalalgia 2018;38(1):1–211.
16. Aboulezz AO, Sartor K, Geyer CA, et al. Position of cerebellar tonsils in the normal population and in patients with chiari malformation. J Comput Assist Tomogr 1985;9(6):1033–6.
17. Barkovich AJ, Wippold FJ, Sherman JL, et al. Significance of cerebellar tonsillar position on MR. AJNR Am J Neuroradiol 1986;7(5):795–9.
18. Jansen PR, Dremmen M, Berg A van den, et al. Incidental findings on brain imaging in the general pediatric population. N Engl J Med 2017;377(16):1593–5.
19. Sullivan EV, Lane B, Kwon D, et al. Structural brain anomalies in healthy adolescents in the NCANDA cohort: relation to neuropsychological test performance, sex, and ethnicity. Brain Imaging Behav 2017;11(5):1302–15.
20. Aitken LA, Lindan CE, Sidney S, et al. Chiari type I malformation in a pediatric population. Pediatr Neurol 2009;40(6):449–54.
21. Strahle J, Muraszko KM, Kapurch J, et al. Chiari malformation Type I and syrinx in children undergoing magnetic resonance imaging: clinical article. J Neurosurg Pediatr 2011;8(2):205–13.
22. Tubbs RS, Lyerly MJ, Loukas M, et al. The pediatric Chiari I malformation: a review. Child's Nerv Syst 2007;23(11):1239–50.
23. Smith BW, Strahle J, Bapuraj JR, et al. Distribution of cerebellar tonsil position: implications for understanding Chiari malformation: Clinical article. J Neurosurg 2013;119(3):812–9.
24. Tubbs RS, Beckman J, Naftel RP, et al. Institutional experience with 500 cases of surgically treated pediatric Chiari malformation Type I: Clinical article. J Neurosurg Pediatr 2011;7(3):248–56.
25. Tubbs RS, McGirt MJ, Oakes WJ. Surgical experience in 130 pediatric patients with Chiari I malformations. J Neurosurg 2003;99(2):291–6.
26. Milhorat TH, Chou MW, Trinidad EM, et al. Chiari I malformation redefined: clinical and radiographic

findings for 364 symptomatic patients. Neurosurgery 1999;44(5):1005–17.

27. Newton EJ. Syringomyelia as a manifestation of defective fourth ventricular drainage. Ann Roy Coll Surg 1969;44(4):194–213.

28. Rusbridge C, Greitz D, Iskandar BJ. Syringomyelia: current concepts in pathogenesis, diagnosis, and treatment. J Vet Intern Med 2006;20(3):469–79.

29. Iskandar BJ, Hedlund GL, Grabb PA, et al. The resolution of syringohydromyelia without hindbrain herniation after posterior fossa decompression. Neurosurg Focus 2000;8(3):1–5.

30. Kyoshima K, Kuroyanagi T, Oya F, et al. Syringomyelia without hindbrain herniation: tight cisterna magna: report of four cases and a review of the literature. J Neurosurg Spine 2002;96(2):239–49.

31. Tubbs RS, Elton S, Grabb P, et al. Analysis of the posterior fossa in children with the chiari 0 malformation. Neurosurgery 2001;48(5):1050–5.

32. Sekula RF, Jannetta PJ, Casey KF, et al. Dimensions of the posterior fossa in patients symptomatic for Chiari I malformation but without cerebellar tonsillar descent. Cerebrospinal Fluid Res 2005;2(1):11.

33. Markunas CA, Tubbs RS, Moftakhar R, et al. Clinical, radiological, and genetic similarities between patients with Chiari Type I and Type 0 malformations: clinical article. J Neurosurg Pediatr 2012;9(4):372–8.

34. Tubbs RS, Chern JJ, Muhleman M, et al. Lateral compression of the foramen magnum with the Chiari I malformation: case illustrations. Child's Nerv Syst 2013;29(3):495–8.

35. Kim IK, Wang KC, Kim IO, et al. Chiari 1.5 Malformation : An Advanced Form of Chiari I Malformation. J Korean Neurosurg S 2010;48(4):375–9.

36. McLone DG, Naidich TP. Developmental morphology of the subarachnoid space, brain vasculature, and contiguous structures, and the cause of the Chiari II malformation. AJNR Am J Neuroradiol 1992;13(2):463–82.

37. Meadows J, Kraut M, Guarnieri M, et al. Asymptomatic Chiari Type I malformations identified on magnetic resonance imaging. J Neurosurg 2000;92(6):920–6.

38. Bollo RJ, Riva-Cambrin J, Brockmeyer MM, et al. Complex Chiari malformations in children: an analysis of preoperative risk factors for occipitocervical fusion: clinical article. J Neurosurg Pediatr 2012;10(2):134–41.

39. Gardner WJ, Goodall RJ. The surgical treatment of arnold-chiari malformation in adults: an explanation of its mechanism and importance of encephalography in diagnosis. J Neurosurg 1950;7(3):199–206.

40. Fons K, Jnah AJ. Arnold-chiari malformation: core concepts. Neonatal Netw 2021;40(5):313–20.

41. Deans AE, Barkovich AJ. The Chiari Malformations. Published online 2013:153-169. doi:10.1007/978-1-4614-6369-6_12

42. Penfield W, Coburn DF. Arnold-chiari malformation and its operative treatment. Arch Neurol Psychiatry 1938;40(2):328–36.

43. McLone DG, Dias MS. The Chiari II malformation: cause and impact. Child's Nerv Syst 2003;19(7–8):540–50.

44. Blount JP. The Chiari Malformations. Published online 2013:283-289. doi:10.1007/978-1-4614-6369-6_25

45. Ocal E, Irwin B, Cochrane D, et al. Stridor at birth predicts poor outcome in neonates with myelomeningocele. Child's Nerv Syst 2012;28(2):265–71.

46. Rath GP, Bithal PK, Chaturvedi A. Atypical presentations in Chiari II malformation. Pediatr Neurosurg 2006;42(6):379–82.

47. McLone DG, Knepper PA. The cause of Chiari II malformation: a unified theory. Pediatr Neurosurg 1989;15(1):1–12.

48. Adzick NS, Thom EA, Spong CY, et al. A randomized trial of prenatal versus postnatal repair of myelomeningocele. N Engl J Med 2011;364(11):993–1004.

49. Grabb PA, Vlastos EJ, Lundy PA, et al. Significant brainstem dysfunction in neonates with myelomeningoceles: a comparison of prenatal versus postnatal closure. J Neurosurg Pediatr 2022;29(5):497–503.

50. Tubbs RS, Oakes WJ. The Chiari Malformations. J Pediatr Neurosci 2013;15(4):1–3. https://doi.org/10.1007/978-1-4614-6369-6_1.

51. Elbaroody M, Mostafa HE, Alsawy MFM, et al. Outcomes of chiari malformation III: a review of literature. J Pediatr Neurosci 2020;15(4):358–64.

52. Smith AB, Gupta N, Otto C, et al. Diagnosis of Chiari III malformation by second trimester fetal MRI with postnatal MRI and CT correlation. Pediatr Radiol 2007;37(10):1035–8.

53. Ivashchuk G, Loukas M, Blount JP, et al. Chiari III malformation: a comprehensive review of this enigmatic anomaly. Child's Nerv Syst 2015;31(11):2035–40.

54. Cakirer S. Chiari III malformation Varieties of MRI appearances in two patients. Clin Imag 2003;27(1):1–4.

55. Poretti A, Boltshauser E, Huisman TAGM. Chiari Malformations and Syringohydromyelia in Children. Semin Ultrasound Ct Mri 2016;37(2):129–42.

56. Hentati A, Badri M, Bahri K, et al. Acquired Chiari I malformation due to lumboperitoneal shunt: A case report and review of literature. Surg Neurol Int 2019;10:78.

57. Wang J, Alotaibi NM, Samuel N, et al. Acquired chiari malformation and syringomyelia secondary to space-occupying lesions: a systematic review. World Neurosurg 2017;98:800–8.e2.

Epidemiology of Chiari I Malformation and Syringomyelia

Katherine G. Holste, MD*, Karin M. Muraszko, MD, Cormac O. Maher, MD

KEYWORDS

- Chiari • Epidemiology • Syringomyelia • Imaging

KEY POINTS

- Determining the incidence and prevalence of Chiari I malformation and syringomyelia is difficult, and many estimates of prevalence rely on imaging.
- Asymptomatic Chiari I malformation is common, and symptomatic Chiari I malformation is less so.
- Syringomyelia associated with Chiari I malformation is more likely to occur with a lower tonsillar position below the foramen magnum and usually occurs in the cervical spine.
- Age, sex, race, ethnicity, and socioeconomic status are important factors in reported Chiari I malformation and syringomyelia frequency and presentation.
- The natural history of Chiari I malformation is benign. Most asymptomatic or minimally symptomatic patients will not require surgery.

EPIDEMIOLOGY OF CHIARI I MALFORMATION

Chiari I malformation (CM) is a common condition seen by neurosurgeons.[1–6] It has historically been defined as cerebellar tonsillar position greater than or equal to 5 mm (mm) below the level of the foramen magnum.[7,8] With the increased utilization of MRI over time, incidental findings of CM are discovered more frequently.[9–11] With this increased frequency of incidentally diagnosed CMs, greater pressure is put on clinicians to determine if the degree of MRI findings have any truly pathologic consequence. Understanding the difference between disease prevalence and imaging prevalence as well as the prevalence of asymptomatic versus symptomatic CM is crucial for patient management.

Determining the prevalence of CM and an associated spinal syrinx is challenging. To establish the true population prevalence of CM, all individuals of the target population would require evaluation, which is not feasible. Instead, most epidemiologic studies of CM report the prevalence based on retrospectively analyzed images.[5,10,12,13] This is an imperfect estimation as these imaging studies are affected by potential detection bias. Physicians usually obtain MRIs to evaluate neurologic symptoms or disease, such as headaches, weakness, or seizures. When the condition of interest is associated with symptoms, this group of patients is more likely to be imaged. When the condition is asymptomatic, the imaging prevalence is more likely to reflect the true prevalence. Conversely, surgical series are biased toward the symptomatic cases. These are the patients who were selected for surgery and are more symptomatic; therefore, these studies are more likely to overestimate the true prevalence.[14–16] To mitigate detection bias, a few studies have used the images of healthy adult volunteers.[9,17,18] For example, Vernooij and colleagues found 0.9% of the healthy, asymptomatic adults over the age of 45 years who volunteered to undergo an MRI had an incidental CM based on the measurement of tonsillar position.[9] This likely underestimates the true prevalence of

Department of Neurosurgery, University of Michigan, 1500 East Medical Center Drive, Room 3552 TC, Ann Arbor, MI 48109-5338, USA
* Corresponding author.
E-mail address: holsteka@med.umich.edu
Twitter: @kholsteMD (K.G.H.); @CormacOMaher (C.O.M.)

Neurosurg Clin N Am 34 (2023) 9–15
https://doi.org/10.1016/j.nec.2022.08.001
1042-3680/23/© 2022 Elsevier Inc. All rights reserved.

CM as symptomatic cases and the pediatric population are excluded. Care must be taken to understand the potential bias and limitations when interpreting the results of the available epidemiologic studies.

Crowding of the foramen magnum causing abnormal cerebrospinal fluid movement is thought to be the main contributor to CM symptoms and syringomyelia. As crowding is difficult to quantify on imaging, tonsillar position of at least 5 mm below the basion-opisthion line has been used as a surrogate. This number was based on a few small series utilizing the early MRI technology.[19,20] The 5-mm cutoff was found to have a 92% sensitivity and 100% specificity for CM in the early radiologic research.[7] Since then, radiologic studies have demonstrated that cerebellar tonsil position generally follows a normal distribution (**Fig. 1**).[21] Five millimeters below the foramen magnum falls along the low end of the normal distribution and may or may not be associated with pathologic consequences for that individual. It is not unreasonable, then, to see those diagnosed with CM on MRI as outliers along the normally distributed tonsil position distribution curve.

Differentiating between the asymptomatic and symptomatic prevalence of CM is crucial. Imaging studies estimate CM prevalence to be between 0.24% and 3.6%.[9,10,22] Of those diagnosed with CM on imaging, symptomatic cases vary greatly from 32% to 63%.[5,12,23] Few true epidemiologic studies have been performed in CM and associated syringomyelia, likely due to the resources required to analyze such a large cohort.[12,23–26] One such study of all children enrolled in the Kaiser Permanente health care system in Northern California found the prevalence of symptomatic CM to be 7:100,000.[12] Countries or regions with smaller populations may find this more feasible. A study of both children and adults in northwestern Italy found the prevalence of symptomatic CM to be 7.74:100,000 with an incidence of 3.08:100,000.[23] In the Republic of Tatarstan, the prevalence of symptomatic CM was found to be more than double that of prior studies, 20:100,000.[24] Multiple factors influence the reported prevalence of both asymptomatic and symptomatic CM. Age, sex, ethnicity, race, and socioeconomic status are important factors when discussing CM and associated syringomyelia epidemiology.

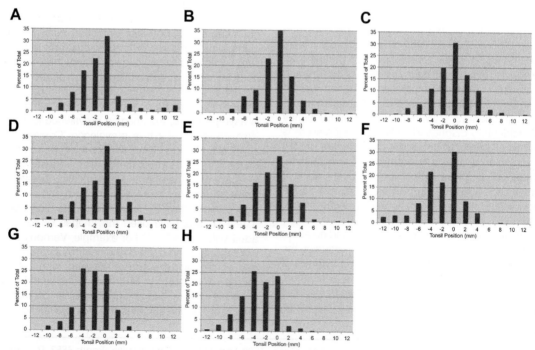

Fig. 1. Graphical representations of the distributions of the mean lowest tonsil position measurement below the foramen magnum for the following age groups: 0 to 10 years (*A*), 11 to 20 years (*B*), 21 to 30 years (*C*), 31 to 40 years (*D*), 41 to 50 years (*E*), 51 to 60 years (*F*), 61 to 70 years (*G*), and 71 years or older (*H*). Negative numbers equate to a more rostral tonsil location below the foramen magnum. (*From* Smith BW, Strahle J, Bapuraj JR, Muraszko KM, Garton HJ, Maher CO. Distribution of cerebellar tonsil position: implications for understanding Chiari malformation. *J Neurosurg.* 2013;119(3):812-819. doi: 10.3171/2013.5.jns121825)

EPIDEMIOLOGY OF SYRINGOMYELIA ASSOCIATED WITH CHIARI MALFORMATION

Syringomyelia associated with CM is a well-described phenomenon.[27–31] Determining the prevalence of syringomyelia in CM patients is challenging for the same reasons as mentioned earlier. Imaging studies are prone to detection bias as patients with neurologic symptoms are more likely to have spinal imaging obtained and a syrinx diagnosed.[5,12,16] This is especially true in operative series in which a CM-related syrinx is reported in up to 85% of cases.[32,33] As surgeons are more likely to recommend surgery when a syrinx is present, the true prevalence of syringomyelia in this population is definitely substantially lower.[5,34] In 1 large single-center radiologic study of 14,116 children, 23% of patients with CM were found to have an associated syrinx, about 0.83% of the total population.[5] Others have found a lower prevalence in pediatric and mixed populations, 12%[12] and 4.6%,[35] respectively. In the northern Italian epidemiologic study, the prevalence of a symptomatic syrinx was 4.84:100,000, and the incidence was 0.82:100,000.[23] Again age likely plays a role in the significant variation of syrinx prevalence. More research is needed to clarify the prevalence and incidence of syringomyelia associated with CM.

The risk of developing a syrinx with CM appears to be related to relative foramen magnum stenosis.[31] Patients found to have a syrinx had a lower tonsillar position on imaging.[5,36] Furthermore, a pegged tonsil morphology, suggestive of foramen magnum compression, was also associated with increased syrinx frequency; only 6% of patients with rounded tonsils developed a syrinx.[5] Although a lower tonsillar position was associated with the presence of a syrinx, it was not associated with syrinx width or length.[5] The cervical spine is the most frequently affected region for a syrinx associated with CM; 86% of patients had the rostral end of the syrinx in the cervical spine.[5,31] The fourth to sixth cervical vertebral levels were the most commonly affected levels in the cervical and thoracic spine in 1 study of 68 patients.[8] Isolated thoracic or lumbar spine syrinxes are less common.

AGE AND CHIARI MALFORMATION AND SYRINGOMYELIA

Age plays a significant role in the prevalence and presentation of CM and syringomyelia. Imaging studies of purely pediatric populations have found 0.97% to 3.6% of children to have a CM,[5,12] whereas purely adult and mixed populations have a prevalence of 0.9%[9] and 0.77%,[13]

respectively. This is in part because of the normal age-related changes in tonsil position. A radiologic study of 221 patients with an age range of 5 months to 89 years found tonsil position moved rostrally with increasing age.[37] This was confirmed by an even larger study of 2400 patients, which found increasing age in adults was associated with decreased likelihood of tonsillar position greater than or equal to 5 mm below the foramen magnum. Interestingly, tonsil position descended during childhood and young adulthood to reach a nadir between 21 and 30 years of age. In general, the tonsil position for each age group followed a normal distribution (**Fig. 2**).[21] Age also appears to affect the frequency of associated syringomyelia. In 1 systematic review of CM patients who were selected for surgery, 69% of adults and 40% of pediatric patients had an associated syrinx.[14] Children were found to have an age-related higher rate of syringomyelia in the first 5 years of life, but the rate plateaued after that.[5]

Age also plays a role in presenting symptoms. In the pediatric population, older children were more likely to be symptomatic at the time of CM diagnosis.[5] This may be because it is challenging to elicit a history of CM symptoms from young children. Infants with CM often present with atypical symptoms such as irritability, crying, or back arching.[38] Oropharyngeal dysfunction such as dysphagia, choking, gagging, snoring, sleep apnea, or vocal cord palsy were seen in 62.5% of patients with CM under 3 years of age in a single-center surgical series.[39] Additionally, the elderly were also less likely to be symptomatic from CM; patients older than 60 years made up only 19% of the northern Italian cohort of CM.[23] This seems to echo the bimodal distribution of age, 8 to 9 years old and 41 to 46 year old, seen at presentation for operative cases.[16] The prevalence and presentation of CM and syringomyelia differ between the pediatric and adult populations.

Sex Determinants in Chiari Malformation and Syringomyelia

Sex also plays a significant role in the prevalence and presentation of CM and syringomyelia. Most cohorts report a female predominance in the CM population, but the ratio of female to male patients varies. Female predominance has been reported from 1.3:1 to 4:1.[5,8,13,16,34,40,41] This predominance is present in both pediatric and adult populations.[25,34] The exact etiology for the sex difference is not well understood. One reason may be an increased likelihood for lower tonsil position in females than in males, as seen across age groups.[21] There is also a female predominance in

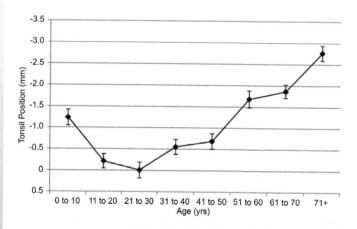

Fig. 2. Mean lowest tonsil position by age. Negative numbers equate to a more rostral tonsil position below the foramen magnum. (*From* Smith BW, Strahle J, Bapuraj JR, Muraszko KM, Garton HJ, Maher CO. Distribution of cerebellar tonsil position: implications for understanding Chiari malformation. *J Neurosurg*. 2013;119(3):812-819. doi: 10.3171/2013.5.jns121825)

CM-associated syrinxes; 1 mixed-age study found 64% of symptomatic syrinxes occurred in female patients. Radiologically, syringomyelia was found more commonly in girls than in boys in a pediatric cohort.[5]

Sex also influences the presentation of CM. In Strahle and colleagues' radiologic study of 14,116 children, girls were more likely to be symptomatic at presentation from their CM than boys.[5] This is in contrast to a mixed-age cohort, in which males with CM were more likely to present with more significant tonsillar herniation and more severe symptoms. The authors postulated that this may be because CM is less common in males, so symptoms must be severe for imaging to be obtained and a diagnosis made.[40] Alternatively, this may be a sample size issue as only 17.1% of their cohort of 287 patients were male. Although females had a higher rate of CM and syringomyelia, the data remain mixed on severity of symptoms on presentation.

Ethnic, Racial, and Socioeconomic Determinants in Chiari Malformation and Syringomyelia

Ethnic, racial, and socioeconomic status variations in CM and syringomyelia prevalence are new areas of study. A retrospective study of all patients diagnosed with CM-associated syringomyelia in northern New Zealand found the prevalence was 3.9 and 8.8 times greater in the Maori and Pacific populations, respectively, than in Caucasians.[26] Their reported total population prevalence was very similar to that of the northern Italian study, 4.84:100,000, even though the makeup of the Italian cohort was 99% Caucasian.[23] In a nationwide survey of patients in Japan, the prevalence of CM-associated syringomyelia was found to be 0.93:100,000, which is significantly lower than that

in the Italian and New Zealand studies.[25] Variation in prevalence occurs not only between countries, but within regions. In the Republic of Tatarstan, patients in the Baltasy district were 10 times more likely to be diagnosed with CM than the rest of the country. The authors propose this may be due to familial clustering.[24]

In the United States, race and socioeconomic status appear to have an impact on CM prevalence and presentation. Krucoff and colleagues dichotomized their cohort of 287 patients into white and African American as well as public and private insurance groups.[40] Other racial groups were excluded due to low number, and 76.7% of their cohort was white. African American patients were more likely to have greater tonsillar herniation at presentation and to present with a syrinx. They were also more likely to present with extremity weakness, whereas white patients had a higher frequency of back pain, ataxia, and syncope. Both groups had an equivalent time from onset of symptoms to diagnosis. The authors postulated that access to health care or acknowledgment of symptoms may contribute to the differences in presentation. Age at presentation was significantly older in the public insurance group, but differences in tonsillar herniation and frequency of syrinxes were not significant. It can be difficult to parse out the exact role of socioeconomic status, especially since African American patients were more likely to have public insurance, so race could be a confounder.[40] Using the Park-Reeves Syringomyelia Research Consortium, Akbari and colleagues examined racial disparities in a larger operative cohort.[42] This population was dichotomized into non-white and white groups. Non-white patients and those with public insurance were more likely to be older at diagnosis and present with signs and symptoms of cerebellar dysfunction. In this study, non-white patients had statistically longer time from symptom onset until diagnosis.[42] Further research is needed with nonoperative cohorts to determine if these same racial differences are seen.

NATURAL HISTORY

The natural history of CM appears to be quite benign for most individuals. Tonsil position does not tend to change dramatically over time. In 1 prospective study of conservatively managed patients imaged annually, 50% had stable tonsil position, and 36% had improved tonsillar position over the course of 12 years.[43] Symptoms also appear to be largely stable over time as well.[44] In a study of 226 patients, only 4 developed new associated symptoms, and 1 developed a new syrinx after the initial neurosurgical evaluation.[45] Syrinx width and length remained stable for the conservatively managed patients in another cohort.[44] Unsurprisingly, very few patients require surgery if they are asymptomatic or minimally symptomatic at the time of presentation.[3,44,46] In a large cohort of 427 patients with CM and without a syrinx initially managed conservatively, only 15 patients required surgery at a median time of 21 months after presentation.[46] Similarly, in other studies of pediatric patients with or without syrinx managed conservatively, 3.5% to 18.8% later underwent surgery.[43–45,47] The most common indication for both early, less than 6 months after presentation, and late, greater than 6 months after presentation, surgeries was syringomyelia. Additionally, the likelihood of requiring surgery 5 and 9 years after presentation changed very little.[47] The natural history of asymptomatic or minimally symptomatic CM appears to be quite benign over time in most cases.

SUMMARY

- Asymptomatic CM is a common incidental imaging finding. Of the patients with CM on imaging, a fraction are symptomatic.
- Determining the prevalence and incidence of CM and syringomyelia is challenging. Imaging studies are affected by detection bias.
- The level of the cerebellar tonsils follows a normal distribution, and 5 mm below the foramen magnum represents one end of this spectrum. This should not be considered a threshold with clear pathologic implications, as many asymptomatic patients have tonsil position that meets or exceeds this imaging criterion.
- Syrinx formation is increasingly likely with increasingly lower tonsillar position.

- Age, sex, ethnicity, race, and socioeconomic status play a role in CM and syringomyelia detection, prevalence, and presentation.
- The natural history of CM is benign, with few patients experiencing significant worsening after an initial asymptomatic or minimally symptomatic presentation.

CLINICS CARE POINTS

- Asymptomatic Chiari I malformation (CM) is a common incidental imaging finding. Of the patients with CM on imaging, a fraction are symptomatic.
- Determining the prevalence and incidence of CM and syringomyelia is challenging. Imaging studies are affected by detection bias.
- The level of the cerebellar tonsils follows a normal distribution, and 5 mm below the foramen magnum represents one end of this spectrum. This should not be considered a threshold with clear pathologic implications, as many asymptomatic patients have tonsil position that meets or exceeds this imaging criterion.
- Syrinx formation is increasingly likely with increasingly lower tonsillar position.
- Age, sex, ethnicity, race, and socioeconomic status play a role in CM and syringomyelia detection, prevalence, and presentation.
- The natural history of CM is benign, with few patients experiencing significant worsening after an initial asymptomatic or minimally symptomatic presentation.

DISCLOSURE

The authors have nothing to disclose.

REFERENCES

1. Armonda RA, Citrin CM, Foley KT, et al. Quantitative cine-mode magnetic resonance imaging of Chiari I malformations: an analysis of cerebrospinal fluid dynamics. Neurosurgery 1994;35(2):214–23 [discussion 223-214].
2. Cahan LD, Bentson JR. Considerations in the diagnosis and treatment of syringomyelia and the Chiari malformation. J Neurosurg 1982;57(1):24–31.
3. Chatrath A, Marino A, Taylor D, et al. Chiari I malformation in children-the natural history. Childs Nerv Syst 2019;35(10):1793–9.
4. Nishizawa S, Yokoyama T, Yokota N, et al. Incidentally identified syringomyelia associated with Chiari

I malformations: is early interventional surgery necessary? Neurosurgery 2001;49(3):637–40 [discussion 640-631].

5. Strahle J, Muraszko KM, Kapurch J, et al. Chiari malformation Type I and syrinx in children undergoing magnetic resonance imaging. J Neurosurg Pediatr 2011;8(2):205–13.

6. Abdallah A, Çınar İ, Gündağ Papaker M, et al. The factors affecting the outcomes of conservative and surgical treatment of chiari i adult patients: a comparative retrospective study. Neurol Res 2022; 44(2):165–76.

7. Barkovich AJ, Wippold FJ, Sherman JL, et al. Significance of cerebellar tonsillar position on MR. AJNR Am J Neuroradiol 1986;7(5):795–9.

8. Elster AD, Chen MY. Chiari I malformations: clinical and radiologic reappraisal. Radiology 1992;183(2): 347–53.

9. Vernooij MW, Ikram MA, Tanghe HL, et al. Incidental findings on brain MRI in the general population. N Engl J Med 2007;357(18):1821–8.

10. Morris Z, Whiteley WN, Longstreth WT Jr, et al. Incidental findings on brain magnetic resonance imaging: systematic review and meta-analysis. Bmj 2009;339:b3016.

11. Trost MJ, Robison N, Coffey D, et al. Changing Trends in Brain Imaging Technique for Pediatric Patients with Ventriculoperitoneal Shunts. Pediatr Neurosurg 2018;53(2):116–20.

12. Aitken LA, Lindan CE, Sidney S, et al. Chiari type I malformation in a pediatric population. Pediatr Neurol 2009;40(6):449–54.

13. Meadows J, Kraut M, Guarnieri M, et al. Asymptomatic Chiari Type I malformations identified on magnetic resonance imaging. J Neurosurg 2000;92(6): 920–6.

14. Arnautovic A, Splavski B, Boop FA, et al. Pediatric and adult Chiari malformation Type I surgical series 1965-2013: a review of demographics, operative treatment, and outcomes. J Neurosurg Pediatr 2015;15(2):161–77.

15. Tubbs RS, Beckman J, Naftel RP, et al. Institutional experience with 500 cases of surgically treated pediatric Chiari malformation Type I. J Neurosurg Pediatr 2011;7(3):248–56.

16. Wilkinson DA, Johnson K, Garton HJ, et al. Trends in surgical treatment of Chiari malformation Type I in the United States. J Neurosurg Pediatr 2017;19(2):208–16.

17. Weber F, Knopf H. Cranial MRI as a screening tool: findings in 1,772 military pilot applicants. Aviat Space Environ Med 2004;75(2):158–61.

18. Yue NC, Longstreth WT Jr, Elster AD, et al. Clinically serious abnormalities found incidentally at MR imaging of the brain: data from the Cardiovascular Health Study. Radiology 1997;202(1):41–6.

19. Aboulezz AO, Sartor K, Geyer CA, et al. Position of cerebellar tonsils in the normal population and in patients with Chiari malformation: a quantitative approach with MR imaging. J Comput Assist Tomogr 1985;9(6):1033–6.

20. Ishikawa M, Kikuchi H, Fujisawa I, et al. Tonsillar herniation on magnetic resonance imaging. Neurosurgery 1988;22(1 Pt 1):77–81.

21. Smith BW, Strahle J, Bapuraj JR, et al. Distribution of cerebellar tonsil position: implications for understanding Chiari malformation. J Neurosurg 2013; 119(3):812–9.

22. Dangouloff-Ros V, Roux CJ, Boulouis G, et al. Incidental Brain MRI Findings in Children: A Systematic Review and Meta-Analysis. AJNR Am J Neuroradiol 2019;40(11):1818–23.

23. Ciaramitaro P, Garbossa D, Peretta P, et al. Syringomyelia and Chiari Syndrome Registry: advances in epidemiology, clinical phenotypes and natural history based on a North Western Italy cohort. Ann Ist Super Sanita 2020;56(1):48–58.

24. Bogdanov EI, Faizutdinova AT, Mendelevich EG, et al. Epidemiology of Symptomatic Chiari Malformation in Tatarstan: Regional and Ethnic Differences in Prevalence. Neurosurgery 2019;84(5):1090–7.

25. Sakushima K, Tsuboi S, Yabe I, et al. Nationwide survey on the epidemiology of syringomyelia in Japan. J Neurol Sci 2012;313(1–2):147–52.

26. Brickell KL, Anderson NE, Charleston AJ, et al. Ethnic differences in syringomyelia in New Zealand. J Neurol Neurosurg Psychiatr 2006;77(8):989–91.

27. Blagodatsky MD, Larionov SN, Manohin PA, et al. Surgical treatment of "hindbrain related" syringomyelia: new data for pathogenesis. Acta Neurochir (Wien) 1993;124(2–4):82–5.

28. Bogdanov EI, Mendelevich EG. Syrinx size and duration of symptoms predict the pace of progressive myelopathy: retrospective analysis of 103 unoperated cases with craniocervical junction malformations and syringomyelia. Clin Neurol Neurosurg 2002;104(2):90–7.

29. Eule JM, Erickson MA, O'Brien MF, et al. Chiari I malformation associated with syringomyelia and scoliosis: a twenty-year review of surgical and nonsurgical treatment in a pediatric population. Spine (Phila Pa 1976) 2002;27(13):1451–5.

30. Hida K, Iwasaki Y, Koyanagi I, et al. Pediatric syringomyelia with chiari malformation: its clinical characteristics and surgical outcomes. Surg Neurol 1999;51(4):383–90 [discussion 390-381].

31. Oldfield EH, Muraszko K, Shawker TH, et al. Pathophysiology of syringomyelia associated with Chiari I malformation of the cerebellar tonsils. Implications for diagnosis and treatment. J Neurosurg 1994; 80(1):3–15.

32. Tubbs RS, Webb DB, Oakes WJ. Persistent syringomyelia following pediatric Chiari I decompression: radiological and surgical findings. J Neurosurg 2004;100(5 Suppl Pediatrics):460–4.

33. Menezes AH. Chiari I malformations and hydromyelia–complications. Pediatr Neurosurg 1991;17(3): 146–54.

34. Greenberg JK, Olsen MA, Yarbrough CK, et al. Chiari malformation Type I surgery in pediatric patients. Part 2: complications and the influence of co-morbid disease in California, Florida, and New York. J Neurosurg Pediatr 2016;17(5):525–32.

35. Horn SR, Shepard N, Vasquez-Montes D, et al. Chiari malformation clusters describe differing presence of concurrent anomalies based on Chiari type. J Clin Neurosci 2018;58:165–71.

36. Halvorson KG, Kellogg RT, Keachie KN, et al. Morphometric Analysis of Predictors of Cervical Syrinx Formation in the Setting of Chiari I Malformation. Pediatr Neurosurg 2016;51(3):137–41.

37. Mikulis DJ, Diaz O, Egglin TK, et al. Variance of the position of the cerebellar tonsils with age: preliminary report. Radiology 1992;183(3):725–8.

38. Carew CL, Prasad A, Tay KY, et al. Unusual presentation of Chiari I in toddlers: case reports and review of the literature. Childs Nerv Syst 2012;28(11): 1965–70.

39. Grahovac G, Pundy T, Tomita T. Chiari type I malformation of infants and toddlers. Childs Nerv Syst 2018;34(6):1169–76.

40. Krucoff MO, Cook S, Adogwa O, et al. Racial, Socioeconomic, and Gender Disparities in the Presentation, Treatment, and Outcomes of Adult Chiari I Malformations. World Neurosurg 2017;97:431–7.

41. Vedantam A, Mayer RR, Staggers KA, et al. Thirty-day outcomes for posterior fossa decompression in children with Chiari type 1 malformation from the US NSQIP-Pediatric database. Childs Nerv Syst 2016;32(11):2165–71.

42. Akbari SHA, Rizvi AA, CreveCoeur TS, et al. Socioeconomic and demographic factors in the diagnosis and treatment of Chiari malformation type I and syringomyelia. J Neurosurg Pediatr 2021;1–10.

43. Whitson WJ, Lane JR, Bauer DF, et al. A prospective natural history study of nonoperatively managed Chiari I malformation: does follow-up MRI surveillance alter surgical decision making? J Neurosurg Pediatr 2015;16(2):159–66.

44. Strahle J, Muraszko KM, Kapurch J, et al. Natural history of Chiari malformation Type I following decision for conservative treatment. J Neurosurg Pediatr 2011;8(2):214–21.

45. Carey M, Fuell W, Harkey T, et al. Natural history of Chiari I malformation in children: a retrospective analysis. Childs Nerv Syst 2021;37(4):1185–90.

46. Leon TJ, Kuhn EN, Arynchyna AA, et al. Patients with "benign" Chiari I malformations require surgical decompression at a low rate. J Neurosurg Pediatr 2019;23(4):498–506.

47. Davidson L, Phan TN, Myseros JS, et al. Long-term outcomes for children with an incidentally discovered Chiari malformation type 1: what is the clinical significance? Childs Nerv Syst 2021;37(4):1191–7.

Sociodemographics of Chiari I Malformation

Syed Hassan Abbas Akbari, MD, MSCI

KEYWORDS

- Chiari I malformation • Sociodemographics • Syringomyelia • Race • Cost • Insurance

KEY POINTS

- Socioeconomic and demographic factors affect neurosurgical care for patients with Chiari I malformation.
- Careful patient selection, treatment selection, postoperative protocols, and varying payment structures can help reduce costs for the surgical treatment of Chiari I malformation.
- Racial differences exist for age at diagnosis and treatment, presentation, and surgical complexity between non-white and white patients, whereas insurance status does not seem to affect preoperative, operative, or postoperative characteristics.
- Greater neurosurgical access and outreach to community physicians can help achieve greater parity for the care of patients with Chiari I malformation.

INTRODUCTION

Socioeconomic status (SES) and demographic factors affect a variety of disease processes. Much of the literature regarding the impact of race, insurance, and SES has been conducted in medical specialties, such as cardiology,[1,2] obesity,[3,4] and oncology.[5,6] However, only few studies have been performed in the neurosurgical literature. Most of the studies pertaining to SES and demographic factors in neurosurgery pertain to spine disorders,[7–9] whereas scoliosis and craniofacial surgery have been a focus in the pediatric neurosurgical literature. A study of 400 patients with idiopathic scoliosis found a difference in disease severity at a presentation by race,[10] whereas another study of almost 10,000 patients found that white patients and those with private insurance were more likely to undergo surgical treatment and be admitted to larger teaching hospitals.[11] Recent studies on craniofacial surgery reveal that patients with private insurance or who were self-pay were more likely to undergo strip craniectomy compared with calvarial vault remodeling.[12] Another study showed that non-white patients were more likely to be older at the time of surgery and had higher hospital costs.[13]

Chiari I malformation (CM-I) with or without syringomyelia can be associated with significant symptoms and morbidity. Treatment by posterior fossa decompression with (PFDD) or without (PFD) duraplasty can lead to significant symptom reduction. However, the effects of SES and demographic factors in the care of CM-I have only recently been investigated. In this article, we review current literature pertaining to socioeconomic and demographic factors associated with the care and management of CM-I, especially concerning cost, race, and insurance status.

COST
The Cost of Chiari I Malformation Treatment

The total financial impact of CM-I is challenging to define. Although many studies have analyzed the cost of surgical treatment of CM-I, little data exist regarding the financial impact of lost school or work days, repeat doctor visits, repeated imaging studies, and more in patients treated either surgically or conservatively. For a disease with an

Disclosures: No disclosures.
Johns Hopkins University School of Medicine, Johns Hopkins All Children's Hospital, 601 5th Street South, Suite 511, St. Petersburg, FL 33705, USA
E-mail address: sakbari3@jhu.edu

Neurosurg Clin N Am 34 (2023) 17–23
https://doi.org/10.1016/j.nec.2022.08.004
1042-3680/23/© 2022 Elsevier Inc. All rights reserved.

estimated prevalence of up to 4% in children obtaining MRI scans,[14–17] the overall disease burden on society may be quite substantial.

Studies have described the financial impact of surgical treatment of CM-I. Greenberg and colleagues[18] used the State Inpatient Databases from California, Florida, and New York to retrospectively study approximately 2000 adult patients undergoing surgery for CM-1. Using a risk-adjusted model, the authors found an average hospital cost of $19,420 for the index admission, $22,530 at 30 days after surgery, and $24,852 at 90 days postoperatively. As expected, resource use was greater in patients encountering surgical ($46,264) or medical complications ($65,679) compared with those without complications ($18,880). Length of hospitalization was greater in those with a surgical (16.3 days) or medical (21.9 days) complication compared with those without complications (4.7 days), which contributed to these differences.

Elsamadicy and colleagues[19] found similar effects of the length of hospital stay on the overall cost for surgical treatment of adult CM-I. Using the National Inpatient Sample, the authors identified almost 30,000 patients undergoing treatment of CM-1. They found that patients with an extended length of stay (defined as >4 days) had a higher complication rate (29.1% vs 10.6%) and higher overall costs ($25,324 vs $14,959) of treatment. Hydrocephalus and other complications along with race and insurance status were associated with an extended hospital stay.

Lam and colleagues[20] tried to define the costs associated with CM-I treatment in the pediatric population. Using the Kids' Inpatient Database for the year 2009, the authors found an average surgical cost of $13,484 for CM-I with an average length of hospitalization of 3.8 days. Factors associated with higher costs included hydrocephalus-related complications, surgical complications, and medical complications. Device-dependent comorbidities were a significant contributor to increased costs. Patients treated at children's hospitals incurred higher costs compared with those treated at non-children's hospitals by approximately $5000. Higher nurse-patient ratios, a higher level of acuity, and greater complexity are all factors that may be contributing to the higher cost incurred at children's hospitals. The authors posit that bundled payments for Chiari I surgery and other novel payment models may be effective cost-reducing strategies for the care of these patients.

Another study of approximately 4000 patients using the Kids' Inpatient Database over multiple time points found an average surgical cost of approximately $19,000.[21] The authors further analyzed the cost difference between those treated at children's hospitals compared with those treated at other hospitals. Although the length of stay was not significantly different between groups, approximately 4 days for both groups, the overall cost was significantly different. The cost of treatment at children's hospitals was $23,131 compared with $16,535 for those treated at other hospitals using both multivariate and propensity-score analysis ($p < 0.0001$). Furthermore, the authors found that the cost of CM-I treatment has been increasing since 2003 and at a higher rate at children's hospitals compared with non-children's hospitals. Surgical urgency and complexity were implicated as possible contributors to this difference.

Reducing the Cost of Chiari I Malformation Treatment

Various studies have looked at reducing the cost of CM-I treatment. Medical and surgical complications as well as hydrocephalus are major factors contributing to cost and length of stay.[18,19] This highlights the necessity of appropriate patient selection and the mitigation of other contributing factors before pursuing surgical intervention for CM-I to minimize the risk of complications. In addition, although costs are greater at a dedicated children's hospital, it remains to be seen whether the overall economic burden is different after factoring in the need for reoperation or poorer overall outcomes at non-children's hospitals.

Numerous centers have applied specific protocols to decrease the cost of CM-1 care. For example, dural splitting has been used as a way to reduce complications, reduce the length of stay, and reduce hospital costs. Comparing 63 patients undergoing dural splitting with 50 patients undergoing duraplasty, Limonadi and Selden,[22] and Litvak and colleagues[23] found that dural splitting was associated with approximately an hour less operating time, a shorter length of stay, and a reduction in cost by approximately $2000 to $3000 without sacrificing outcomes. In addition, Mazur-Hart and colleagues[24] found that a dedicated protocol for postoperative pain management including diazepam, dexamethasone, ketorolac, and rapid urinary catheter removal and ambulation led to a reduction in hospital stay, more patients being discharged on postoperative day 1, and a cost reduction of almost $2000 per surgery.

Perhaps the most controversial factor determining the cost of CM-I treatment is the type of surgery performed between PFD and PFDD.

Shweikeh and colleagues[25] conducted a study using the Kids' Inpatient Database to assess for differences between PFD and PFDD. With roughly 1500 patients treated with PFD and 1000 patients treated with PFDD, the authors found that patients undergoing PFDD were more likely to undergo immediate reoperations, had more complications, had a greater length of hospital stay, and had a higher treatment cost by approximately $4000. More recently, Akbari and colleagues[26] used the Park-Reeves Syringomyelia Research Consortium (PRSRC) database to identify 692 pediatric patients with CM-I and syringomyelia. The 575 patients undergoing PFDD had greater operating room time, greater blood loss, longer hospital stays, and a greater complication rate (24.3% versus 13.7%) compared with those undergoing PFD. However, PFD was associated with a higher revision rate (17.9% vs 8.3%). Although the study did not directly address hospital cost due to limitations of the database, operating room time, hospital stays, and complication rates are associated with higher overall cost. Although the data seem to suggest a higher overall cost associated with PFDD versus PFD, it remains to be seen how the higher revision rate in PFD affects the overall cost for the care of CM-1. It is important to note, however, that the higher revision rate in the PFD group may reflect issues with patient selection as opposed to true treatment failure.[26]

Cost reduction in CM-I treatment is ultimately a multifaceted issue involving preoperative, operative, and postoperative factors. Patient selection can dramatically reduce costs associated with surgical treatment while treatment by skilled neurosurgeons with a low complication profile can reduce cost as well. Coupling this with appropriate treatment selection to reduce predicted complications or the need for future reoperation may help substantially reduce cost further. The use of postoperative pain and mobilization protocols can lead to more rapid discharges and lower resource utilization. Finally, varying cost models such as bundled payment or flat-rate treatments may help to make surgery more cost-effective in the treatment of CM-I.

SOCIODEMOGRAPHIC FACTORS

Sociodemographic factors affect the treatment of neurosurgical disease. A systematic review of 38 studies revealed that non-white patients, patients with public insurance, and patients from lower SES had reduced access and worse outcomes in pediatric neurosurgical diseases.[27] The authors also found that non-white patients were typically older at the age of diagnosis, presented with more severe disease, and had greater morbidity and mortality, whereas underinsured patients had greater delays in surgical referral, were less likely to undergo treatment, and had greater inpatient mortality. This study highlights the racial and socioeconomic disparities in pediatric neurosurgical care. This section will address the significant sociodemographic disparities for adult and pediatric CM-I.

Race

Recently, racial differences in the presentation, treatment, and outcomes of CM-I treatment have been explored. Krucoff and colleagues analyzed the charts of over 600 adult patients with CM-I. They found that white patients were more likely to present with back pain, whereas African American patients were more likely to present with lower extremity weakness, worse tonsillar herniation, and higher rates of syringomyelia.[28] In the study performed by Elsamadicy and colleagues[19] cited earlier, the authors found that black race and Hispanic ethnicity among other parameters were independently associated with an increased length of stay among adults treated for CM-1. Meanwhile, Wilkinson and colleagues[17] found that among adult and pediatric CM-I patients, surgical patients were more likely to be white and to be from households with a net worth greater than $250,000

Much of the research on racial disparities in the treatment of CM-I has been conducted in the pediatric population. One study looking at the natural history of benign CM-I touched upon some of these disparities.[29] In this single-institution study, the authors followed approximately 420 patients with CM-I without syringomyelia who presented asymptomatically. Patients who required surgery more than 9 months after their initial visit were deemed to have progressed, which was often due to the development of headaches. Fifteen patients required delayed surgery in this fashion, but significantly, all of these patients were white, raising concerns about racial disparities in the population. This prompted further analysis of the single-institutional cohort using area-level measures of SES.[30] In this study, Akbari and colleagues analyzed 665 pediatric patients treated at the same institution for CM-I. Outcome measures included surgical versus conservative treatment, type of surgery performed, and presenting symptoms. Area-level socioeconomic disadvantage was measured using the Area Deprivation Index (ADI), which creates a composite score for an area based on multiple factors aggregated to US Census blocks, with higher scores indicating greater levels of disadvantage.[31,32] Area-level rurality was determined by the US Department of Agriculture 2010 Rural-Urban Commuting Area (RUCA) codes that classify census tracts based on population density, daily commuting, and urbanization, with higher scores indicating greater rurality.[33] Distance to the hospital, race/ethnicity, and insurance status were also collected.

The authors found that 82% of the cohort was non-Hispanic white and 74% had private insurance.[30] Out of their cohort, 472 did not require surgery and 153 underwent surgical intervention within 9 months of initial presentation. Forty patients underwent surgery beyond 9 months from initial presentation and were labeled as "delayed symptomatic" patients. Non-white patients were less likely to use private insurance (54.1% vs 78.5%), had higher levels of disadvantage by ADI score (5.6 vs 3.8), and were less likely to be from rural areas by RUCA score (1.6 vs 2.4) compared with non-Hispanic white patients. There were no differences in distance to hospital, treatment type received, age at surgery, operative time, length of stay, or presenting symptoms. Interestingly, the delayed symptomatic group, or those requiring surgery for progression of disease beyond 9 months from the initial visit, were more likely to be white (92.5%), more likely to be from more affluent areas (ADI 3.2 vs 4.1), and were more likely to be from more urban areas (RUCA 1.8 vs 2.3). Overall, non-white patients were more likely to reside in disadvantaged urban neighborhoods and have public health insurance. However, the lack of difference in terms of treatment type, rates of surgery, or outcomes seems to indicate relative racial parity once patients present to a neurosurgeon. Therefore, the findings may point to a disparity in terms of primary care referral or referral to a neurosurgeon. This is highlighted by the relative disparity of non-white patients treated at this institution compared with the demographics of the institution's catchment area.[30] In addition, patients in the delayed symptomatic group were more likely to be white and from more affluent urban areas, pointing to a socioeconomic and racial disparity in terms of follow-up for patients with initially asymptomatic CM-I in this population. The findings may point to racial and socioeconomic disparities resulting from poorer follow-up care, loss to follow-up, decreased access to care, or decreased primary care reengagement of neurosurgical services once symptoms develop.

Addressing issues of race in pediatric patients with CM-I on a national scale, Shweikeh and colleagues[25] analyzed the Kids' Inpatient Database for CM-I patients undergoing PFD or PFDD.

Across over 2500 patients, the authors found that patients undergoing PFDD were more likely to be white (81.2%) compared with patients undergoing PFD (75.6%). These data seem to indicate a racial disparity with respect to treatment. To analyze the nation-wide effects of race on the treatment of pediatric CM-I with syringomyelia, Akbari and colleagues[34] conducted a retrospective analysis using the PRSRC database. The PRSRC is a multicenter research collaborative involving 42 contributing centers with data collected both retrospectively and prospectively on patients with CM-I and syringomyelia. In this study, 637 pediatric patients with at least one year of follow-up data were identified. The authors analyzed presenting demographic information, symptoms, physical examination findings, imaging characteristics, and surgical parameters. They grouped patients into non-white and non-Hispanic white groups. "Low-volume centers" were those in the lowest quartile of patient volume, and "high-volume centers" were those in the highest quartile of patient volume.

The authors found that non-white patients were more likely to use non-private insurance (57.8%) compared with white patients (20.2%).[34] Non-white patients were also older at the age of diagnosis (median age 11.5 years vs 9.3 years). Interestingly, there were no differences from the time of symptom onset to diagnosis. Non-white patients were also more likely to present to low-volume centers (38.7%) compared with high-volume centers (15.2%). In terms of presenting symptoms, non-white patients were more likely to present with gait ataxia and tremor, were more likely to have preexisting skull malformations, and were more likely to have cranial nerve and cerebellar signs such as nystagmus, dysconjugate gaze, hearing loss, gait instability, and dysmetria. Non-white patients were more likely to have platybasia or basilar invagination on imaging. There were no differences in the number of preoperative imaging studies obtained, syrinx size, or extent of tonsillar descent. In terms of treatment, non-white patients were older at the surgery by about 2 years (12.1 years vs 9.8 years). Non-white patients tended to have longer surgeries associated with greater blood loss and longer hospital stays. However, there were no differences in terms of type of treatment performed (PFD vs PFDD), surgical complications, or delayed complications except for a higher rate of hydrocephalus in non-white patients (17.1% vs 5.3%). There were no differences in clinical improvement or new symptom development.

Together, the results point to the possibility of delayed diagnosis and greater surgical complexity in non-white patients compared with non-Hispanic white patients. Non-white patients were older at diagnosis and at treatment and were more likely to have underlying skull malformations, cranial nerve dysfunction, and cerebellar dysfunction as a result. These differences in presentation correlated with longer operative times and greater blood loss potentially due to greater surgical complexity from a delayed diagnosis. An alternative explanation is that there are differences in the pathophysiology of CM-I with syringomyelia by race. Differences in operative parameters may also be explained by the fact that non-white patients were more likely to present to low-volume centers. This highlights the need for patients to be referred to skilled pediatric neurosurgeons at high-volume centers. Interestingly, there were no differences in the number of preoperative and postoperative imaging studies, follow-up visits, type of surgery performed, or outcomes suggesting that patients receive equivocal treatment once referred to a pediatric neurosurgeon. Moreover, the difference in age at diagnosis and age at treatment by race emphasizes socioeconomic disparities in care before neurosurgical referral. The disparity may be due to differences in patients' or families' desire to seek medical care, pediatrician familiarity with CM-I and syringomyelia, or a referral bias against those with decreased access to care. Less severely affected non-white patients may not be properly referred, resulting in disease progression that finally necessitates neurosurgical referral at an older age with greater disease complexity. These challenges may be overcome through greater pediatrician education regarding CM-I signs and symptoms as well as greater access to pediatric neurosurgeons. Nearly a quarter of children in the United States live more than 60 miles from a pediatric neurosurgeon, and these families are typically uninsured and below the poverty level.[35] Therefore, it is important for neurosurgeons to work on dissemination and implementation of neurosurgical research and policy changes to bridge the racial divide. Remote clinics in underserved areas may also help to increase accessibility to pediatric neurosurgical care.

Insurance Status

Fortunately, across a variety of studies, insurance status has not seemed to affect the care of patients with CM-I significantly. In Greenberg and colleagues's[18] study using the State Inpatient Database, Medicaid insurance only correlated with medical complications for the treatment of adult CM-I. Meanwhile, Elsamadicy and colleagues[19] and Krucoff and colleagues[28] found that private insurance was associated with a reduced length of hospital stay and public insurance was associated with a greater length of stay for adults with CM-I, respectively. In the pediatric population, Lam and colleagues[20] found no link between insurance status and the cost of care, and Lane and colleagues[21] found that patients with Medicaid were more likely to be treated at children's hospitals compared with those with commercial insurance. Akbari and colleagues,[30] in their single-institution study cited earlier, found that surgical and non-surgical patients had similar rates of private insurance use, and insurance status did not affect the type of surgery performed. There was no effect of insurance status on time to surgery or on the number of follow-up images. Private insurance was only associated with having fewer overall postoperative follow-up visits, which may indicate that neurosurgeons have a bias in following uninsured patients more closely so as not to lose them to follow-up. Of note, however, the proportion of patients treated with Medicaid was lower in the study population than the proportion in the general population, which may indicate difficulties with access to neurosurgical care or a deficiency in referrals to a pediatric neurosurgeon. Finally, Akbari and colleagues's[34] study involving the PRSRC database found no differences based on insurance group for any factors pertaining to presentation, treatment, outcomes, or complications in surgically treated pediatric patients with CM-I and syringomyelia. These later two studies did show that non-white patients were more likely to use public insurance than were non-Hispanic white patients.[30,34] Overall, the studies in the pediatric population show that once patients are referred to a pediatric neurosurgeon, insurance status is not a significant barrier to treatment, outcomes, and cost. This is likely because patients without private insurance usually have access to Medicaid and full care at children's hospitals. However, uninsured or underinsured patients may have difficulty gaining access to pediatric neurosurgeons in the first place, potentially due to deficiencies in pediatric primary care, limited referrals, or socioeconomic barriers.

SUMMARY

CM-Is are common diagnoses for the adult and pediatric neurosurgeon. Careful patient and treatment selection, the use of postoperative pain protocols, minimizing complications, and different payment schemes may help to reduce costs for the surgical treatment of this condition. Meanwhile, racial differences pertaining to the age at presentation, severity of symptoms, and surgical complexity highlight disparities in neurosurgical referrals. Fortunately, there do not seem to be substantial differences in treatment, outcomes, and complications between race and insurance groups, emphasizing the need for neurosurgical outreach and improved access to neurosurgical care.

CLINICS CARE POINTS

- Socioeconomic and demographic factors affect neurosurgical care for Chiari I malformation.
- Careful patient selection, treatment selection, postoperative protocols, and varying payment structures can help reduce costs for the surgical treatment of Chiari I malformation.
- Racial differences exist in age at diagnosis and treatment, presentation, and surgical complexity for non-white compared with white patients. Greater neurosurgical access and outreach to community physicians can help achieve greater parity for the care of patients with Chiari I malformation.
- Insurance status does not seem to affect outcomes once patients are referred to a neurosurgeon, and therefore increasing access to insurance can help further the care of patients with Chiari I malformation.

REFERENCES

1. Bild DE. Multi-ethnic study of atherosclerosis: objectives and design. Am J Epidemiol 2002;156(9):871–81.
2. Feng TR, White RS, Gaber-Baylis LK, et al. Coronary artery bypass graft readmission rates and risk factors - A retrospective cohort study. Int J Surg Lond Engl 2018;54(Pt A):7–17.
3. Byrd AS, Toth AT, Stanford FC. Racial disparities in obesity treatment. Curr Obes Rep 2018;7(2):130–8.
4. Patterson ML, Stern S, Crawford PB, et al. Sociodemographic factors and obesity in preadolescent black and white girls: NHLBI's Growth and Health Study. J Natl Med Assoc 1997;89(9):594–600.
5. Keegan THM, Li Q, Steele A, et al. Sociodemographic disparities in the occurrence of medical conditions among adolescent and young adult Hodgkin lymphoma survivors. Cancer Causes Control CCC 2018;29(6):551–61.
6. Lau SKM, Gannavarapu BS, Carter K, et al. Impact of socioeconomic status on pretreatment weight loss and survival in non-small-cell lung cancer. J Oncol Pract 2018;14(4):e211–20.
7. Katz J. Lumbar disc disorders and low-back pain: socioeconomic factors and consequences. J Bone Joint Surg Am 2006;88(Suppl 2).
8. Bernstein DN, Merchan N, Fear K, et al. Greater socioeconomic disadvantage is associated with worse symptom severity at initial presentation in patients seeking care for lumbar disc herniation. Spine 2021;46(7):464–71.
9. Derakhshan A, Miller J, Lubelski D, et al. The impact of socioeconomic status on the utilization of spinal imaging. Neurosurgery 2015;77(5):746–53 [discussion: 753-754].
10. Zavatsky J, Peters A, Nahvi F, et al. Disease severity and treatment in adolescent idiopathic scoliosis: the impact of race and economic status. Spine J 2015;15(5). https://doi.org/10.1016/j.spinee.2013.06.043.
11. Nuño M, Drazin DG, Acosta FL. Differences in treatments and outcomes for idiopathic scoliosis patients treated in the United States from 1998 to 2007: impact of socioeconomic variables and ethnicity. Spine J 2013;13(2):116–23.
12. Mozaffari MA, Hauc SC, Junn AH, et al. Socioeconomic disparities in the surgical management of craniosynostosis. J Craniofac Surg 2022;33(1):294–7.
13. Shweikeh F, Foulad D, Nuño M, et al. Differences in surgical outcomes for patients with craniosynostosis in the US: impact of socioeconomic variables and race. J Neurosurg Pediatr 2016;17(1):27–33.
14. Aitken LA, Lindan CE, Sidney S, et al. Chiari type I malformation in a pediatric population. Pediatr Neurol 2009;40(6):449–54.
15. Meadows J, Kraut M, Guarnieri M, et al. Asymptomatic Chiari Type I malformations identified on magnetic resonance imaging. J Neurosurg 2000;92(6):920–6.
16. Strahle J, Muraszko KM, Kapurch J, et al. Chiari malformation Type I and syrinx in children undergoing magnetic resonance imaging. J Neurosurg Pediatr 2011;8(2):205–13.
17. Wilkinson DA, Johnson K, Garton HJL, et al. Trends in surgical treatment of Chiari malformation Type I in the United States. J Neurosurg Pediatr 2017;19(2):208–16.
18. Greenberg J, Ladner T, Olsen M, et al. Complications and resource use associated with surgery for chiari malformation type 1 in adults: a population perspective. Neurosurgery 2015;77(2).
19. Elsamadicy AA, Koo AB, Lee M, et al. Risk factors portending extended length of stay after suboccipital decompression for adult chiari I malformation. World Neurosurg 2020;138:e515–22.
20. Lam SK, Mayer RR, Luerssen TG, et al. Hospitalization cost model of pediatric surgical treatment of chiari type 1 malformation. J Pediatr 2016;179:204–10.e3.

21. Lane J, Schilling AL, Hollenbeak C, et al. Cost of chiari i malformation surgery: comparison of treatment at children's hospitals versus non-children's hospitals. Cureus 2021;13(1):e12866.

22. Limonadi FM, Selden NR. Dura-splitting decompression of the craniocervical junction: reduced operative time, hospital stay, and cost with equivalent early outcome. J Neurosurg 2004;101(SUPPL. 2): 184–8.

23. Litvack ZN, Lindsay RA, Selden NR. Dura splitting decompression for Chiari I malformation in pediatric patients: clinical outcomes, healthcare costs, and resource utilization. Neurosurgery 2013;72(6): 922–8 [discussion: 928-929].

24. Mazur-Hart DJ, Bowden SG, Pang BW, et al. Standardizing postoperative care for pediatric intradural Chiari decompressions to decrease length of stay. J Neurosurg Pediatr 2021;28(5):579–84.

25. Shweikeh F, Sunjaya D, Nuno M, et al. National trends, complications, and hospital charges in pediatric patients with chiari malformation type i treated with posterior fossa decompression with and without duraplasty. Pediatr Neurosurg 2015;50(1):31–7.

26. Akbari SHA, Yahanda AT, Ackerman LL, et al. Complications and outcomes of posterior fossa decompression with duraplasty versus without duraplasty for pediatric patients with Chiari malformation type I and syringomyelia: a study from the Park-Reeves Syringomyelia Research Consortium. J Neurosurg Pediatr 2022;1–13. https://doi.org/10.3171/2022.2. PEDS21446.

27. Lechtholz-Zey E, Bonney PA, Cardinal T, et al. Systematic Review of Racial, Socioeconomic, and Insurance Status Disparities in the Treatment of Pediatric Neurosurgical Diseases in the United States. World Neurosurg 2022;158:65–83.

28. Krucoff MO, Cook S, Adogwa O, et al. Racial, socioeconomic, and gender disparities in the presentation, treatment, and outcomes of adult chiari I malformations. World Neurosurg 2017;97:431–7.

29. Leon TJ, Kuhn EN, Arynchyna AA, et al. Patients with "benign" Chiari I malformations require surgical decompression at a low rate. J Neurosurg Pediatr 2019;23(4):498–506.

30. Akbari SHA, Oates GR, Gonzalez-Sigler I, et al. Care for Chiari malformation type I: the role of socioeconomic disadvantage and race. J Neurosurg Pediatr 2021;29(3):305–11.

31. Kind AJH, Buckingham WR. Making neighborhood-disadvantage metrics accessible — the neighborhood atlas. N Engl J Med 2018;378(26):2456–8.

32. University of Wisconsin School of Medicine and Public Health. Area Deprivation Index v2.0. 2015. Available at: https://www.neighborhoodatlas. medicine.wisc.edu. Accessed May 26, 2022.

33. US Department of Agriculture Economic Research Service. Rural-Urban Communting Area Codes. US Department of Agriculture. Available at: https://www. ers.usda.gov/data-products/rural-urban-commuting-area-codes/. Accessed May 26, 2022.

34. Akbari SHA, Rizvi AA, CreveCoeur TS, et al. Socioeconomic and demographic factors in the diagnosis and treatment of Chiari malformation type I and syringomyelia. J Neurosurg Pediatr 2021;3:1–10.

35. Ahmed AK, Duhaime AC, Smith TR. Geographic proximity to specialized pediatric neurosurgical care in the contiguous United States. J Neurosurg Pediatr 2018;21(4):434–8.

Clinical Manifestations of Chiari I Malformation

Ziyad Makoshi, MBBS, MSc, FRCSC[a,b], Jeffrey R. Leonard, MD[a,c,d],*

KEYWORDS

- Chiari 1 malformation • Syringomyelia • Syrinx • Scoliosis • Headache • Cervicomedullary junction
- Craniocervical junction • Oropharyngeal dysfunction

KEY POINTS

- Asymptomatic Chiari 1 malformation (CM1) patients often remain so over time. Those with mild symptoms are likely to remain stable and may improve.
- The most common clinical presentation of CM1 in children involves headaches, syringomyelia, and/or scoliosis.
- The most common headache associated with CM1 are occipital/suboccipital headaches, worsened by Valsalva-like maneuvers, and lasting less than 5 minutes.
- Oropharyngeal dysfunction is one of the most common findings in symptomatic CM1 among children aged younger than 3 years.
- Sensorimotor deficits, lower cranial nerve dysfunction, and respiratory changes in CM1 relate to syringomyelia and compression at the cervicomedullary junction.

INTRODUCTION

The definition of Chiari 1 malformation (CM1) continues to evolve. Diagnosis is often based on imaging features and include herniation of the cerebellar tonsils (one or both) 5 mm or more below a line drawn from the basion to the opisthion (McRae's line), herniations of 3 to 5 mm in the presence of syringomyelia, or if there is a peg-like rather than rounded appearance to the tonsils.[1] Tonsillar impaction occurring at the foramen magnum with consequent disruption of cerebrospinal fluid (CSF) flow dynamics and compression of structures at the cervicomedullary junction leads to signs and symptoms of CM1.[2–7] The clinical features of CM1 can differ based on the extent of these disruptions, the age at presentation, and from one individual to another. Here, we present possible clinical manifestations of CM1 in order to better recognize and care for individuals with CM1.

APPROACH

A complete history and physical examination are necessary when assessing children with CM1. History from the child should be obtained whenever possible; localization and association with certain activities can be extremely informative. The first important consideration is to distinguish *incidental* from *symptomatic CM1*. The second is to recognize the *associated features* of CM1 (eg, syringomyelia and scoliosis) and to look for *secondary causes* of tonsillar herniation (ie, acquired Chiari malformation) where different management strategies may be indicated. Secondary causes can include mass lesions,[8] craniosynostosis,[9] intracranial hypertension (eg, idiopathic intracranial hypertension),[10] intracranial hypotension (eg, CSF leak or lumboperitoneal shunting),[11,12] and less understood associations such as hydrocephalus[13] and tethered cord.[14]

---

[a] Division of Neurological Surgery, Nationwide Children's Hospital, Columbus, OH, USA; [b] Division of Neurosurgery, The Ottawa Hospital, 1053 Carling Avenue, Ottawa, ON K1Y 4E9, Canada; [c] Department of Neurological Surgery, The Ohio State University College of Medicine, The Ohio State University Wexner Medical Center, Columbus, OH, USA; [d] Nationwide Children's Hospital, The Ohio State College of Medicine, 700 Children's Drive, Columbus, OH 43205, USA
* Corresponding author. Nationwide Children's Hospital, The Ohio State College of Medicine, 700 Children's Drive, Columbus, OH 43205.
E-mail address: Jeffrey.Leonard@nationwidechildrens.org

Neurosurg Clin N Am 34 (2023) 25–34
https://doi.org/10.1016/j.nec.2022.09.003
1042-3680/23/© 2022 Elsevier Inc. All rights reserved.

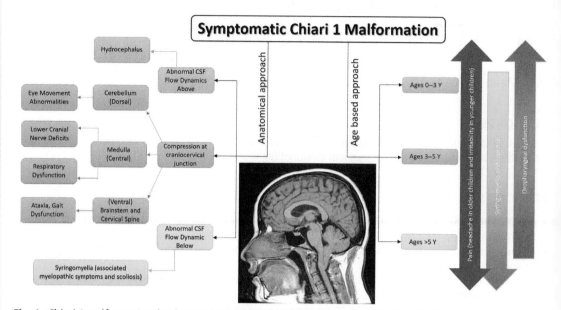

Fig. 1. Chiari 1 malformation (midsagittal MRI scan of head and upper cervical spine). Age-based and anatomic approaches to manifestations of Chiari 1 malformation. CSF, cerebrospinal fluid.

ASYMPTOMATIC CHIARI 1 MALFORMATION

An incidental CM1 may be seen in children undergoing MRI for other reasons approximately 0.2% to 1.3% of the time.[15,16] These radiological findings may improve or even resolve as the child grows, and progression of symptoms is infrequent.[15,17] Approximately 15% to 37% of pediatric patients with radiographic evidence of inferior cerebellar tonsillar ectopia may be asymptomatic, based on large retrospective reviews.[18–20] The natural clinical history of these individuals continues to be studied but mounting evidence suggests that asymptomatic children largely remain so during long-term follow-up,[21] and even those with mild features of CM1 are likely to remain stable or improve with time.[18,22–24] Therefore, recognizing the clinical features of CM1 is important for clinical decision-making.

SYMPTOMATIC CHIARI 1 MALFORMATION

Patients with CM1 usually present between the ages of 3 and 13 years.[17,18,21–26] Symptoms tend to be present for variable time points before finding a CM1.[26] In symptomatic patients with CM1, the following characteristics should be recognized[27]:

- Clinical presentation (symptoms and signs) varies with respect to age and
- Younger patients tend to present with shorter symptom duration than older patients.

Age-based and anatomic approaches are shown in **Fig. 1**.

Chiari Headaches

Headaches are one of the most common types of pain in children with a reported prevalence of 20% to 88%.[28] These are often tension type headaches and migraines and can occur in patients with CM1.[29,30] Headaches are a significant component of the clinical presentation in 27% to 81% of children with symptomatic CM1.[3–6,19,27,31] No specific criteria exists for diagnosing a "Chiari headache" and its characteristics continue to be updated in the International Headache Society Classification.[32] However, 3 aspects can aid the clinician in suspecting a headache caused by CM1[32]:

- Evidence of CM1 on imaging (cerebellar tonsillar herniation or crowding of the subarachnoid space around the cervicomedullary junction),
- Common headache characteristics described in CM1 (see later discussion), and
- Presence of associated symptoms and signs of CM1 (eg, intermittent dizziness, symptoms related to syringomyelia and/or scoliosis, symptoms related to compression of structures at the cervicomedullary junction).

Classically, headaches in adolescents and adults with CM1 demonstrate the following characteristics[2,3,5,6,18,19,33–36]:

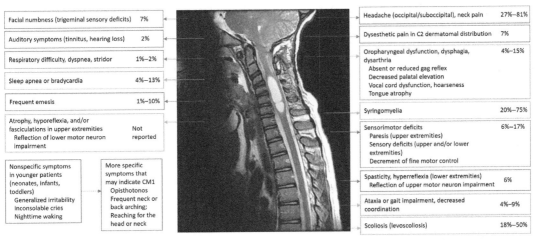

Facial numbness (trigeminal sensory deficits)	7%
Auditory symptoms (tinnitus, hearing loss)	2%
Respiratory difficulty, dyspnea, stridor	1%–2%
Sleep apnea or bradycardia	4%–13%
Frequent emesis	1%–10%
Atrophy, hyporeflexia, and/or fasciculations in upper extremities Reflection of lower motor neuron impairment	Not reported

| Nonspecific symptoms in younger patients (neonates, infants, toddlers)
Generalized irritability
Inconsolable cries
Nighttime waking | More specific symptoms that may indicate CM1
Opisthotonos
Frequent neck or back arching;
Reaching for the head or neck |

Headache (occipital/suboccipital), neck pain	27%–81%
Dysesthetic pain in C2 dermatomal distribution	7%
Oropharyngeal dysfunction, dysphagia, dysarthria Absent or reduced gag reflex Decreased palatal elevation Vocal cord dysfunction, hoarseness Tongue atrophy	4%–15%
Syringomyelia	20%–75%
Sensorimotor deficits Paresis (upper extremities) Sensory deficits (upper and/or lower extremities) Decrement of fine motor control	6%–17%
Spasticity, hyperreflexia (lower extremities) Reflection of upper motor neuron impairment	6%
Ataxia or gait impairment, decreased coordination	4%–9%
Scoliosis (levoscoliosis)	18%–50%

Fig. 2. Chiari 1 malformation with associated cervical syrinx. Common symptoms (blue) and signs (green) and their reported frequency (prevalence estimates are based on frequencies reported in peer-reviewed publications, and likely represent upper estimates in most cases). (*Data from* Refs.[3,4,18,19,27,31,34–36,44,57])

- Most often occipital or suboccipital,
- Provoked or intensified by Valsalva-type maneuvers,
- Last less than 5 minutes, and
- Frequent and severe.

Various functions or activities that induce a Valsalva-type response, consistent with childhood behavior, include the following[27]:

- Sneezing, coughing;
- Laughing, screaming;
- Defecation; and
- Running, repetitive jumping.

The description of the headache is variable (eg, pounding, crushing, pressure-like, pulsatile, radiating to vertex, behind the eyes, or to the neck and shoulders), and other aggravating factors reported include head movement (eg, turning, extending), change in position, and physical exertion. It is important to note that most patients with symptomatic CM1 tend to exhibit more than one symptom rather than headache in isolation (although this can occur)[26,37] and that those with the "classic" headache characteristics are more likely to respond to surgical decompression.[37] However, a retrospective study suggests that some individuals with CM1 may present with poorly localized headaches or frontotemporal headaches and still benefit from surgical decompression (although less frequently).[38] Additionally, younger patients (ie, neonates, infants, toddlers) may fail to demonstrate or adequately communicate these classic headache descriptors,[19] and therefore other symptoms and signs should be recognized as will be discussed.

Scoliosis and Syringomyelia

In addition to headaches and/or neck pain, the most common radiographic associations with CM1 are syringomyelia and scoliosis (most commonly levoscoliosis), common signs and symptoms and their frequency are shown in **Fig. 2**.[3,18,19,27,34,36] In children undergoing craniospinal MRI scans (most common indications were scoliosis and pain) and found to have a syrinx, CM1 was the most common concurrent diagnosis in 43%.[39]

Syringomyelia in CM1 demonstrates predilection for the following regions[2,3]:

- Cervical spinal cord (15%–21%),
- Cervicothoracic spinal cord (12%–25%),
- Thoracic spinal cord (15%–16%),
- Lumbar spinal cord (3%–4%), and
- Holocord (39%–44%).

Classic symptoms and physical examination signs suggesting syringomyelia include the following[5,27,35]:

- Upper extremity weakness, prominently affecting intrinsic muscles of the hand,
- Pain and temperature sensory loss (functions served by the spinal cord anterolateral spinothalamic tracts) in a "cape-like" distribution,
- Preservation of light touch sensation and proprioception (functions served by the spinal cord dorsal columns), and
- Absence of superficial abdominal reflexes ipsilateral to the convexity of scoliosis.

Characterized objectively by Cobb angles, scoliosis demonstrates a strong association with syringomyelia in CM1.[6,7,27,34,36] Scoliosis can be identified in 31% of children with CM1 and syringomylia.[25] In general, the following rules apply[3,7,34]:

- Most (but not all) pediatric patients with CM1 with scoliosis have underlying syringomyelia and
- Not all patients with CM1 with syringomyelia have scoliosis.

These patients may report back or shoulder pain, paresthesias, gait disturbance, and/or clumsiness. Alternatively, physical examination findings of cosmetic irregularity along the spine, asymmetry of the shoulders or pelvis, subtle sensorimotor deficits, or hyperreflexia may reflect underlying scoliosis or syringomyelia.

COMPRESSION OF THE CERVICOMEDULLARY JUNCTION

Less common but concerning symptoms of CM1 include those related to compression of structures around the cervicomedullary junction[2–4,27,35,36]:

- *Medullary compression* may adversely affect respiratory function and lead to sleep apnea,
- *Brainstem or cervical spinal cord compression* can cause sensorimotor deficits (eg, hemiparesis, upper extremity paraparesis, quadriparesis), spasticity, or bladder dysfunction,
- *Lower cranial nerve deficits* (present in up to 10% of pediatric patients with CM1) can cause dysphagia, absent gag reflex, dysarthria, vocal cord dysfunction, or abnormal extraocular motility (eg, esotropia owing to cranial nerve VI paresis)[2,3,5,27,36];
- *Cerebellar flocculus compression* may present as gaze-evoked nystagmus in up to 30% of young adults with CM1,[36] or less commonly other neuro-ophthalmological findings,[40] and its incidence in the pediatric population is not as well defined but reported[41], and
- Up to 10% of those with CM1 may also present with *hydrocephalus* owing to fourth ventricular outlet obstruction.[3,27]

These symptoms occur with less frequency in the modern era likely owing to the advent of MRI offering earlier diagnosis, before neurologic disability occurs.[2,27] However, lower cranial nerve dysfunction is a predominant presentation in children aged younger than 3 years with symptomatic CM1.[36] Medullary compression symptoms are also seen more commonly in children with complex CM1 that includes basilar invagination and/or instability with ventral compression of the cervicomedullary junction.[2,42]

CLINICAL PRESENTATION DURING THE NEONATAL PERIOD AND INFANCY (AGE 0–3 YEARS)

The symptoms and signs of CM1 in this population are more commonly related to pain and features of compression at the craniocervical junction. Pain can present as generalized irritability, inconsolable cries, and nighttime waking in most patients.[3–5,18,27,43] Additional clinical signs can provide further localization, and include the following[3–5,18,27,36]:

- Opisthotonos,
- Frequent neck or back extension/arching, and
- Crying spells with behavioral patterns suggesting head discomfort (eg, reaching for the head or neck).

Oropharyngeal dysfunction, caused by medullary compression and lower cranial nerve compromise, is one of the most common presenting symptoms in approximately 62% to 78% of children aged 0 to 2 years with CM1.[34,36,43] Clinical manifestations can include the following[4,5,20,27,34,36,42]:

- Dysphagia, choking, or aspiration;
- Poor feeding, failure to thrive;
- Gastroesophageal reflux;
- Persistent cough;
- Snoring or episodic sleep apnea;
- Stridor; and
- Recurrent respiratory infections.

Less common symptoms include abdominal pain and vomiting.[36] These more dramatic presentations are typically observed in the setting of significant ventral compression owing to basilar invagination, retroflexion of the dens, and/or frank cervical instability.[42,44] Diagnosis of CM1 in this age group is low and likely reflects delayed identification among other factors. It is not uncommon for these children to undergo gastrointestinal investigations and interventions (eg, feeding tubes), or assessments for vocal cord paralysis that require tracheostomies before the identification of CM1.[36,45]

Clinical presentations with syringomyelia and/or scoliosis are possible in the neonatal and infant populations but occur less frequently than in older children.[4,34,36] In this and other age groups, there does not seem to exist a correlation between the extent of tonsillar herniation and the presence or absence of syringomyelia.[34] Long tract signs can also be present in this age group such as spasticity and gait instability.[43]

CLINICAL PRESENTATION IN TODDLERS (AGE 3–5 YEARS)

As patients develop improved ability to communicate and localize their pain, they may be able to more effectively verbalize complaints attributable to the presence of an underlying CM1. Toddlers with adequate verbal skills may report headache pain or discomfort in the upper neck. Occipital headaches represent a component of the clinical presentation of CM1 in up to 40% to 78% of patients during the toddler stages and early childhood.[3,4,34,36,46] Children aged 3 to 5 years with CM1 frequently present with syringomyelia and/or scoliosis (the latter present in 14%–38% of pediatric patients).[4,27,31,34,36] As with neonates and infants, symptoms or signs of medullary and lower cranial nerve dysfunction (eg, sleep apnea, oropharyngeal dysphagia, dysarthria, absent gag reflex) may be present in toddlers with CM1.[19,27,34,36]

CLINICAL PRESENTATION DURING CHILDHOOD AND ADOLESCENCE (AGE 5 YEARS AND OLDER)

As they mature into the childhood and adolescent years, pediatric patients more frequently and reliably report the classic symptoms of CM1. Most commonly, patients note occipital headaches and/or neck pain, often induced by Valsalva-type maneuvers (eg, straining for a bowel movement, laughing, coughing, sneezing) and of short duration (typically <5 minutes).[3] To warrant surgical consideration, these headaches should be severe and frequent enough to impact activities of daily living (eg, missing school) or quality of life.[5] Some children present with frontotemporal or poorly localized headaches and still benefit from decompression but with lower success rates reported.[38] As with younger patients, older children and adolescents with CM1 may also experience oropharyngeal dysfunction, although less frequently.

Scoliosis, typically associated with syringomyelia (present in 19%–76% of patients with CM1), represents another important component of the clinical presentation in this group of patients.[2–4,7,31,34,36] Syringomyelia with scoliosis may lead to back or shoulder pain.[3] Children may also present with myelopathic features (shown in **Fig. 3**) in the absence of any headache.[38] The constellation of CM1, syringomyelia,

and/or scoliosis may produce multiple physical examination findings that are easier to elicit or observe within older children and adolescents (**Fig. 4**).

CLINICAL PRESENTATION IN ADULTS

In adults with CM1, symptoms in order of frequency include headaches (cough-induced, migrainous, or others), paresthesia, ataxia, and less frequently oropharyngeal and cranial nerve dysfunction. Available, although, limited studies suggest that asymptomatic and mildly symptomatic adults with CM1 have a benign natural history. Indications for intervention vary but include Chiari headaches affecting the quality of life, neurologic symptoms attributed to brainstem compression, and symptomatic or enlarging syrinx.[47]

CLINICAL CONDITIONS ASSOCIATED WITH CHIARI I MALFORMATION

In addition to scoliosis, other, less common spinal or craniocervical osseous abnormalities may occur in the pediatric CM1 population (**Table 1**).[2–6,27,31,34,42,44,48] CM1 represents a common finding (up to 33%–38%) in patients with craniovertebral junction abnormalities such as basilar invagination.[2] A variety of other clinical conditions and syndromes have been associated with CM1, many of which may be incidental or displacement of the tonsils occurs secondary to the primary disease.[49] Common associated conditions include the following[3–5,27,34]:

- Hydrocephalus (8%–10%),[3,27]
- Craniosynostosis,[50]
- Neurofibromatosis type I (up to 5%),[3,27]
- Ehlers Danlos syndrome type 3,[51,52] and
- Growth hormone deficiency (idiopathic; around 4%).[3,27]

RARE AND ACUTE PRESENTATIONS OF CHIARI I MALFORMATION IN CHILDREN

In addition to the common clinical presentations of CM1 described, more obscure presentations exist based on their acuity, rapid progression, or rarity of symptomatology. In unusual circumstances, pediatric patients with CM1 can present acutely in distress and require urgent operative intervention. Previously reported acute onset or rapidly progressive symptoms and signs include the following[3,53–56]:

- Dysphagia,
- Isolated upper or upper and lower extremity weakness or paralysis,
- Paresthesias,

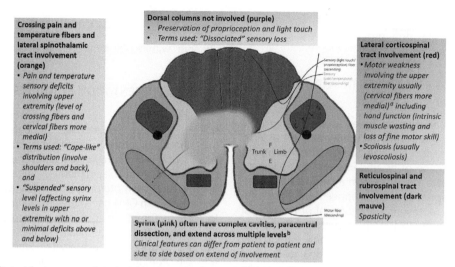

Fig. 3. Clinical features associated with syringomyelia. Authors' depiction of cervical spinal cord cross section with select tracts represented. [a]This anatomic pathophysiology has recently been challenged.[58] [b]Pathological features of syrinx from Ref.[59] C, cervical; E, extensors; F, flexors; L, lumbar; S, sacral; T, thoracic.

- Respiratory distress,
- Gait dysfunction,
- Foot drop, and
- Anisocoria.

These presentations tend to have the following commonality in addition to CM1[56]:

- Often (but not always) have an inciting event (eg, trauma, infection, breath holding),
- Often (but not always) associated with spinal cord changes (syringomyelia or "presyrinx") in cases of sensorimotor deficits,

- Most respond well to surgical decompression, and
- These events are rare.

These acutely presenting or rapidly progressive symptoms and signs reflect pathologic compression of the brainstem and/or spinal cord long tracts.[53] Although the specific symptoms may not represent rare findings given their appearance as chronic symptoms in other patients with CM1, their rapid presentation or progression defy common patterns. Several rare presentations of CM1 have been reported in the literature and are summarized in **Table 2**.[3–5,19,20,27,31,34–36,53]

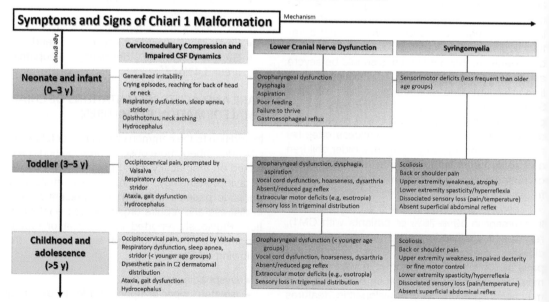

Fig. 4. Prominent symptoms and signs of Chiari I malformation and syringomyelia in children, based on mechanism and age. CSF, cerebrospinal fluid; Yrs, years.

Table 1
Abnormalities associated and/or reported with Chiari I malformation (list not exhaustive)[3,4,8–14,60]

Type/Location	Association
Cranial vault	Craniosynostosis Decreased volume of posterior fossa
Intracranial	Hydrocephalus Idiopathic intracranial hypertension Mass lesions
Skull base	Fibrous dysplasia and McCune-Alright syndrome Achondroplasia
Craniocervical junction	Basilar invagination Platybasia Atlas assimilation
Cervical spine	Odontoid process retroversion/retroflexion Klippel–Feil anomaly or variants
Vertebral column/spine	Hemivertebra Butterfly vertebra Tethered cord
Skeletal	Cervical rib Sprengel deformity
Syndromes	Neurofibromatosis type 1 Ehler's Danlos syndrome
Others	Idiopathic growth hormone deficiency Epilepsy

Table 2
Rare presentations of Chiari I malformation in children

Severity of Presentation	Clinical Finding
Mild	Nystagmus (typically down-beating) Chronic hiccups Chronic cough Cerebellar or cerebellovestibular dysfunction (eg, vertigo)
Moderate	Focal sensorimotor deficits (mononeuropathy; eg, plantar flexion weakness) Urinary incontinence Torticollis Trigeminal or glossopharyngeal neuralgia Sensorineural hearing loss
Severe	Syncopal episodes, drop attacks Acute spinal cord injury after trauma (eg, quadriplegia) Respiratory failure requiring mechanical ventilation Cardiorespiratory arrest, sudden death

SUMMARY

Incidental CM1 is common and likely to remain asymptomatic in most cases. When symptomatic, it most often presents with headaches that are typically occipital or suboccipital, provoked or worsened by Valsalva-like maneuvers, and of relatively short duration. CM1 is most commonly associated with syringomyelia with or without scoliosis at presentation in the pediatric population. CM1 and syringomyelia may be associated with a wide spectrum of signs and symptoms in children, which can differ in presentation between older and the very young children. In those younger than 3 years, in addition to pain symptoms, oropharyngeal symptoms seem to predominate more so than syringomyelia or scoliosis. Other symptoms related to compression at the cervicomedullary junction include respiratory dysfunction, lower cranial nerve deficits, ataxia, and nystagmus. CM1 is also associated with osseous abnormalities and certain genetic syndromes. Although most patients with CM1 with symptoms tend to have a longer duration of symptoms and benign course, acute neurologic changes have been reported and are rare.

CLINICS CARE POINTS

- Evaluation of children referred for incidental or asymptomatic CM1 should rule out associated findings and management should consider that most children will remain asymptomatic over time.

- The nature of the headache in symptomatic CM1, its effect on daily activities, and other signs and symptoms related to CM1 should be elicited on history and examination to identify patients that are likely to benefit from surgical decompression.
- There should be a high clinical suspicion for cervicomedullary compression, including CM1, in patients younger than 3 years presenting with pain symptoms, oropharyngeal dysfunction, and signs such as opisthotonos, neck/back arching, or reaching for the head or neck.
- Syringomyelia and scoliosis are highly associated with CM1 and signs and symptoms (eg, sensorimotor deficits, shoulder or back pain, asymmetry of the shoulder, chest, or pelvis) should be elicited during assessment.

DISCLOSURE

The authors have no commercial or financial conflicts of interest to report. There were no funding sources for the completion of this study.
Acknowledgments

REFERENCES

1. Massimi L, Peretta P, Erbetta A, et al. Diagnosis and treatment of Chiari malformation type 1 in children: the International Consensus Document. Neurol Sci 2022;43(2):1311–26.
2. Menezes AH. Craniovertebral junction abnormalities with hindbrain herniation and syringomyelia: regression of syringomyelia after removal of ventral craniovertebral junction compression. J Neurosurg 2012; 116(2):301–9.
3. Tubbs RS, Beckman J, Naftel RP, et al. Institutional experience with 500 cases of surgically treated pediatric Chiari malformation Type I. J Neurosurg Pediatr 2011;7(3):248–56.
4. Tubbs RS, McGirt MJ, Oakes WJ. Surgical experience in 130 pediatric patients with Chiari I malformations. J Neurosurg 2003;99(2):291–6.
5. Tubbs R, Griessenauer C, Oakes W. Chiari malformations. In: Albright A, Pollack I, Adelson P, editors. Principles and practice of pediatric neurosurgery. 3rd edition. New York: Thieme; 2015. p. 217–32.
6. Milhorat TH, Chou MW, Trinidad EM, et al. Chiari I malformation redefined: clinical and radiographic findings for 364 symptomatic patients. Neurosurgery 1999;44(5):1005–17.
7. Muhonen MG, Menezes AH, Sawin PD, et al. Scoliosis in pediatric Chiari malformations without myelodysplasia. J Neurosurg 1992;77(1):69–77.
8. Wang J, Alotaibi NM, Samuel N, et al. Acquired Chiari Malformation and Syringomyelia Secondary to Space-Occupying Lesions: A Systematic Review. World Neurosurg 2017;98:800–8.e2.
9. Cinalli G, Spennato P, Sainte-Rose C, et al. Chiari malformation in craniosynostosis. Childs Nerv Syst 2005;21(10):889–901.
10. Fagan LH, Ferguson S, Yassari R, et al. The Chiari pseudotumor cerebri syndrome: symptom recurrence after decompressive surgery for Chiari malformation type I. Pediatr Neurosurg 2006;42(1):14–9.
11. Chumas PD, Armstrong DC, Drake JM, et al. Tonsillar herniation: the rule rather than the exception after lumboperitoneal shunting in the pediatric population. J Neurosurg 1993;78(4):568–73.
12. Schievink WI. Spontaneous spinal cerebrospinal fluid leaks and intracranial hypotension. JAMA 2006;295(19):2286–96.
13. Massimi L, Pennisi G, Frassanito P, et al. Chiari type I and hydrocephalus. Childs Nerv Syst 2019;35(10):1701–9.
14. Milano JB, Barcelos ACES, Onishi FJ, et al. The effect of filum terminale sectioning for Chiari 1 malformation treatment: systematic review. Neurol Sci 2020;41(2):249–56.
15. Dangouloff-Ros V, Roux CJ, Boulouis G, et al. Incidental Brain MRI Findings in Children: A Systematic Review and Meta-Analysis. AJNR Am J Neuroradiol 2019;40(11):1818–23.
16. Li Y, Thompson WK, Reuter C, et al. Rates of Incidental Findings in Brain Magnetic Resonance Imaging in Children. JAMA Neurol 2021;78(5):578–87.
17. Whitson WJ, Lane JR, Bauer DF, et al. A prospective natural history study of nonoperatively managed Chiari I malformation: does follow-up MRI surveillance alter surgical decision making? J Neurosurg Pediatr 2015;16(2):159–66.
18. Benglis D, Covington D, Bhatia R, et al. Outcomes in pediatric patients with Chiari malformation Type I followed up without surgery. J Neurosurg Pediatr 2011;7(4):375–9.
19. Aitken LA, Lindan CE, Sidney S, et al. Chiari type I malformation in a pediatric population. Pediatr Neurol 2009;40(6):449–54.
20. Chambers KJ, Setlur J, Hartnick CJ. Chiari type I malformation: presenting as chronic cough in older children. Laryngoscope 2013;123(11):2888–91.
21. Leon TJ, Kuhn EN, Arynchyna AA, et al. Patients with "benign" Chiari I malformations require surgical decompression at a low rate. J Neurosurg Pediatr 01 04 2019;23(4):498–506.
22. Carey M, Fuell W, Harkey T, et al. Natural history of Chiari I malformation in children: a retrospective analysis. Childs Nerv Syst 04 2021;37(4):1185–90.
23. Strahle J, Muraszko KM, Kapurch J, et al. Natural history of Chiari malformation Type I following

decision for conservative treatment. J Neurosurg Pediatr 2011;8(2):214–21.

24. Pomeraniec IJ, Ksendzovsky A, Awad AJ, et al. Natural and surgical history of Chiari malformation Type I in the pediatric population. J Neurosurg Pediatr 2016;17(3):343–52.

25. Strahle JM, Taiwo R, Averill C, et al. Radiological and clinical predictors of scoliosis in patients with Chiari malformation type I and spinal cord syrinx from the Park-Reeves Syringomyelia Research Consortium. J Neurosurg Pediatr 2019;1–8.

26. Toldo I, Tangari M, Mardari R, et al. Headache in children with Chiari I malformation. Headache 2014;54(5):899–908.

27. Rozzelle CJ. Clinical presentation of pediatric Chiari I malformations. In: The Chiari malformations. New York, NY: Springer; 2013. p. 247–51.

28. Nieswand V, Richter M, Gossrau G. Epidemiology of Headache in Children and Adolescents-Another Type of Pandemia. Curr Pain Headache Rep 2020; 24(10):62.

29. Curone M, Valentini LG, Vetrano I, et al. Chiari malformation type 1-related headache: the importance of a multidisciplinary study. Neurol Sci 2017; 38(Suppl 1):91–3.

30. Pascual J, Oterino A, Berciano J. Headache in type I Chiari malformation. Neurology 1992;42(8):1519–21.

31. Greenlee J, Garell PC, Stence N, et al. Comprehensive approach to Chiari malformation in pediatric patients. Neurosurg Focus 1999;6(6):E6.

32. Headache Classification Committee of the International Headache Society (IHS) The International Classification of Headache Disorders, 3rd edition. Cephalalgia. 01 2018;38(1):1-211.

33. Taylor FR, Larkins MV. Headache and Chiari I malformation: clinical presentation, diagnosis, and controversies in management. Curr Pain Headache Rep 2002;6(4):331–7.

34. Greenlee JD, Donovan KA, Hasan DM, et al. Chiari I malformation in the very young child: the spectrum of presentations and experience in 31 children under age 6 years. Pediatrics 2002;110(6):1212–9.

35. Laufer I, Engel M, Feldstein N, et al. Chiari malformation presenting as a focal motor deficit. Report of two cases. J Neurosurg Pediatr 2008;1(5):392–5.

36. Albert GW, Menezes AH, Hansen DR, et al. Chiari malformation Type I in children younger than age 6 years: presentation and surgical outcome. J Neurosurg Pediatr 2010;5(6):554–61.

37. Grangeon L, Puy L, Gilard V, et al. Predictive Factors of Headache Resolution After Chiari Type 1 Malformation Surgery. World Neurosurg 2018;110:e60–6.

38. Greenberg JK, Yarbrough CK, Radmanesh A, et al. The Chiari Severity Index: a preoperative grading system for Chiari malformation type 1. Neurosurgery 2015;76(3):279–85 [discussion: 285].

39. Strahle J, Muraszko KM, Garton HJ, et al. Syrinx location and size according to etiology: identification of Chiari-associated syrinx. J Neurosurg Pediatr 2015;16(1):21–9.

40. Shaikh AG, Ghasia FF. Neuro-ophthalmology of type 1 Chiari malformation. Expert Rev Ophthalmol 2015; 10(4):351–7.

41. Nash DL, Diehl NN, Mohney BG. Incidence and Types of Pediatric Nystagmus. Am J Ophthalmol 2017;182:31–4.

42. Bollo RJ, Riva-Cambrin J, Brockmeyer MM, et al. Complex Chiari malformations in children: an analysis of preoperative risk factors for occipitocervical fusion. J Neurosurg Pediatr 2012;10(2):134–41.

43. Grahovac G, Pundy T, Tomita T. Chiari type I malformation of infants and toddlers. Childs Nerv Syst 2018;34(6):1169–76.

44. Goel A. Basilar invagination, Chiari malformation, syringomyelia: a review. Neurol India 2009;57(3): 235–46.

45. Jang M, Biggs P, North L, et al. Management and outcomes of pediatric vocal cord paresis in Chiari malformation. Int J Pediatr Otorhinolaryngol 2018; 115:49–53.

46. Chae JK, Greenfield JP. Revision Chiari Surgery in Young Children: Predictors and Outcomes. Pediatr Neurosurg 2021;56(6):529–37.

47. Langridge B, Phillips E, Choi D. Chiari Malformation Type 1: A Systematic Review of Natural History and Conservative Management. World Neurosurg 2017; 104:213–9.

48. Goel A, Desai K, Bhatjiwale M, et al. Basilar invagination and Chiari malformation associated with cerebellar atrophy: report of two treated cases. J Clin Neurosci 2002;9(2):194–6.

49. Loukas M, Shayota BJ, Oelhafen K, et al. Associated disorders of Chiari Type I malformations: a review. Neurosurg Focus 2011;31(3):E3.

50. Strahle J, Muraszko KM, Buchman SR, et al. Chiari malformation associated with craniosynostosis. Neurosurg Focus 2011;31(3):E2.

51. Milhorat TH, Bolognese PA, Nishikawa M, et al. Syndrome of occipitoatlantoaxial hypermobility, cranial settling, and chiari malformation type I in patients with hereditary disorders of connective tissue. J Neurosurg Spine 2007;7(6):601–9.

52. Sadler B, Kuensting T, Strahle J, et al. Prevalence and Impact of Underlying Diagnosis and Comorbidities on Chiari 1 Malformation. Pediatr Neurol 2020; 106:32–7.

53. Wellons JC, Tubbs RS, Bui CJ, et al. Urgent surgical intervention in pediatric patients with Chiari malformation type I. Report of two cases. J Neurosurg 2007;107(1 Suppl):49–52.

54. Jayamanne C, Fernando L, Mettananda S. Chiari malformation type 1 presenting as unilateral

progressive foot drop: a case report and review of literature. BMC Pediatr 2018;18(1):34.

55. McMillan HJ, Sell E, Nzau M, et al. Chiari 1 malformation and holocord syringomyelia presenting as abrupt onset foot drop. Childs Nerv Syst 2011; 27(1):183–6.

56. Talamonti G, Marcati E, Gribaudi G, et al. Acute presentation of Chiari 1 malformation in children. Childs Nerv Syst 2020;36(5):899–909.

57. Dahdaleh NS, Menezes AH. Incomplete lateral medullary syndrome in a patient with Chiari malformation Type I presenting with combined trigeminal and vagal nerve dysfunction. J Neurosurg Pediatr 2008;2(4):250–3.

58. Morecraft RJ, Stilwell-Morecraft KS, Ge J, et al. Lack of somatotopy among corticospinal tract fibers passing through the primate craniovertebral junction and cervical spinal cord: pathoanatomical substrate of central cord syndrome and cruciate paralysis. J Neurosurg 2021;1–15.

59. Milhorat TH, Capocelli AL, Anzil AP, et al. Pathological basis of spinal cord cavitation in syringomyelia: analysis of 105 autopsy cases. J Neurosurg 1995; 82(5):802–12.

60. Furtado SV, Reddy K, Hegde AS. Posterior fossa morphometry in symptomatic pediatric and adult Chiari I malformation. J Clin Neurosci 2009;16(11): 1449–54.

Chiari I Malformation and Sleep-Disordered Breathing

Alexandria C. Marino, MD, PhD[a,b,*], Faraz Farzad, BA[c], John A. Jane Jr, MD[a]

KEYWORDS

● Chiari I ● Sleep apnea ● Posterior fossa decompression ● Pediatric neurosurgery

KEY POINTS

● The rate of sleep-disordered breathing (SDB) is higher in patients with Chiari I than in healthy patients.
● SDB can be obstructive or central. Obstructive sleep apnea occurs more frequently than patients with central Chiari I but both obstructive and central patterns are observed.
● Polysomnography should be completed to characterize SDB in patients aged younger than 6 years, patients with symptoms of snoring, excessive sleepiness, or nighttime apneas, or patients with significant tonsillar descent.
● Surgical decompression is associated with improvement in SDB.
● Recurrence of SDB can herald recurrence of Chiari I.

INTRODUCTION

The primary anatomic abnormality in Chiari type 1 malformations is the descent of the cerebellar tonsils through the foramen magnum. This descent has multiple potentially serious clinical consequences. Symptoms can include headaches, central cord syndrome, and scoliosis due to syringomyelia resulting from deranged cerebrospinal fluid dynamics, nystagmus, dysphagia, and sleep-disordered breathing (SDB) due to medullary and cranial nerve involvement, ataxia due to cerebellar dysfunction, and hydrocephalus. SDB is characterized by abnormal apneas and/or hypopneas during sleep and can lead to hypoxia and sleep disruption that can lead to disruptive daytime sleepiness. SDB can be characterized as obstructive, in which inspiratory effort is attempted by fails due to an obstructed pharyngeal passage, or central, in which inspiratory effort does not occur. SDB in neurologic disease results from disruptions of medullary centers involved in respiratory control and is more frequent and severe in patients with Chiari II than in Chiari I malformations[1,2] but SDB in Chiari I is increasingly recognized. SDB is a relatively common pathologic condition in children regardless of craniocervical junction pathologic condition but is more common and especially important in children with Chiari malformations. It is crucial for clinicians to consider brainstem compromise when evaluating patients with SDB, and for neurosurgeons to evaluate patients with Chiari I for SDB, because this may inform surgical decision-making. Here key issues associated with SDB in patients with Chiari I are reviewed, including demographics, diagnosis, pathophysiology, and management.

Case

A 13-month-old male infant with macrocephaly, hypotonia, and developmental delay was referred

[a] Department of Neurological Surgery, University of Virginia Health System, Charlottesville, VA, USA; [b] Department of Neurological Surgery, University of Virginia Health Sciences Center, PO Box 800212, Charlottesville, VA 22908, USA; [c] University of Virginia School of Medicine, Charlottesville, VA, USA
* Corresponding author. Department of Neurological Surgery, University of Virginia Health Sciences Center, PO Box 800212, Charlottesville, VA 22908.
E-mail address: acm7sp@hscmail.mcc.virginia.edu

Neurosurg Clin N Am 34 (2023) 35–41
https://doi.org/10.1016/j.nec.2022.08.005
1042-3680/23/© 2022 Elsevier Inc. All rights reserved.

to neurosurgery. His head circumference increased from 50th percentile at birth to 97th percentile at presentation. He was able to pull to stand and stand with support at 13 months but unable to take independent steps. His mother noted drooling and difficulty swallowing. He frequently snored and did not sleep through the night but his mother did notice apneic events. Aside from hypotonia in bilateral lower extremities, his physical examination was unremarkable. Brain MRI showed Chiari I malformation with mild-to-moderate ventriculomegaly and 7 mm of tonsillar descent (**Fig. 1**A). MRI of the cervical spine showed subtle T2 hyperintense signals within the dorsal upper cervical cord at C2-C3 concerning for early presyrinx. The patient was referred for neurosurgical consultation and polysomnography. Polysomnography revealed significant SDB with central sleep apneas (CSAs; **Table 1**). The apnea/hypopnea index (AHI) was 12.3 events per hour. He also had intermittent desaturations to a low of 77% with apneic events, and he snored 50% of the time. He underwent posterior fossa decompression with dural splitting and C1 laminectomy as well as concurrent adenoidectomy by the otolaryngology team. There were no significant surgical complications.

Polysomnography completed 6 weeks postoperatively showed significant improvement. The AHI improved to 3.5 events per hour. His mean oxygen saturation was 98.3% with rare desaturations to a low of 87%. He did not snore. Postoperative MRI showed resolution of ventriculomegaly and expected postoperative changes at the level of the foramen magnum (**Fig. 1**B).

Demographics, Presentation, and Natural History

Chiari I malformation is usually defined as greater than 5 mm descent of cerebellar tonsils below the foramen magnum. The average age at diagnosis is around 25 years of age,[3] and although true prevalence is difficult to estimate due to the frequency of asymptomatic disease, it is likely that greater than 200,000 Americans have Chiari I malformations.[3] Approximately 40% of patients diagnosed are children.[4] Evidence of Chiari I is found in 1% of children who undergo cranial imaging,[5] which is comparable to 0.8% prevalence in adult imaging.[6] Often, Chiari I malformations are found incidentally; however, pediatric case series report that 65% to 69% of patients with Chiari I that present to neurosurgeons and are ultimately managed conservatively are symptomatic.[7,8]

The most common presenting symptom in children with Chiari I is suboccipital headache.[9,10]

Tubbs and colleagues published the largest cohort of children undergoing surgery for Chiari I; of the 500 children included, 40% presented with head or neck pain. Other common presenting symptoms included scoliosis, apnea/bradycardia, upper extremity pain/numbness, dysphagia, ataxia, vocal hoarseness or altered tone and emesis.[10] Fifty-seven percent of patients were noted to have syringomyelia.[10]

The natural history of Chiari I has been informed by case series of patients who underwent conservative management. In these cohorts, 0% to 27% of children had progressive symptoms during 1 year of follow-up.[11,12] However, because the conservative management is not prescribed in a randomized fashion, these patients are likely less symptomatic than patients who were treated with surgery and therefore do not necessarily accurately represent all patients with Chiari I. No study has randomized patients to surgical intervention; one pediatric cohort compared surgical intervention to observation and found better symptom improvement with surgery but the surgical cohort was not assumed to match the nonsurgical cohort.[8]

SDB occurs in 24% to 70% of patients with Chiari I,[13] which is higher than the rate of SDB observed in general pediatric cohorts.[14] A small number of series have quantified SDB specifically in children with Chiari I. A recent series by Moore and colleagues reviewed 465 patients with Chiari I, of whom 44% had symptoms of SDB characterized by snoring or apneas. Of these, 75 children underwent sleep studies, and 23 of these were diagnosed with SDB. Sixteen patients had obstructive sleep apnea (OSA), 6 had CSA, and 1 had mixed sleep apnea with both obstructive and central events.[15] Another series of 26 patients who underwent polysomnography showed a 61.5% rate of SDB. Seventy-five percent of the children with sleep apnea showed an obstructive pattern.[16] As in healthy patients, higher body mass index is associated with higher incidence of sleep apnea in the setting of Chiari I.[16] Although these estimates provide a reference point, they may not be representative of the true prevalence of SDB in patients with Chiari I because not all center conduct routine polysomnography, and those that do may use different indications for sleep study referrals because there is not a widely agreed-upon threshold for polysomnography. Clinicians should be aware that SDB can sometimes be the only presenting symptoms of Chiari I malformation,[17] although it is difficult to discern from current literature how commonly SDB represents this isolated symptom in children presenting with Chiari I.

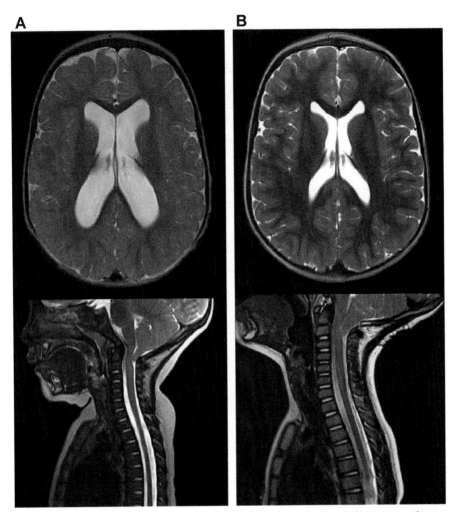

Fig. 1. Preoperative and postoperative MRI of patient with Chiari I with central sleep apnea that resolved with posterior fossa decompression. (*A*) Preoperative T2-weighted MRI. Axial slice at the level of the lateral ventricles showing mild-to-moderate ventriculomegaly. Midsagittal slice of the cervical spine showing Chiari 1 malformation with 7 mm cerebellar tonsillar ectopy. Subtle hyperintensity in the dorsal midline of the cord at the C2/C3 disc level, which may represent an early presyrinx. (*B*) A 17-month postoperative T2-weighted MRI. Axial slice at the level of the lateral ventricles showing improved ventriculomegaly. Midsagittal slice of the cervical spine showing Chiari 1 malformation with postsurgical changes.

PATHOPHYSIOLOGY

Normal ventilation maintains blood pH, arterial $PaCO_2$ and PaO_2 within a physiologic range. SDB in Chiari I malformation can be multifactorial and can result from disruption of afferent sensory signals, intrinsic brainstem circuits, and/or efferent ventilatory signals.

Multiple afferent inputs to the central nervous system modulate breathing. Signals from peripheral chemoreceptors in the carotid bodies, located the junction of the internal and external carotid arteries, send signals via Hering's nerve as part of cranial nerve IX. These carotid bodies respond specifically to PaO_2 and to hydrogen ion concentration (which serves as a proxy signal for $PaCO_2$) and primarily lead to modulation of tidal volume. Another population of chemoreceptors in the ventral medulla responds to hypercapnia and acidemia by sensing CSF H^+ ions but is less responsive to hypoxia.[18] These receptors lead to modulations in respiratory rate.[19] Other afferent signals that influence ventilation include input from pulmonary receptors in the lungs that send signals via the vagus as well as muscle proprioceptors in the chest wall that project to medullary respiratory centers via the anterior reticulospinal tract. There are several intrinsic brainstem areas in the medulla that are involved in various aspects of respiratory control. The site of the central

Table 1
Preoperative and postoperative polysomnography metrics

	Preoperative	6 Weeks Postoperative	57 Months Postoperative
Sleep Architecture			
Total sleep time (minutes)	371	376	400
Sleep efficiency (%)	88	89	91
Respiratory parameters			
Central apneas	63	22	26
Obstructive apneas	0	0	0
Mixed apneas	0	0	0
Hypopneas	13	0	0
Apnea-hypopnea index (events/hour)	12.3	3.5	3.9
Mean oxygen saturation (%) [minimum]	97.8 [77]	98.3 [87]	96.7 [90]

pattern generator that generates efferent signals lies in the dorsal respiratory group in the nucleus solitarius. This dorsal respiratory group sends signals that drive the diaphragm via the phrenic nerve as well as accessory muscles of inspiration.[20] Other medullary structures involved in respiration include retrotrapezoid and parafacial nuclei, Botzinger and pre-Botzinger complexes, and rostral and caudal respiratory groups.[21] The pontine pneumotaxic center also regulates the duration of inspiration and expiration but is less likely to be affected by Chiari I due to its rostral location.[18] Cerebral cortical signals can also influence breathing but this is less important during sleep.[22] Efferent signals involved in respiration travel via the phrenic nerve, which innervates the diaphragm. Efferent signals carried by cranial nerves IX and X also affect pharyngeal tone and can therefore impair respiration by allowing obstruction of the airway.

Even in normal subjects, the onset of sleep leads to blunted responses to hypoxia and hypercapnia as well as reduced muscle tone in pharyngeal and airway dilator muscles, leading to the unmasking of apneic episodes during sleep in predisposed patients. Sleep apnea can be characterized as obstructive or central. Obstructive apneic occur when diaphragmatic and thoracic muscular activity exerts negative pressure against an airway that is obstructed. Central apneic episodes are characterized by an absence of diaphragmatic or thoracic contraction that is associated with a prolonged pause in respiration.

OSA is promoted by decreased tone of pharyngeal muscles. This localizes to cranial nerves IX and X as well as the dorsal motor nuclei of the vagus or nucleus ambiguus. Increased pharyngeal

tissue or a smaller airway can also predispose to OSA.[13] CSA can occur due to various mechanisms. These include direct dysfunction of medullary respiratory centers due to compression or ischemia, dysfunction of cranial nerve IX, which impairs chemoreception and therefore blunts responses to hypoxia or hypercapnia, compression of phrenic motor neurons due to syringomyelia, or decreased medullary responsiveness to chemosensory signals.[13] The exact cause of CSA is not often determined in patients with Chiari I, perhaps in part, because surgical decompression is the common treatment regardless of the cause of CSA. Individual case reports provide some insight into mechanisms for specific patients. For instance, OSA has been linked to the loss of pharyngeal sensation.[23] In other patients, failure to increase respiration in response to hypercapnia has been demonstrated,[24] whereas other patients with Chiari I with sleep apnea demonstrate a failure to increase respiratory rate in response to hypoxia.[25] Direct compression of medullary structures, and indeed the severity of CSA correlates both with effacement of the perimedullary subarachnoid space as well as with extent of tonsillar descent.[26,27]

EVALUATION

A diagnosis of SDB in the setting of Chiari I can be suggested by witnessed snoring, apneas, or daytime sleepiness. Clinicians can use clinical tools such as the Epworth sleepiness scale to screen for SDB in patients that are old enough.[28] However, definitive diagnosis requires an overnight sleepy study, or polysomnogram. Current consensus guidelines suggest referral for polysomnography in all symptomatic patients aged younger than 6 years, in patients exhibiting signs or symptoms of SDB, or in patients with severe tonsillar descent.[29] Polysomnograms allow the quantification of apneas, defined as a reduction in airflow of greater than 90% for at least 10 seconds, as well as hypopneas, defined as a reduction in airflow greater than 30% or a reduction in oxygen saturation of 3% or more, although criteria for hypopneas have evolved over time.[30] Apneas and hypopneas are further characterized as obstructive if they occur in the setting of inspiratory effort or central if no inspiratory effort occurs. The number of apneas and hypopneas occurring per hour is reported as the AHI, which is normal when less than 5 per hour.[13]

MANAGEMENT

Noninvasive positive pressure ventilation is often trialed for SDB. However, in some patients with Chiari I, even with OSA, this does not reliably improve symptoms.[31] Systematic data on the frequency of noninvasive ventilation in patients with Chiari I and its success rate are lacking.

Adenoidectomy is undertaken to address OSA before posterior fossa decompression, in some cases, because the Chiari I malformation is undiagnosed. However, at least in some cases, this fails to improve SDB[27,32] or improves only the obstructive component, unmasking CSA.[33] This approach does not address the underlying craniocervical stenosis, although some parents may be interested in pursuing adenoidectomy due to the impression of decreased surgical risk in comparison to posterior fossa decompression. Although no studies directly compare adenoidectomy to posterior fossa decompression, multiple case reports exist of improvement after posterior fossa decompression when adenoidectomy failed.[27,32] Patients should be counseled regarding the likelihood of needing posterior fossa decompression even if adenoidectomy is completed.

Consensus guidelines have not addressed how the diagnosis of SDB should guide decision-making around surgical decompression,[29] and detailed guidelines will require further reporting and meta-analysis of outcomes. Case reports and small case series suggest that the majority of children with CSA will show improvement or resolution after foramen magnum decompression[32,34,35]; this is comparable to the improvement in SDB observed in adult patients with Chiari I.[36,37] Improvement occurs with both duroplasty and dural splitting.[38] However, the decision to operate must be considered in the context of the natural history of Chiari I. Strahle

and colleagues[11] found that a significant number of patients showed improvement of various Chiari I symptoms with watchful waiting, although improvement in SDB was not specifically reported. Case reports have shown improvement of CSA with watchful waiting.[39] Therefore, it may be reasonable to observe patients with mild SDB. However, children with more severe SDB should be offered decompression because SDB can become quite severe and even life threatening in some cases and can predict more severe presentations of respiratory illnesses such as pneumonia.[25,40] Surgical decompression consisting of posterior fossa decompression with duraplasty or dural splitting is relatively safe, with 2.5% complication rate reported and 0.8% life-threatening complication rate reported.[10] Acute respiratory failure can occasionally be the only presenting symptom in patients with Chiari I, and urgent surgical decompression can lead to reversal of symptoms.[40] Clinicians should also be aware that, similar to other Chiari symptoms, SDB can recur and can sometimes be the only sign of recurrence.[41] Continued follow-up and monitoring of snoring and nighttime apneas is warranted regardless of whether surgical decompression is undertaken.

SUMMARY

SDB is a consequential symptom of Chiari I and occurs in a sizable number of patients. The cause of SDB is multifactorial and can result from disruption of afferent or efferent signals as well as intrinsic medullary circuits. OSA is slightly more common than CSA in children with Chiari I, and definitive characterization requires polysomnography. Posterior fossa decompression is a promising treatment and many children show improvement in sleep apnea after decompression.

CLINICS CARE POINTS

- SDB is an increasingly recognized feature of Chiari I and can manifest as obstructive or central sleep apnea due to medullary compression or cranial nerve dysfunction.
- Clinicians should maintain a high degree of suspicion for SDB in patients with known Chiari I malformations and should maintain a high degree of suspicion for Chiari I malformation or other causes of brainstem compression in the setting of SDB in children.

- Diagnosis and characterization of SDB requires polysomnography, and should be pursued in all symptomatic patients with Chiari I aged younger than 6 years, in patients with signs or symptoms of SDB such as snoring, excessive sleepiness, or nighttime breathing irregularities, or in patients with severe tonsillar descent.
- Case series suggest that surgical decompression improves SBD, whereas isolated adenoidectomy in patients with Chiari I with obstructive sleep apnea may unmask central sleep apnea.
- Recurrence of Chiari I malformation can be heralded by recurrence of SDB, and so clinicians should continue to monitor for symptoms of SDB postoperatively.

DISCLOSURE

The authors have no funding or conflicts of interest to declare.

REFERENCES

1. Choi SS, Tran LP, Zalzal GH. Airway abnormalities in patients with Arnold-Chiari malformation. Otolaryngol Head Neck Surg 1999;121(6):720–4.
2. Dauvilliers Y, Stal V, Abril B, et al. Chiari malformation and sleep related breathing disorders. J Neurol Neurosurg Psychiatr 2007;78(12):1344–8.
3. Speer MC, Enterline DS, Mehltretter L, et al. Review article: chiari type I malformation with or without syringomyelia: prevalence and genetics. J Genet Couns 2003;12(4):297–311.
4. Gilmer HS, Xi M, Young SH. Surgical decompression for chiari malformation type I: An age-based outcomes study based on the chicago chiari outcome scale. World Neurosurg 2017;107:285–90.
5. Aitken LA, Lindan CE, Sidney S, et al. Chiari type I malformation in a pediatric population. Pediatr Neurol 2009;40(6):449–54.
6. Meadows J, Kraut M, Guarnieri M, et al. Asymptomatic Chiari Type I malformations identified on magnetic resonance imaging. J Neurosurg 2000;92(6):920–6.
7. Benglis D Jr, Covington D, Bhatia R, et al. Outcomes in pediatric patients with Chiari malformation Type I followed up without surgery. J Neurosurg Pediatr 2011;7(4):375–9.
8. Pomeraniec IJ, Ksendzovsky A, Awad AJ, et al. Natural and surgical history of Chiari malformation Type I in the pediatric population. J Neurosurg Pediatr 2016;17(3):343–52.
9. Milhorat TH, Chou MW, Trinidad EM, et al. Chiari I malformation redefined: clinical and radiographic findings for 364 symptomatic patients. Neurosurgery 1999;44(5):1005–17.
10. Tubbs RS, Beckman J, Naftel RP, et al. Institutional experience with 500 cases of surgically treated pediatric Chiari malformation Type I. J Neurosurg Pediatr 2011;7(3):248–56.
11. Strahle J, Muraszko KM, Kapurch J, et al. Natural history of Chiari malformation Type I following decision for conservative treatment. J Neurosurg Pediatr 2011;8(2):214–21.
12. Saletti V, Farinotti M, Peretta P, et al. The management of Chiari malformation type 1 and syringomyelia in children: a review of the literature. Neurol Sci 2021;42(12):4965–95.
13. Abel F, Tahir MZ. Role of sleep study in children with Chiari malformation and sleep disordered breathing. Childs Nerv Syst 2019;35(10):1763–8.
14. Redline S, Tishler PV, Schluchter M, et al. Risk factors for sleep-disordered breathing in children. Associations with obesity, race, and respiratory problems. Am J Respir Crit Care Med 1999;159(5 Pt 1):1527–32.
15. Moore M, Fuell W, Jambhekar S, et al. Management of sleep apnea in children with chiari i malformation: a retrospective study. Pediatr Neurosurg 2022;57(3):175–83.
16. El-Kersh K, Cavallazzi R, Fernandez A, et al. Sleep disordered breathing and magnetic resonance imaging findings in children with chiari malformation type I. Pediatr Neurol 2017;76:95–6.
17. Hershberger ML, Chidekel A. Arnold-Chiari malformation type I and sleep-disordered breathing: an uncommon manifestation of an important pediatric problem. J Pediatr Health Care 2003;17(4):190–7.
18. Nogues MA, Roncoroni AJ, Benarroch E. Breathing control in neurological diseases. Clin Auton Res 2002;12(6):440–9.
19. Caruana-Montaldo B, Gleeson K, Zwillich CW. The control of breathing in clinical practice. Chest 2000;117(1):205–25.
20. Berger AJ, Mitchell RA, Severinghaus JW. Regulation of respiration: (second of three parts). N Engl J Med 1977;297(3):138–43.
21. Spyer KM. To breathe or not to breathe? That is the question. Exp Physiol 2009;94(1):1–10.
22. Horn EM, Waldrop TG. Suprapontine control of respiration. Respir Physiol 1998;114(3):201–11.
23. Doherty MJ, Spence DP, Young C, et al. Obstructive sleep apnoea with Arnold-Chiari malformation. Thorax 1995;50(6):690–1 [discussion: 696-697].
24. Rabec C, Laurent G, Baudouin N, et al. Central sleep apnoea in Arnold-Chiari malformation: evidence of pathophysiological heterogeneity. Eur Respir J 1998;12(6):1482–5.
25. Bokinsky GE, Hudson LD, Weil JV. Impaired peripheral chemosensitivity and acute respiratory failure in Arnold-Chiari malformation and syringomyelia. N Engl J Med 1973;288(18):947–8.

26. Dhamija R, Wetjen NM, Slocumb NL, et al. The role of nocturnal polysomnography in assessing children with Chiari type I malformation. Clin Neurol Neurosurg 2013;115(9):1837–41.

27. Katwa U, Sisniega C, McKeon M, et al. Sleep endoscopy-directed management of Arnold-Chiari malformation: a child with persistent obstructive sleep apnea. J Clin Sleep Med 2020;16(2):325–9.

28. Johns MW. A new method for measuring daytime sleepiness: the Epworth sleepiness scale. Sleep 1991;14(6):540–5.

29. Massimi L, Peretta P, Erbetta A, et al. Diagnosis and treatment of Chiari malformation type 1 in children: the International Consensus Document. Neurol Sci 2022;43(2):1311–26.

30. Malhotra RK, Kirsch DB, Kristo DA, et al. Polysomnography for obstructive sleep apnea should include arousal-based scoring: an american academy of sleep medicine position statement. J Clin Sleep Med 2018;14(7):1245–7.

31. Tran K, Hukins CA. Obstructive and central sleep apnoea in Arnold-Chiari malformation: resolution following surgical decompression. Sleep Breath 2011;15(3):611–3.

32. Aarts LA, Willemsen MA, Vandenbussche NL, et al. Nocturnal apnea in Chiari type I malformation. Eur J Pediatr 2011;170(10):1349–52.

33. Yoshimi A, Nomura K, Furune S. Sleep apnea syndrome associated with a type I Chiari malformation. Brain Dev 2002;24(1):49–51.

34. Khatwa U, Ramgopal S, Mylavarapu A, et al. MRI findings and sleep apnea in children with Chiari I malformation. Pediatr Neurol 2013;48(4):299–307.

35. Furtado SV, Thakar S, Hegde AS. Correlation of functional outcome and natural history with clinicoradiological factors in surgically managed pediatric Chiari I malformation. Neurosurgery 2011;68(2):319–27 [discussion: 328].

36. Botelho RV, Bittencourt LR, Rotta JM, et al. The effects of posterior fossa decompressive surgery in adult patients with Chiari malformation and sleep apnea. J Neurosurg 2010;112(4):800–7.

37. Gagnadoux F, Meslier N, Svab I, et al. Sleep-disordered breathing in patients with Chiari malformation: improvement after surgery. Neurology 2006;66(1):136–8.

38. Pomeraniec IJ, Ksendzovsky A, Yu PL, et al. Surgical history of sleep apnea in pediatric patients with chiari type 1 malformation. Neurosurg Clin N Am 2015;26(4):543–53.

39. Del-Rio Camacho G, Aguilar Ros E, Moreno Vinues B, et al. Reversible central sleep events in type I Chiari malformation. Sleep Med 2016;20:134–7.

40. Alvarez D, Requena I, Arias M, et al. Acute respiratory failure as the first sign of Arnold-Chiari malformation associated with syringomyelia. Eur Respir J 1995;8(4):661–3.

41. Zolty P, Sanders MH, Pollack IF. Chiari malformation and sleep-disordered breathing: a review of diagnostic and management issues. Sleep 2000;23(5):637–43.

Orthostatic Intolerance and Chiari I Malformation

Lindsay S. Petracek, BSc, Peter C. Rowe, MD*

KEYWORDS

- Chiari malformation • Orthostatic intolerance • Postural tachycardia syndrome
- Neurally mediated hypotension • Syncope • Cervical spinal stenosis • Craniocervical instability
- Joint hypermobility

KEY POINTS

- Patients with Chiari malformation can present with recurrent syncope.
- *Non-syncopal* orthostatic intolerance also can be a component of the presentation of Chiari malformation.
- Connective tissue laxity is a risk factor for both Chiari malformation and orthostatic intolerance; joint hypermobility and Ehlers–Danlos syndrome are more common in both.
- Be alert to postoperative orthostatic headaches as a feature of orthostatic intolerance rather than a problem stemming from the neurosurgical repair.

INTRODUCTION

It is well-documented that individuals with Chiari malformation can present with symptoms of fatigue, lightheadedness, and syncope[1–10]—the cardinal features of orthostatic intolerance. It is less well appreciated that orthostatic intolerance can complicate the clinical course following Chiari decompression. The presence of orthostatic intolerance in patients with Chiari malformation is not surprising given the location of the major circulatory control centers and their pathways in the brainstem. Other contributory factors for associated orthostatic intolerance include the potential for Chiari malformations to create direct compression of neural structures to interfere with normal cerebrospinal fluid flow, impose adverse mechanical tension within the spinal cord and in the setting of complex Chiari, and to be associated with excessive rotational movement between C1 and C2 or excessive translation in the anteroposterior dimension.[11–13] This article reviews the normal physiologic response to upright posture and the common forms of orthostatic intolerance encountered in clinical practice. The authors describe the association of orthostatic intolerance with Chiari and other complex craniocervical abnormalities and provide suggestions regarding the evaluation and management of these autonomic disorders.

THE NORMAL AND ABNORMAL RESPONSES TO ORTHOSTATIC STRESS

In a healthy adolescent or adult, on standing there is an approximately 500 to 1000 mL shift of blood volume to below the level of the heart.[14] This gravitational pooling of blood causes a drop in blood pressure (BP), buffered in large part by the baroreceptor reflex. Afferent impulses from the aortic arch baroreceptors are transmitted through the vagus nerve, whereas those from the carotid sinus travel through the glossopharyngeal nerve. Baroreceptor input converges in the nucleus tractus solitarius in the posterolateral medulla and lower pons.[15] After integrated input from the vasomotor center, the initial drop in BP with standing is followed by an increase in sympathetic neural output, leading to increased norepinephrine-mediated vasoconstriction and the adrenal release of epinephrine. The sympathetic response is

Department of Pediatrics, Division of Adolescent and Young Adult Medicine, The Johns Hopkins University School of Medicine, Baltimore, MD, USA
* Corresponding author. 200 N. Wolfe Street, Room 2077, Baltimore, MD 21287.
E-mail address: prowe@jhmi.edu

Neurosurg Clin N Am 34 (2023) 43–54
https://doi.org/10.1016/j.nec.2022.09.002
1042-3680/23/© 2022 Elsevier Inc. All rights reserved.

accompanied by reduced vagal input to the sino-atrial and atrioventricular nodes, increasing heart rate. Taken together, these changes improve venous return to the heart, and result in a modest 10 to 20 bpm increase in heart rate, as well as a normalization of BP. The ultimate effect is to improve blood flow reaching the cerebral circulation during upright posture.

Orthostatic intolerance refers to a group of circulatory disorders defined by the provocation of symptoms with assuming or maintaining upright posture and the improvement in those symptoms with recumbency.[16] These disorders occur when the autonomic nervous system adjustments described above are dysfunctional. Although multiple complex and interdependent physiologic responses to upright posture are involved, the three most important contributors to orthostatic intolerance are excessive dependent pooling of blood, low blood volume, and an exaggerated catecholamine response, as illustrated in **Fig. 1**. **Table 1** describes the diagnostic criteria for the most common forms of orthostatic intolerance.

Symptoms of Orthostatic Intolerance

Symptoms of orthostatic intolerance (**Table 2**) can be aggravated by prolonged sitting or standing, low-impact activities such as shopping or visiting a museum, and warm environments. Some orthostatic symptoms, like lightheadedness, resolve promptly on lying down. Others, such as fatigue and cognitive dysfunction, can persist for hours, even after assuming recumbency. This phenomenon of prolonged fatigue after vasovagal syncope has been appreciated at least since 1932 when Sir Thomas Lewis described a soldier who was tired and tremulous for 36 hours after fainting.[25]

Among the pathophysiologic factors that contribute to increased gravitational pooling of blood are venous insufficiency in the pelvis or lower limbs,[26] prolonged sitting or standing, alcohol, excessive histamine release,[27] and vasodilating medications. Some studies have shown defects in vasoconstrictor reserve among those with syncope.[28]

Evidence has shown that some individuals with orthostatic intolerance have a reduced circulating blood volume.[29–31] In some instances, this is associated with lower antidiuretic hormone levels[32] or renin angiotensin system abnormalities, including a reduced aldosterone response to standing.[30] Reductions in blood volume can also be associated with physical inactivity. Complete bed rest, such as might be relevant in patients with a slow recovery from surgery, can be followed by worse hemodynamic responses to upright posture.[33] In those with increased gravitational pooling of blood, low blood volume or both assuming and maintaining upright posture is associated with lower return of blood to the heart, lower cerebral blood flow, and a markedly increased catecholamine response.[34,35] Goldstein and colleagues have proposed that the relative balance of epinephrine to norepinephrine can influence the phenotype of the circulatory response.[36] Patients with more norepinephrine can maintain BP longer due to its vasoconstricting effects, but the high circulating levels have a chronotropic effect. In contrast, epinephrine causes dilation of the skeletal muscle vasculature and can therefore promote hypotension. Epinephrine is often elevated immediately before the onset of neurally mediated syncope. Individuals who meet criteria for POTS during the first 10 minutes upright can develop neurally mediated hypotension (NMH) as the orthostatic stress becomes more prolonged, demonstrating that these two conditions are not mutually exclusive.[37,38] Fortunately, however, the treatments of postural tachycardia syndrome (POTS), NMH, and low orthostatic tolerance overlap almost completely.

More recently, extracranial Doppler can be used to measure blood flow in each internal carotid and each vertebral artery over a 2 to 3 minute span. Adding the flow through these four vessels can provide a measure of total cerebral blood inflow and allows comparison between supine and upright postures. Even in the absence of POTS or hypotension, individuals with symptoms of orthostatic intolerance can have clinically and statistically significant reductions in cerebral blood inflow. For example, among those with myalgic encephalomyelitis/chronic fatigue syndrome, there is a mean reduction of 26% in cerebral blood flow during 30 minutes of head-up tilt testing compared with supine values. In contrast, healthy controls have only a 7% reduction when upright.[24] These findings emphasize the limitations of our current methods of classifying orthostatic intolerance using heart rate and BP differences. As these techniques for measuring cerebral blood flow become more widely available, they will allow an improved ability to accurately identify those with orthostatic intolerance.

Orthostatic intolerance can accompany a variety of clinical conditions including those in **Table 3**. Individuals with connective tissue laxity may be predisposed to orthostatic intolerance because their vessel walls are more compliant, and in response to hydrostatic pressure during upright posture, they accommodate increased peripheral pooling of blood.[39]

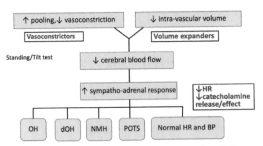

Fig. 1. Major physiologic influences on the different hemodynamic types of orthostatic intolerance and (in red) the categories of treatments needed to counteract them. BP, blood pressure; dOH, delayed orthostatic hypotension; HR, heart rate; NMH, neurally mediated hypotension; OH, orthostatic hypotension; POTS, postural tachycardia syndrome.

PRESENTATION OF ORTHOSTATIC INTOLERANCE IN CHIARI MALFORMATION

The modern emphasis on syncope as a presenting feature of Chiari malformation includes articles from several groups. Dobkin reported a 44-year-old man with Chiari malformation and recurrent syncope who experienced a complete resolution of fainting postoperatively.[2] A report by Hampton described three patients with syncope and Chiari malformation who underwent cranioverterbral decompression.[3] Two of the three had a complete resolution of syncope and a marked improvement in their symptoms.

A report from Weig and colleagues described two patients with recurrent syncope and Chiari malformation.[4] One patient's syncopal episodes occurred with neck movement, the other's occurred with coughing. The former patient also experienced vertigo and changes in heart rate and BP on standing.

Despite the emphasis on syncope, other symptoms of orthostatic intolerance also have been reported in association with Chairi malformation. Prilipko and colleagues described a 42-year-old woman with orthostatic intolerance and Chiari malformation.[1] Her symptoms included occipital headaches, nausea, vomiting, chronic fatigue, recurrent syncope, tachycardia, palpitations, pallor, diaphoresis, and diplopia. With a standing test, she had an increase in heart rate from 72 bpm supine to a peak of 130 bpm after 3 minutes upright. The test was stopped because of imminent syncope at 5 minutes. She had a reproduction of her usual symptoms of vertigo, diplopia, and diaphoresis. After surgical decompression for Chiari malformation, she experienced a complete resolution of symptoms. On repeat standing 3 months postoperatively, she was able to tolerate 20 minutes upright and was asymptomatic throughout. Her heart rate increased from 69 supine to an average of 83 bpm throughout the 20-min standing test, providing objective confirmation of the subjective improvement. The case presented in **Box 1** illustrates the potential for comorbid orthostatic intolerance to affect the postoperative outcomes following Chiari decompression surgery.

Although it is unclear whether the association of Chiari malformation with syncope and other forms of orthostatic intolerance is caused by the Chiari malformation, the improvement in syncope after surgical decompression would be most consistent with a causal relationship. Similarly, other neuroanatomic abnormalities also can be associated with orthostatic intolerance. These include cervical stenosis,[40] odontoid abnormalities,[50,51] basilar invagination,[5] anterior displacement of the C1 posterior arch,[52] atlanto-occipital assimilation,[6,7] and craniocervical or C1–C2 instability.[11] In the case series describing a group 20 patients with Ehlers–Danlos syndrome or hypermobility spectrum disorder and atlanto-axial instability, Henderson and colleagues reported a significant reduction in the frequency of lightheadedness, pre-syncope, and syncope after surgical fusion of C1–C2 instability when compared with preoperative status.[12] They suggested that neuroanatomic abnormalities should be considered when orthostatic symptoms can be aggravated by neck flexion, extension, or lateral rotation, if the head feels heavy and unsupported, and if syncope occurs rapidly without prodromal lightheadedness or warning. However, further study is needed to define these relationships and any role for surgical stabilization.

Other studies have confirmed that orthostatic intolerance can be a treatable contributor to symptoms in those with Chiari malformation and syringomyelia. Nogués and colleagues described a 45-year-old woman who had undergone surgical decompression of Chiari malformation and a cervico-thoracic syrinx, then later developed episodic palpitations, lightheadedness, nausea, dyspnea, and associated anxiety.[8] Tilt table testing provoked a marked tachycardia and eventually syncope associated with a relative bradycardia, consistent with both POTS early and neurally mediated syncope later during the test. She had a complete resolution in symptoms when treated with atenolol 12.5 mg twice daily and fludrocortisone 0.1 mg daily. A repeat tilt test on medications showed resolution of the postural tachycardia and no evidence of persistent syncope.

Table 1 The common types of orthostatic intolerance	
Initial orthostatic hypotension	Transient drop of >40 mm Hg in Systolic blood pressure (SBP) or >20 mm Hg Diastolic blood pressure (DBP) within 15 s of standing, accompanied by lightheadedness and reflex tachycardia, with hypotension lasting for <1 minute.[17] Syncope is uncommon. This condition is more common in adolescents. Pharmacologic treatment is not necessary unless there is impairment in overall function on a chronic basis.
Classical orthostatic hypotension (cOH)	A sustained 20 mm Hg drop in SBP or a 10 mm Hg drop in DBP within the first 3 minutes of standing or head-up tilt.[18] This is more common in adults, but can be seen in children with acute dehydration, anorexia nervosa, or in response to certain medications (eg, tricyclic antidepressants, prochlorperazine, quetiapine).
Delayed orthostatic hypotension (dOH)	dOH involves the same drop in blood pressure as in cOH but occurring after 3 min upright.[18]
Neurally mediated hypotension (NMH)	Characterized by an abrupt drop in blood pressure and frequently a relative bradycardia at the time of hypotension, often associated with recurrent syncope or pre-syncope in day-to-day life. However, syncope in daily life is not universal in this group, so we refer to this circulatory pattern as NMH, the physiology of which is identical to reflex syncope, often termed vasovagal syncope, neurocardiogenic syncope, and neurally mediated syncope.[19–21] Symptoms can be present soon after assuming an upright posture, but hypotension usually is not detected unless the orthostatic stress is prolonged.
Postural tachycardia syndrome (POTS)	In adolescents, POTS is characterized by a sustained heart rate increment of at least 40 beats/min (30 beats/min in adults) within 10 min of standing or head-up tilt testing, in the absence of cOH in the first 3 min upright, and in association with chronic orthostatic symptoms. The onset is insidious for some, but it often appears after infection, immunization, surgery, and trauma.[22]
Inappropriate sinus tachycardia	Characterized by a sinus rhythm with a heart rate >100 bpm at rest.[23] The symptoms are similar to those of POTS.
Low orthostatic tolerance	Characterized by prominent orthostatic symptoms without the heart rate and blood pressure changes of OH, NMH, or POTS.[24]

Prevalence

Although these case reports establish the association of orthostatic intolerance with skull-base and cervical spinal abnormalities, they do not identify the true prevalence of orthostatic intolerance in patients with Chiari malformation. Estimates of that prevalence have varied widely in the literature. Nogués described only four with orthostatic intolerance out of 100 adult patients with syringomyelia (two-thirds of whom had Chiari malformation).[9] In contrast, Milhorat and colleagues reported on 364 patients with Chiari malformation, 257 of whom had not had surgery and 107 of whom had already undergone surgery for Chiari or syringomyelia.[10] There was a substantial overlap of presenting symptoms of Chiari and the presenting symptoms of orthostatic intolerance. Common symptoms for both conditions included fatigue (61%), dizziness (60%), blurred vision (50%), impaired memory (41%), tremors (28%), palpitations (27%), vertigo (20%), nausea or

Table 2
Symptoms of orthostatic intolerance

Due to Reduced Cerebral Blood Flow	Due to Secondary Hyperadrenergic Response
Lightheadedness	Dyspnea
Syncope	Chest discomfort
Diminished concentration	Palpitations
	Tremulousness
Headache	Anxiety
Blurred vision	Diaphoresis
Fatigue	Nausea
Exercise intolerance	

vomiting (19%), and syncope (13%). The prevalence of symptoms in the postoperative versus preoperative group was not reported.

One study has examined the prevalence of Chiari malformation among those with confirmed autonomic dysfunction. From a sample of 55 adults with POTS being evaluated in a tertiary care autonomic specialty clinic, Garland and colleagues identified 23 female patients who had

Table 3
Conditions associated with orthostatic intolerance

Conditions	References
Neuroanatomic	
Atlanto-axial instability	12
Cervical stenosis	40,41
Chiari malformation	1
Craniocervical instability	11
Retroflexed odontoid	11
Vascular	
May–Thurner syndrome/pelvic venous insufficiency/pelvic congestion syndrome	26
Median arcuate ligament syndrome	42
Thoracic outlet syndrome	43
Others	
Allergies/mast cell activation syndrome	27,44
Autoimmune disorders	45
Infection (including SARS-CoV-2)	46
Joint hypermobility/hypermobile and classical Ehlers–Danlos syndrome	39,47,48
Myalgic encephalomyelitis/chronic fatigue syndrome	19,24,49

undergone a brain MRI.[53] Of these, three (13%) had cerebellar tonsillar descent of at least 3 mm, similar to the prevalence in a comparison group of 46 patients who had undergone a brain MRI to investigate other neurologic symptoms. This study is limited by several methodologic problems. The patients with orthostatic intolerance were not representative of the entire orthostatic intolerance population, as the study entry criteria required a dramatic increase in plasma norepinephrine levels on standing. Only 23 of 55 (42%) of the group with POTS had an MRI available. Moreover, the 95% confidence interval on the 13% estimate of those with cerebellar tonsillar descent was wide (4% to 33%), indicating a need for larger studies of this issue.

Methodologic Factors

Several methodologic factors would be important to consider in future studies of the prevalence of orthostatic intolerance in those with Chiari malformation. An important one would be the referral bias that would apply both to neurosurgical Chiari clinics and to subspecialty autonomic clinics. Patients with asymptomatic Chiari malformation would be unlikely to undergo confirmatory MRI studies and therefore would not be evaluated in neurosurgery clinics. Studies performed in tertiary autonomic clinics with long waiting lists might not identify those with progressive acute symptoms that require more immediate attention. Studies of autonomic dysfunction might have other enrollment criteria that would bias against inclusion of those with neuroanatomic problems. In both groups, there might be differential ascertainment of the important physical examination findings (incomplete neurologic examinations in those being evaluated for orthostatic intolerance and incomplete ascertainment of orthostatic symptoms and hemodynamics in neurosurgical clinics).

EVALUATION OF ORTHOSTATIC INTOLERANCE

Although syncope is dramatic and rarely overlooked, other clinical features of orthostatic intolerance are less obvious. Because not everyone with orthostatic intolerance reports lightheadedness, it is important to ask how people feel in specific settings such as waiting in line, shopping, standing at a reception or in a choir, in a hot shower or bath, or in hot weather. It is important to ask if patients feel unwell when standing for more than 5 minutes. Without knowing why, affected individuals often adopt postural counter maneuvers that help return blood to the heart, including shifting their weight when standing,

Box 1
Case presentation

A 15-year-old woman was energetic and active until age 14, when she developed bitemporal, non-pounding headaches. These symptoms fluctuated over the next 6 months, at which point her headaches increased in frequency. She felt some numbness in her left arm and mouth and often felt the need to lie down. Nine months after the onset, she experienced her first syncopal episode. Continuous headaches prevented her from attending school. On examination, she had nystagmus and a positive Romberg sign. An MRI showed cerebellar tonsillar descent 10 mm below the level of the foramen magnum, without a syrinx, consistent with Chiari malformation.

After craniectomy, C1 laminectomy, and a duraplasty, she experienced an initial resolution of her headaches for 3 weeks before they returned, associated with lightheadedness and vertigo. Vestibular testing was normal. Her vertigo initially was attributed to migraines. Trials of amitriptyline, topiramate, propranolol, sumatriptan, and acupuncture yielded no improvement. Three months after surgery, the headaches were daily, starting mid-morning and lasting the rest of the day. They were bitemporal, achy, and rated as having a 4 to 7/10 severity. Aggravating factors were warm environments and riding in the car or bus. Although she developed visual blackouts several times a day, she did not endorse lightheadedness except during and soon after a hot bath. She also reported feeling less sharp mentally and often had to reread texts.

A repeat neurologic examination was normal. She had no further nystagmus. She had some posterior neck muscle tightness. Based on the lightheadedness, visual blackouts, cognitive fogginess, and warm environments as an aggravating factor, we suspected orthostatic intolerance and performed a passive standing test, described in the Testing section later in this article. Her response to standing (**Fig. 2**) was consistent with neurally mediated hypotension.

Multimodal treatment consisted of the following:

1. Salt tablets decreased the frequency of her headaches.
2. Fludrocortisone was added to improve blood volume. She tolerated a dose of 0.05 mg daily, but 0.1 mg daily was associated with adverse effects (nightmares), so she returned to the 0.05-mg dose.
3. Midodrine, an alpha-1 agonist vasoconstrictor, led to a prompt improvement in symptoms such that she was able to participate on her summer swim team.
4. Pindolol 2.5 to 5 mg twice daily was added to help with residual lightheadedness and responses to stress.
5. Physical therapy was helpful for neck muscle tightness.

On this combination of fludrocortisone, midodrine, and pindolol, she completed high school, college, and medical school, and eventually was able to discontinue the fludrocortisone.

Comment: This patient had a very brief improvement after surgical decompression before developing recurrent headaches along with intolerance of quiet upright posture. The standing test confirmed an orthostatic provocation of symptoms. After 9 minutes upright, she developed presyncope. A recognition of the orthostatic intolerance directed attention away from the hypothesis that she had migraines and also away from consideration of a surgical cause of the symptoms. She did not have cerebellar ptosis, a cerebrospinal fluid leak, or other neurosurgical reasons for symptoms. Her case emphasizes the importance of considering orthostatic intolerance in the differential diagnosis of persistent symptoms post-decompression, especially when those symptoms include lightheadedness, fatigue, and cognitive dysfunction, and when they worsen with quiet upright posture or in warm environments.

standing with the legs crossed, studying in a reclining position, and bringing the knees to the chest when seated.

Physical Examination

Along with a thorough general physical examination and a detailed neurologic examination, we recommend looking for several specific findings among those with orthostatic intolerance. Skin color changes can include facial pallor and also peripheral acrocyanosis, which refers to a red/purple diffuse discoloration of the dependent limbs, distinguished from Raynaud's phenomenon by the absence of blanching. Because joint hypermobility is a risk factor for Chiari malformation, as well as for ligamentous instability at the skull-base and in the cervical spine, we recommend performance of a Beighton score or similar hypermobility screening test.[48]

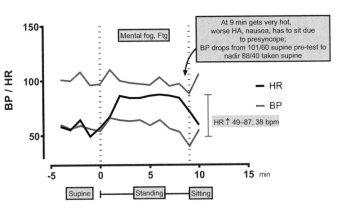

At 9 min gets very hot, worse HA, nausea, has to sit due to presyncope; BP drops from 101/60 supine pre-test to nadir 88/40 taken supine

Mental fog, Ftg

HR ↑ 49–87, 38 bpm

— HR
— BP

Supine ⊢—Standing—⊢—Sitting

Fig. 2. Standing test results. BP, blood pressure; Ftg, fatigue; HA, headache; HR, heart rate.

Testing

As described in **Box 2**, the most common tests used to evaluate for orthostatic intolerance are (1) active and passive standing tests and (2) head-up tilt table tests. Lower body negative pressure testing is a method of simulating orthostatic stress when patients are positioned supine, but this method is usually confined to research studies.

Several methodologic factors can affect the outcome of testing, described elsewhere.[23,49,58,59] More detailed autonomic tests are available in specific situations, reviewed by Goodman.[60]

Box 2
Orthostatic stress test methods

Standing Tests

Passive Standing Test

The passive standing test is performed with the patient supine for 5 to 15 minutes, then standing for 10 minutes with the feet positioned at shoulder width, approximately 6 inches from a wall, with the upper back leaning against the wall.[54] Heart rate and blood pressure are recorded each minute, and symptoms are recorded on a 0 to 10 scale every 1 to 2 minutes during the standing phase (0 meaning the absence of the symptom and 10 meaning the worst severity imaginable). Some patients have a higher resting heart rate before the test, possible due to apprehension about what is to follow, and have a more representative age-appropriate heart rate in the 2 to 5 minutes supine after the completion of the standing phase. Using the lowest supine heart rate value from either pretest or posttest can improve the rate of detection of POTS.[55] The posttest heart rate cannot be used for this purpose if the individual has developed a neurally mediated hypotensive response to standing, which often involves excessive slowing of the heart rate.

Active Standing Test

In contrast, during an active standing test, the patient is positioned at the bedside, *not* leaning against the wall. The duration of the supine period varies, as does the duration of standing. While standing, the arm with the blood pressure cuff is supported on a table.[56] Both passive and active standing tests need to be supervised due to the potential for syncope to develop.

Tilt Table Tests

The head-up tilt table test is conducted with the patient supine, usually for 15 minutes, after which the table is brought slowly to a head-up position, in most instances 70°. In many autonomic neurology programs, tilt testing is performed for 10 minutes, but this duration will only detect orthostatic hypotension and POTS. In cardiology programs, the usual duration of the first stage of tilt testing is 30 to 45 minutes. If the patient tolerates the first 45 minutes upright, some tilt testing methods involve returning the patient to the supine position for 10 minutes while beginning an infusion of isoproterenol (1–2 mcg/kg/min), then bringing the table upright again for 15 minutes. Another technique is to use nitroglycerine as a way of provoking syncope. A tilt table test is not indicated when the patient has a history that strongly indicates orthostatic intolerance, provided there is a structurally normal heart, and no evidence of a heart rhythm disturbance. Various indications for tilt testing have been published.[23,57,58]

Table 4
The common medications used for treating orthostatic intolerance, along with the usual dosage and indications for use

Medication	Dose	Comments
Vasoconstrictors		
Midodrine	2.5 mg every 4 h while awake. Increase every 3–7 d by 2.5 mg until an optimal dose is achieved. The usual maximum dose is 10–15 mg every 4 h while awake.	Suggested as first-line therapy for those with baseline hypotension.
Stimulants		
Methylphenidate	Immediate-release form: 5–10 mg BID, increasing gradually to 15–40 mg/d. Sustained-release form: start with 10 mg once daily and increase gradually until an optimal effect is found.	Suggested as first-line therapy for those with prominent cognitive dysfunction or a personal or family history of attention-deficit hyperactivity disorder. Doses higher than 40 mg/d are sometimes tolerated.
Dextroamphetamine	Sustained-release form: 5–10 mg in the morning. Increase by 5–10 mg weekly (max. 15–40 mg daily)	
Volume expanders		
Sodium chloride	Oral: 500–1000 mg tablets with meals IV: 1–2 L of 0.9% NaCl over 1–2 h	Oral supplements not always sufficient as the only therapy. IV normal saline is impractical over the longer term, but can help restore baseline function after acute infections or as rescue therapy.
Fludrocortisone	0.05 mg daily for 1 wk, then 0.1 mg daily. Increase gradually as tolerated to a maximum of 0.2 mg daily	Suggested as first-line therapy for those with baseline hypotension or increased salt appetite. Potassium supplementation is needed due to increased urinary potassium excretion (10 mEq of KCl for every 0.1 mg of fludrocortisone). Can aggravate acne.
Hormonal contraceptives	Most are fine. Conventional dosage or continuous pills for 84 d (one period every 3 mo)	Indicated for females with dysmenorrhea or when fatigue and lightheadedness worsen with menses.
Desmopressin acetate	0.1 mg at bedtime, increasing to 0.2 mg daily	Suggested for those with nocturia. Hyponatremia can occur.
Sympathetic tone and heart rate modifiers		
Pyridostigmine bromide	Rapid release: 30 mg daily, increase by 30 mg every 3–7 d to 60 mg BID or TID. Sustained-release: 180 mg daily	Effective in POTS and neurally mediated hypotension. Also helpful for GI motility problems.

(continued on next page)

Table 4
(continued)

Medication	Dose	Comments
Clonidine	0.05 mg at bedtime. Increase after 1 wk to 0.1 mg nightly	Suggested for those with anxiety, ADHD, insomnia, or hyperhidrosis. Increases blood volume in those with orthostatic intolerance.
Ivabradine	Start with 2.5 mg BID Max 10 mg BID	Suggested for those with elevated baseline heart rate, typically above 100 bpm.
Beta adrenergic antagonist		
Atenolol	12.5–25 mg daily, increase by 12.5 mg increments until optimal effect. Usual dose is 25–50 mg.	Suggested as first-line therapy for those with a relatively elevated resting heart rate, anxiety, or headache. Can exacerbate asthma. Relatively contraindicated for diabetics.
Propranolol	0.5–1 mg/kg body weight 3–4 times daily	
SSRI/SNRI		
Escitalopram	5 mg daily for 2–4 wk, increase to 10 mg daily (max. 40 mg daily)	Indicated for dysthymia, depression, or anxiety.
Sertraline	25–100 mg daily	
Duloxetine	20–30 mg daily for 2 wk, increase to max of 60–90 mg daily	Useful if myalgias are prominent.

Abbreviations: ADHD, Attention Deficit Hyperactivity Disorder; GI, Gastrointestinal; SSRI, Selective Serotonin Reuptake Inhibitor; SNRI, Serotonin Norepinephrine Reuptake Inhibitor.

Modified from Rowe PC, Underhill RA, Friedman KJ, et al. Myalgic Encephalomyelitis/Chronic Fatigue Syndrome Diagnosis and Management in Young People: A Primer. Frontiers in Pediatrics. 2017;5(121).

THERAPEUTIC OPTIONS

Management of orthostatic intolerance includes non-pharmacologic and pharmacologic therapies. Non-pharmacologic treatments include an increased salt and fluid intake, compression garments, avoiding aggravating factors, and raising the head of the bed by 10° to 15° (the entire bed frame must be elevated; an adjustable bed or wedge pillow will not have the same effect).[61] Another important component of managing orthostatic intolerance is treating comorbid conditions (**Table 3** and Ref[46]). Most individuals with more severe orthostatic intolerance will not improve sufficiently with non-pharmacologic measures alone. **Table 4** lists the common medications used for orthostatic intolerance.

Although the goal is to use as few medications as possible, some patients will require medications from each of the three main categories: vasoconstrictors, agents that increase blood volume, and agents that attenuate the sympathoadrenal response. Trials of several medications may be necessary before finding a good fit.

SUMMARY

Neuroanatomic problems at the skull base and in the cervical spine, including Chiari malformation, ligamentous instability, and cervical stenosis, can all present with symptoms of orthostatic intolerance, including recurrent syncope. Connective tissue laxity is a risk factor for Chiari malformation and for the ligamentous instability that contributes to complex Chiari. It is also a risk factor for orthostatic intolerance, as the connective tissue laxity in the blood vessel wall promotes excessive gravitational pooling of blood. The mechanisms by which Chiari malformation might contribute to syncope and other forms of orthostatic intolerance are not well established, but an improvement in syncope after surgical decompression would be most consistent with a causal relationship. Further research is needed to define the prevalence of orthostatic intolerance in Chiari and the other disorders. Orthostatic intolerance is a treatable problem that can complicate the clinical course following decompression surgery and should be kept in the differential diagnosis of orthostatic headaches, lightheadedness, and fatigue.

CLINICS CARE POINTS

- Patients with Chiari malformation can present with recurrent syncope. *Non-syncopal* orthostatic intolerance also can be associated with Chiari malformation, both before and after surgical decompression.

- Connective tissue laxity is a shared risk factor for both Chiari malformation and orthostatic intolerance; joint hypermobility and Ehlers-Danlos Syndrome (EDS) are more common in both.

- When recurrent syncope is refractory to conventional medical management, occurs in the absence of a prodromal warning, is provoked by certain neck movements, and the patient presents with pathologic signs on the neurologic examination, a neuroanatomic cause should be considered.

- Be alert to postoperative orthostatic headaches as a feature of orthostatic intolerance rather than a problem stemming from the neurosurgical decompression.

- The resolution of orthostatic symptoms following Chiari decompression surgery suggests that some physiologic disturbance associated with the Chiari malformation is a cause of the autonomic dysfunction.

- The true prevalence of orthostatic intolerance in patients with Chiari malformation remains to be determined.

DISCLOSURE

The authors have nothing to disclose.

REFERENCES

1. Prilipko O, Dehdashti AR, Zaim S, et al. Orthostatic intolerance and syncope associated with Chiari type I malformation. J Neurol Neurosurg Psychiatry 2005;76(7):1034–6.
2. Dobkin BH. Syncope in the adult Chiari anomaly. Neurology 1978;28(7):718–20.
3. Hampton F, Williams B, Loizou LA. Syncope as a presenting feature of hindbrain herniation with syringomyelia. J Neurol Neurosurg Psychiatry 1982;45(10):919–22.
4. Weig SG, Buckthal PE, Choi SK, et al. Recurrent syncope as the presenting symptom of Arnold-Chiari malformation. Neurology 1991;41(10):1673–4.
5. Corbett JJ, Butler AB, Kaufman B. 'Sneeze syncope', basilar invagination and Arnold-Chiari type I malformation. J Neurol Neurosurg Psychiatry 1976;39(4):381–4.
6. Mangubat EZ, Wilson T, Mitchell BA, et al. Chiari I malformation associated with atlanto-occipital assimilation presenting as orthopnea and cough syncope. J Clin Neurosci 2014;21(2):320–3.
7. Oliveira IC, Carvalho J, Oliveira L. Cough Syncope, a Rare Presenting Symptom of Chiari I Malformation and Atlanto-Occipital Assimilation. Eur J Case Rep Intern Med 2020;7(4):001466.
8. Nogués M, Delorme R, Saadia D, et al. Postural tachycardia syndrome in syringomyelia: response to fludrocortisone and beta-blockers. Clin Auton Res 2001;11(4):265–7.
9. Nogues M. Repeated syncopes and extended paediatric hydrosyringomyelia/Chiari I malformation. J Neurol Neurosurg Psychiatry 1998;65(5):805.
10. Milhorat TH, Chou MW, Trinidad EM, et al. Chiari I malformation redefined: clinical and radiographic findings for 364 symptomatic patients. Neurosurgery 1999;44(5):1005–17.
11. Henderson FC, Francomano CA, Koby M, et al. Cervical medullary syndrome secondary to craniocervical instability and ventral brainstem compression in hereditary hypermobility connective tissue disorders: 5-year follow-up after craniocervical reduction, fusion, and stabilization. Neurosurg Rev 2019;42(4):915–36.
12. Henderson FC, Rowe PC, Narayanan M, et al. Refractory syncope and presyncope associated with atlantoaxial instability: preliminary evidence of improvement following surgical stabilization. World Neurosurg 2021;149:e854–65.
13. Brockmeyer DL, Spader HS. Complex Chiari malformations in children: diagnosis and management. Neurosurg Clin N Am 2015;26(4):555–60.
14. Smit AA, Halliwill JR, Low PA, et al. Pathophysiological basis of orthostatic hypotension in autonomic failure. J Physiol 1999;519 Pt 1(Pt 1):1–10.
15. Salman IM. Major Autonomic Neuroregulatory Pathways Underlying Short- and Long-Term Control of Cardiovascular Function. Curr Hypertens Rep 2016;18(3):18.
16. Low PA, Sandroni P, Joyner M, et al. Postural tachycardia syndrome (POTS). J Cardiovasc Electrophysiol 2009;20(3):352–8.
17. Stewart JM, Javaid S, Fialkoff T, et al. Initial orthostatic hypotension causes (transient) postural tachycardia. J Am Coll Cardiol 2019;74(9):1271–3.
18. Freeman R, Wieling W, Axelrod FB, et al. Consensus statement on the definition of orthostatic hypotension, neurally mediated syncope and the postural tachycardia syndrome. Clin Auton Res 2011;21(2):69–72.
19. Bou-Holaigah I, Rowe PC, Kan J, et al. The Relationship Between Neurally Mediated Hypotension and the Chronic Fatigue Syndrome. JAMA 1995;274(12):961–7.

20. Adkisson WO, Benditt DG. Pathophysiology of reflex syncope: a review. J Cardiovasc Electrophysiol 2017;28(9):1088–97.

21. Grubb BP. Neurocardiogenic syncope. N Engl J Med 2005;352(10):1004–10.

22. Vernino S, Bourne KM, Stiles LE, et al. Postural orthostatic tachycardia syndrome (POTS): state of the science and clinical care from a 2019 National Institutes of Health Expert Consensus Meeting - part 1. Auton Neurosci 2021;102828.

23. Sheldon RS, Grubb BP 2nd, Olshansky B, et al. 2015 heart rhythm society expert consensus statement on the diagnosis and treatment of postural tachycardia syndrome, inappropriate sinus tachycardia, and vasovagal syncope. Heart Rhythm 2015;12(6):e41–63.

24. van Campen CMC, Verheugt FWA, Rowe PC, et al. Cerebral blood flow is reduced in ME/CFS during head-up tilt testing even in the absence of hypotension or tachycardia: a quantitative, controlled study using Doppler echography. Clin Neurophysiol Pract 2020;5:50–8.

25. Lewis T. A Lecture on VASOVAGAL SYNCOPE AND THE CAROTID SINUS MECHANISM. Br Med J 1932; 1(3723):873–6.

26. Knuttinen M-G, Zurcher KS, Khurana N, et al. Imaging findings of pelvic venous insufficiency in patients with postural orthostatic tachycardia syndrome. Phlebology 2021;36(1):32–7.

27. Shibao C, Arzubiaga C, Roberts LJ, et al. Hyperadrenergic postural tachycardia syndrome in mast cell activation disorders. Hypertension 2005;45(3):385–90.

28. Sneddon JF, Counihan PJ, Bashir Y, et al. Impaired immediate vasoconstrictor responses in patients with recurrent neurally mediated syncope. Am J Cardiol 1993;71(1):72–6.

29. Hurwitz Barry E, Coryell Virginia T, Parker M, et al. Chronic fatigue syndrome: illness severity, sedentary lifestyle, blood volume and evidence of diminished cardiac function. Clin Sci 2009;118(2):125–35.

30. Okamoto LE, Raj SR, Peltier A, et al. Neurohumoral and haemodynamic profile in postural tachycardia and chronic fatigue syndromes. Clin Sci 2011; 122(4):183–92.

31. Streeten DHP, Bell DS. Circulating blood volume in chronic fatigue syndrome. J Chronic Fatigue Syndr 1998;4(1):3–11.

32. Wyller VB, Evang JA, Godang K, et al. Hormonal alterations in adolescent chronic fatigue syndrome. Acta Paediatr 2010;99(5):770–3.

33. Takenaka K, Suzuki Y, Uno K, et al. Effects of rapid saline infusion on orthostatic intolerance and autonomic tone after 20 days bed rest. Am J Cardiol 2002;89(5):557–61.

34. Rosen SG, Cryer PE. Postural tachycardia syndrome: reversal of sympathetic hyperresponsiveness and clinical improvement during sodium loading. Am J Med 1982;72(5):847–50.

35. Benditt DG, Ermis C, Padanilam B, et al. Catecholamine response during haemodynamically stable upright posture in individuals with and without tilt-table induced vasovagal syncope. Europace 2003; 5(1):65–70.

36. Goldstein DS, Eldadah B, Holmes C, et al. Neurocirculatory Abnormalities in Chronic Orthostatic Intolerance. Circulation 2005;111(7):839–45.

37. Sandroni P, Opfer-Gehrking TL, Benarroch EE, et al. Certain cardiovascular indices predict syncope in the postural tachycardia syndrome. Clin Auton Res 1996;6(4):225–31.

38. Rowe PC, Calkins H, DeBusk K, et al. Fludrocortisone acetate to treat neurally mediated hypotension in chronic fatigue syndrome a randomized controlled trial. JAMA 2001;285(1):52–9.

39. Rowe PC, Barron DF, Calkins H, et al. Orthostatic intolerance and chronic fatigue syndrome associated with Ehlers-Danlos syndrome. J Pediatr 1999; 135(4):494–9.

40. Heffez DS, Ross RE, Shade-Zeldow Y, et al. Clinical evidence for cervical myelopathy due to Chiari malformation and spinal stenosis in a non-randomized group of patients with the diagnosis of fibromyalgia. Eur Spine J 2004;13(6):516–23.

41. Rowe PC, Marden CL, Heinlein S, et al. Improvement of severe myalgic encephalomyelitis/chronic fatigue syndrome symptoms following surgical treatment of cervical spinal stenosis. J Transl Med 2018; 16(1):21.

42. Moak JP, Ramwell C, Fabian R, et al. Median arcuate ligament syndrome with orthostatic intolerance: intermediate-term outcomes following surgical intervention. J Pediatr 2021;231:141–7.

43. Jones MR, Prabhakar A, Viswanath O, et al. Thoracic outlet syndrome: a comprehensive review of pathophysiology, diagnosis, and treatment. Pain Ther 2019;8(1):5–18.

44. Rowe PC, Marden CL, Jasion SE, et al. Cow's milk protein intolerance in adolescents and young adults with chronic fatigue syndrome. Acta Paediatr 2016; 105(9):e412–8.

45. Fedorowski A, Li H, Yu X, et al. Antiadrenergic autoimmunity in postural tachycardia syndrome. Europace 2017;19(7):1211–9.

46. Rowe PC, Underhill RA, Friedman KJ, et al. Myalgic Encephalomyelitis/Chronic Fatigue Syndrome Diagnosis and Management in Young People: A Primer. Front Pediatr 2017;5(121).

47. De Wandele I, Rombaut L, Leybaert L, et al. Dysautonomia and its underlying mechanisms in the hypermobility type of Ehlers–Danlos syndrome. Semin Arthritis Rheum 2014;44(1):93–100.

48. Roma M, Marden CL, De Wandele I, et al. Postural tachycardia syndrome and other forms of orthostatic

intolerance in Ehlers-Danlos syndrome. Auton Neurosci 2018;215:89–96.

49. Committee on the Diagnostic Criteria for Myalgic Encephalomyelitis/Chronic Fatigue Syndrome, Board on the Health of Select Populations, Institute of Medicine. The National Academies Collection: Reports funded by National Institutes of Health. Beyond myalgic encephalomyelitis/chronic fatigue syndrome: Redefining an Illness. Washington (DC): National Academies Press (US)Copyright 2015 by the National Academy of Sciences. All rights reserved; 2015.

50. Buntting CS, Dower A, Seghol H, et al. Os odontoideum: a rare cause of syncope. BMJ Case Rep 2019;12(11).

51. Ford FR. Syncope, vertigo and disturbances of vision resulting from intermittent obstruction of the vertebral arteries due to defect in the odontoid process and excessive mobility of the second cervical vertebra. Bull Johns Hopkins Hosp 1952;91(3): 168–73.

52. Miyakoshi N, Hongo M, Kasukawa Y, et al. Syncope caused by congenital anomaly at the craniovertebral junction: a case report. J Med Case Rep 2014;8(1): 330.

53. Garland EM, Anderson JC, Black BK, et al. No increased herniation of the cerebellar tonsils in a group of patients with orthostatic intolerance. Clin Auton Res 2002;12(6):472–6.

54. Hyatt KH, Jacobson LB, Schneider VS. Comparison of 70 degrees tilt, LBNP, and passive standing as measures of orthostatic tolerance. Aviat Space Environ Med 1975;46(6):801–8.

55. Roma M, Marden CL, Rowe PC. Passive standing tests for the office diagnosis of postural tachycardia syndrome: New methodological considerations. Fatigue: Biomed Health Behav 2018;6(4):179–92.

56. Plash WB, Diedrich A, Biaggioni I, et al. Diagnosing postural tachycardia syndrome: comparison of tilt testing compared with standing haemodynamics. Clin Sci (Lond) 2013;124(2):109–14.

57. Thijs RD, Brignole M, Falup-Pecurariu C, et al. Recommendations for tilt table testing and other provocative cardiovascular autonomic tests in conditions that may cause transient loss of consciousness. Clin Auton Res 2021;31(3):369–84.

58. Strickberger SA, Benson DW, Biaggioni I, et al. AHA/ ACCF scientific statement on the evaluation of syncope: from the American Heart Association Councils on Clinical Cardiology, Cardiovascular Nursing, Cardiovascular Disease in the Young, and Stroke, and the Quality of Care and Outcomes Research Interdisciplinary Working Group; and the American College of Cardiology Foundation In Collaboration With the Heart Rhythm Society. J Am Coll Cardiol 2006;47(2):473–84.

59. Brewster Jordan A, Garland Emily M, Biaggioni I, et al. Diurnal variability in orthostatic tachycardia: implications for the postural tachycardia syndrome. Clin Sci 2011;122(1):25–31.

60. Goodman BP. Evaluation of postural tachycardia syndrome (POTS). Auton Neurosci 2018;215:12–9.

61. Ten Harkel AD, Van Lieshout JJ, Wieling W. Treatment of orthostatic hypotension with sleeping in the head-up tilt position, alone and in combination with fludrocortisone. J Intern Med 1992;232(2): 139–45.

Elucidating the Genetic Basis of Chiari I Malformation

Gabe Haller, PhD[a], Brooke Sadler, PhD[b],*

KEYWORDS

- Chiari I malformation • Syringomyelia • Human genetics • Exome sequencing • De novo mutations
- Endophenotypes

KEY POINTS

- Understanding the genetic basis of Chiari I malformation (CM1) will help us to understand its biological mechanisms.
- Human genetic studies of CM1 are limited and should be expanded.
- Understanding the relationship between CM1 and CM1-related traits will help to define etiologic CM1 subtypes.

BACKGROUND

Chiari malformation type 1 (CM1) affects 1 in 1000 individuals symptomatically although as many as 1 in 100 meet diagnostic criteria,[1,2] making it a common disorder that represents a substantial personal, familial, and societal burden. Patients present with a wide array of symptoms stemming from the compression of neural tissue that is often accompanied by syringomyelia (SM) and/or hydrocephalus.[3] In fact, approximately 25% of CM1 patients develop SM (**Fig. 1**), a fluid-filled cyst in the spinal cord resulting in wasting in hand muscles and loss of sensation, and about 20% of patients develop scoliosis, although this figure jumps to 60% in the context of SM.[4] CM1 is often comorbid with congenital conditions but can also be acquired due to trauma or following lumbar puncture, shunts or space-occupying lesions. However, acquired CM1 is less common than forms thought to either be idiopathic or secondary to another condition involving the brain.[5] Suboccipital decompression surgery, the primary treatment option, is costly and invasive, and depending on the cause of the CM1, it is not always successful.[6] Patients may ultimately require multiple surgeries that are associated with relatively high complication rates at high economic cost to the individual and society.[7,8] However, without surgery, patients may face a lifetime of headaches, visual disturbance, vertigo, muscle weakness, paresthesia, dysphagia, bowel and bladder incontinence, scoliosis, and a host of other symptoms.[9,10] Understanding the underlying causes of CM1 is essential to improve surgical and nonsurgical treatment strategies that will translate into improved quality of life for patients.

HERITABILITY OF CHIARI MALFORMATION TYPE 1

Despite the high incidence of CM1, there have been relatively few studies addressing the genetic basis of this disorder and only one that has demonstrated a cause of isolated CM, implicating rare and de novo variants in chromodomain genes that lead to a macrocephaly-associated form of CM1.[11] Twin studies have reported higher concordance between identical twins compared with fraternal twins, although the numbers were quite small.[1,12,13] A study of 364 patients with CM1 determined that 12% of cases have at least one

a Department of Neurosurgery, Washington University, 660 South Euclid Avenue, St Louis, MO 63110, USA;
b Department of Pediatrics, Washington University, 660 South Euclid Avenue, St Louis, MO 63110, USA
* Corresponding author.
E-mail address: sadler@wustl.edu

Neurosurg Clin N Am 34 (2023) 55–60
https://doi.org/10.1016/j.nec.2022.07.001
1042-3680/23/© 2022 Elsevier Inc. All rights reserved.

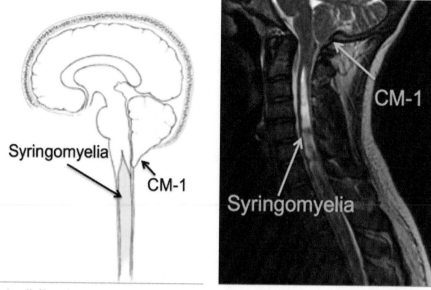

Fig. 1. Drawing (*left*) and T2-weighted sagittal MRI (*right*) demonstrating CM1 and syringomyelia.

affected relative with CM1 or SM.[9] CM1 also segregates within the cavalier King Charles spaniel dog breed, providing further support for a genetic basis.[14] Although CM1 is not fully penetrant in families, MRI measurements from the skulls of family members demonstrated reduced posterior fossa volume, suggesting a heritable malformation of the skull and cervical spine.[15] Interestingly, cerebellar tonsillar herniation was not heritable.

GENETIC EPIDEMIOLOGY OF CHIARI MALFORMATION TYPE 1

Many known genetic disorders that cosegregate with CM1 also involve cartilage or bone, including Klippel-Feil syndrome,[16] achondroplasia,[17] and Hadju-Cheney syndrome.[18] However, most CM1 occur in individuals with no known underlying cause. A subset of isolated CM1 is associated with connective tissue abnormalities. In a study of 2813 patients with CM1, 12.7% met criteria for Ehlers-Danlos syndrome or a related hereditary disorder of connective tissue.[6] Nearly half of the patients with CM1 and joint hypermobility were diagnosed with the hypermobility type of Ehlers-Danlos syndrome, a disorder whose genetic basis has not yet been identified.[19] One study performed retrospective chart review of 612 CM1 patients and categorized them based on their primary comorbidities. They found that nearly 70% of all CM1 patients had isolated (a.k.a. nonsyndromic) Chiari malformation. These patients also had the latest average age at diagnosis.[20] It is typical of many diseases and disorders that in the least

severe patients, these complex traits are the most difficult to unravel.

Previously, the genetic basis of scoliosis has been investigated, which is a disorder that shares many similarities with CM1, including the co-occurrence of both disorders in some patients[10] increased the prevalence of joint hypermobility[6,21] and complex inheritance pattern.[9,22] However, most CM1 patients are isolated[23] and no underlying genetic cause has been identified. It is clear that CM1 has a genetic basis. Posterior fossae measurements have been used as an endophenotype to estimate the heritability of CM1 with heritability estimates ranging from 30% to 70%[24] but this is only one aspect of the disorder. This missing heritability is what genetic studies aim to elucidate. Isolated CM1 patients represent a unique and informative subgroup of all CM1 patients.

PREVIOUS HUMAN GENETICS STUDIES OF CHIARI MALFORMATION TYPE 1

Since 2013, there have been several studies that have attempted to identify genetic factors that contribute to the risk of developing CM1. First, several regions were found to be linked to Chiari in large families with multiple affected individuals. Regions of chromosomes 9 and 15 were linked to connective-tissue-related CM1 and after excluding individuals with connective tissue features, regions on chromosome 8 and 12 were found that segregated with CM1 status. Interestingly, these regions containing growth differentiation factor genes responsible for Klippel-Feil syndrome, a musculoskeletal disorder also associated with CM1.[2] The exact variants responsible for the condition in the reported families were never reported, however. Next, the genetic contribution to posterior fossa morphology was investigated and significant linkage peaks were identified on chromosomes 1 and 22.[24] Causative genes were not identified, however. The study also calculated the heritability of the newly defined posterior fossa morphologic measurements and found several with strong evidence of heritability including the trait, posterior fossa height, which was used to identify the significant linkage peaks. Another study of 58 candidate genes comparing 415 CM1 cases and 524 controls and identified nominal associations in genes involved in somitogenesis and vascular development, although larger studies are required for confirmation.[3] Most recently, Urbizu and colleagues performed exome sequencing on a cohort of 178 CM1 patients and a large Spanish multiplex family and identified an excess of rare, coding variants in extracellular matrix genes,[25] further substantiating the role of connective tissue disorders in the pathophysiology of CM1. The extensive genetic heterogeneity of CM1 and the limited number of genetic associations to date suggests that a comprehensive understanding of the genetic basis of CM1 will require a multicenter study involving thousands of patients. A promising approach to discover the missing heritability in this complex phenotype is to use complementary epidemiologic and genetic methods that consider numerous models of inheritance.

In addition to the genetic association studies mentioned above, there have been 2 whole genome expression studies from human blood and dura mater tissue identifying general pathways of bone development and ribosomal pathways.[26,27] Unfortunately, (1) these studies have small sample sizes and thus a lack of power, (2) no GWAS or replication studies exist, and (3) no studies fully address the phenotypic heterogeneity of CM1. Phenotype is an extremely important variable in a complex condition like CM1. The ability to subclassify CM1 patients based on additional features, more precise brain and skull characteristics, comorbid conditions (ie, craniosynostosis vs hydrocephalus vs Klippel-Feil), combined with large sample size will enable to identify CM1 subclass-specific genetic determinants that are currently not possible to identify due to a lack of statistical power and etiologic understanding of the underlying anatomic and physiologic causes of CM1.

Although CM1 occurs in the context of a myriad of diseases and disorders,[28] as previously noted,

in these cases, CM1 is often not the main pathologic focus. A large proportion of CM1 is isolated[23] but it is often overlooked as either secondary to an unknown other disorder or disregarded as incidental. Somewhat arbitrary diagnostic criteria have also stopped many clinicians from taking a CM1 diagnosis seriously, with many claiming that CM1 is radiological finding unrelated to the symptoms leading to a need for imaging. In the past, CM1 has mainly been diagnosed if the cerebellar tonsil is herniated 5 mm or more through the foramen magnum or if both tonsils are each herniated 3 mm or more. However, these criteria are debated, and there is still a lack of consensus.[26] The true diagnosis is certainly more nuanced than simply presence or absence of a seemingly arbitrary millimeters herniation cutoff because it has been shown that it is possible to have a tonsillar herniation extending more than 5 mm below the foramen magnum and be entirely asymptomatic.[29] Further, patients exist that present with tonsillar herniation of greater than 0 mm but less than 5 mm and SM, suggesting that yet unrecognized factors may play a role in the development and severity of disease. The clinical heterogeneity of CM1 has been described as a major challenge.[26] By understanding the genetic basis of tonsillar herniation, posterior fossa volume and morphometrics, variation in the anatomy of the craniovertebral junction, brain volumetrics, CSF hydrodynamic parameters as quantitative traits or so-called endophenotypes that each may contribute to the risk and severity of CM1 and CM1-related conditions such as SM and scoliosis, we will be able to provide more specific and accurate diagnoses to patients with accompanying improvements in treatment strategies and outcomes.

RECENT GENETIC STUDIES OF CHIARI MALFORMATION TYPE 1

In 2021, the most notable article on CM1 genetics was published.[11] To identify genes that cause Chiari 1 malformation, Sadler and colleagues (2021) performed exome sequencing of 668 people with the condition, as well as 232 of their relatives. Exome sequencing revealed that people with Chiari 1 malformation were significantly more likely to carry genetic variants in a family of genes known as chromodomain genes. Several of the mutations were de novo, meaning the mutation had occurred in the affected person during fetal development and was not present in his or her parents or relatives (**Fig. 2**). In particular, the chromodomain genes *CHD3* and *CHD8* harbored numerous variants associated with CM1.

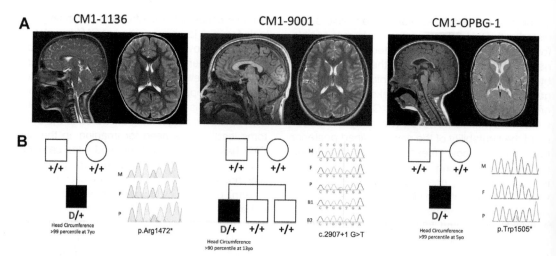

Fig. 2. *CHD8* loss-of-function de novo mutations in individuals with CM1 (*A*) Representative sagittal (*left*) and axial (*right*) brain magnetic resonance images of CM1 probands with de novo CHD8 loss-of-function mutations. (*B*) Pedigrees with Sanger-verified mutated bases for mothers (M), fathers (F), probands (P), and unaffected brothers (B1 and B2).

Chromodomain genes help control access to long stretches of DNA, thereby regulating expression of whole sets of genes. Because appropriate gene expression is crucial for normal brain development, variations in chromodomain genes have been linked to neurodevelopmental conditions such as autism spectrum disorders, developmental delays, and unusually large or small heads. In a zebrafish model, they showed that chd8 heterozygous knockout fish exhibited significantly larger brain volumes in all regions of the brain (forebrain, midbrain, hindbrain) than their wild-type counterparts. It has previously been noted that CM1 patients often have co-occurring overgrowth syndromes such as neurofibromatosis type 1 and Noonan syndrome.[20] Relatedly, this genetic study revealed that even in isolated CM1, children with unusually large heads are 4 times more likely to be diagnosed with Chiari 1 malformation than their peers with normal head circumference, suggesting that increased head circumference in general is a risk factor for CM1. Determining the effect of each of these chromodomain mutations could allow for predicting whether a variant will have a harmful effect for a child, and in what manner.

Another recent study used a trio design and concluded that variants in genes involved in chromatin remodeling were associated with CM1, similar to the conclusions of the CHD gene results. For this study, however, only 16 of the 51 trios were from isolated CM1 cases, and no functionalization of variants was performed.[30] More recently, a small candidate gene study in 12 CM1 patients found several variants in genes associated with craniofacial development; however, the study did not include any controls, and the authors could not determine a direct association between CM1 and bone mineral density.[31]

Overall, the studies of the genetics of CM1 have struggles from small sample sizes and lack of replication. Large families with multiple affected individuals can be a powerful method of identifying disease-causing genes but require more in-depth analysis of the families and ideally some modeling of potentially pathogenic mutations to prove causality. No linkage study in CM1 to date has performed the requisite studies to prove causality for a variant within linked genomic regions. The future of genetic studies in CM1 will require larger numbers of patients, either in a case/control design, large multiplex families with apparent Mendelian transmission or in a trio/quartet study design aimed to identify de novo mutations leading to disease.

FUTURE DIRECTIONS: CHIARI MALFORMATION TYPE 1 GENETICS

The ability to classify CM1 patients by etiologic subtype has the potential to enable a personalized medicine approach to treatment. Although there is likely to be more than one genetic cause of a particular CM1 subtype (ie, CHD3 or CHD8 variants can lead to macrocephaly-associated CM1), the ability to classify a single patient with a specific subtype can provide rationale for new clinical guidelines for treatment. A deeper understanding of the pathogenic mechanisms underlying CM1 and the neurodevelopmental phenotypes in these patients is needed to provide intelligent surgical management. The existence of Mendelian syndromes with CM1 as a frequent symptom and strong familial clustering suggest a strong genetic component. This review of genetic studies of CM1 suggests that genes involved in extracellular matrix structure, chromatin regulation, and various signaling pathways contribute to sporadic CM1. Although some genetic variants have been reported from small cohorts, only one large association studies has been done to date (Sadler, and colleagues, 2021). There are various competing theories regarding the mechanism of CM1 development. Multiple signaling pathways, developmental processes, and cellular functions exist and are suspected to play a role in CM1 pathogenesis. Current literature suggests CM1 is a multigenic malformation, resulting from a dysfunction in one or more neurodevelopmental system (CSF, vasculature, skeleton, brain). Multicenter and collaborative efforts are needed to answer the longstanding questions regarding CM1. With exponentially decreasing sequencing costs, trio-based whole-exome or whole-genome sequencing of large CM1 cohorts will be critical to identify damaging, rare single nucleotide variants and structural variations. This approach, coupled with modern transcriptomics and clinical phenomics, can provide valuable insight into CM1 pathophysiology and produce preventative, diagnostic, and therapeutic benefits for patients and their families.

CLINICS CARE POINTS

- There are likely multiple etiologic subtypes of Chiari I malformation.
- Chiari I malformation is heritable and can be due to underlying conditions or idiopathic in nature.
- Elucidating the genetic basis of Chiari I malformation is important to understand its molecular causes.

DISCLOSURE

The authors have nothing to disclose.

REFERENCES

1. Speer MC, Enterline DS, Mehltretter L, et al. Review Article: Chiari Type I Malformation with or Without Syringomyelia: Prevalence and Genetics. J Genet Couns 2003;12(4):297–311.
2. Markunas CA, Soldano K, Dunlap K, et al. Stratified whole genome linkage analysis of Chiari type I malformation implicates known Klippel-Feil syndrome genes as putative disease candidates. PLoS One 2013;8(4):e61521.
3. Urbizu A, Toma C, Poca MA, et al. Chiari malformation type I: a case-control association study of 58 developmental genes. PLoS One 2013;8(2):e57241.
4. Kelly MP, Guillaume TJ, Lenke LG. Spinal Deformity Associated with Chiari Malformation. Neurosurg Clin N Am 2015;26(4):579–85.
5. Wang J, Alotaibi NM, Samuel N, et al. Acquired Chiari Malformation and Syringomyelia Secondary to Space-Occupying Lesions: A Systematic Review. World Neurosurg 2017;98:800–8.
6. Milhorat TH, Bolognese PA, Nishikawa M, et al. Syndrome of occipitoatlantoaxial hypermobility, cranial settling, and chiari malformation type I in patients with hereditary disorders of connective tissue. J Neurosurg Spine 2007;7(6):601–9.
7. Lam SK, Mayer RR, Luerssen TG, et al. Hospitalization Cost Model of Pediatric Surgical Treatment of Chiari Type 1 Malformation. J Pediatr 2016;179: 204–210 e3.
8. Greenberg JK, Olsen MA, Yarbrough CK, et al. Chiari malformation Type I surgery in pediatric patients. Part 2: complications and the influence of comorbid disease in California, Florida, and New York. J Neurosurg Pediatr 2016;17(5):525–32.
9. Milhorat TH, Chou MW, Trinidad EM, et al. Chiari I malformation redefined: clinical and radiographic findings for 364 symptomatic patients. Neurosurgery 1999;44(5):1005–17.
10. Tubbs RS, Beckman J, Naftel RP, et al. Institutional experience with 500 cases of surgically treated pediatric Chiari malformation Type I. J Neurosurg Pediatr 2011;7(3):248–56.
11. Sadler B, Wilborn J, Antunes L, et al. Rare and de novo coding variants in chromodomain genes in Chiari I malformation. Am J Hum Genet 2021; 108(3):530–1.
12. Herman MD, Cheek WR, Storrs BB. Two siblings with the Chiari I malformation. Pediatr Neurosurg 1990; 16(3):183–4.
13. Cavender RK, Schmidt JH 3rd. Tonsillar ectopia and Chiari malformations: monozygotic triplets. Case report. J Neurosurg 1995;82(3):497–500.
14. Rusbridge C, Knowler SP. Hereditary aspects of occipital bone hypoplasia and syringomyelia (Chiari type I malformation) in cavalier King Charles spaniels. Vet Rec 2003;153(4):107–12.
15. Boyles AL, Enterline DS, Hammock PH, et al. Phenotypic definition of Chiari type I malformation coupled with high-density SNP genome screen shows significant evidence for linkage to regions on chromosomes 9 and 15. Am J Med Genet A 2006;140(24): 2776–85.

16. Khan AA, Bhatti SN, Khan G, et al. Clinical and radiological findings in Arnold Chiari malformation. J Ayub Med Coll Abbottabad 2010;22(2):75–8.

17. Pauli RM, Horton VK, Glinski LP, et al. Prospective assessment of risks for cervicomedullary-junction compression in infants with achondroplasia. Am J Hum Genet 1995;56(3):732–44.

18. Di Rocco F, Oi S. Spontaneous regression of syringomyelia in Hajdu-Cheney syndrome with severe platybasia. Case report. J Neurosurg 2005;103(2 Suppl):194–7.

19. Byers PH, Murray ML. Ehlers-Danlos syndrome: a showcase of conditions that lead to understanding matrix biology. Matrix Biol 2014;33:10–5.

20. Sadler B, Kuensting T, Strahle J, et al. Prevalence and Impact of Underlying Diagnosis and Comorbidities on Chiari 1 Malformation. Pediatr Neurol 2020; 106:32–7.

21. Czaprowski D, Kotwicki T, Pawlowska P, et al. Joint hypermobility in children with idiopathic scoliosis: SOSORT award 2011 winner. Scoliosis 2011;6:22.

22. Riseborough EJ, Wynne-Davies R. A genetic survey of idiopathic scoliosis in Boston, Massachusetts. J Bone Joint Surg Am 1973;55(5):974–82.

23. Strahle J, Muraszko KM, Kapurch J, et al. Chiari malformation Type I and syrinx in children undergoing magnetic resonance imaging. J Neurosurg Pediatr 2011;8(2):205–13.

24. Markunas CA, Enterline DS, Dunlap K, et al. Genetic evaluation and application of posterior cranial fossa traits as endophenotypes for Chiari type I malformation. Ann Hum Genet 2014;78(1):1–12.

25. Urbizu A, Garrett MA, Soldano K, et al. Rare functional genetic variants in COL7A1, COL6A5, COL1A2 and COL5A2 frequently occur in Chiari Malformation Type 1. PLoS One 2021;16(5): e0251289.

26. Markunas CA, Lock E, Soldano K, et al. Identification of Chiari Type I Malformation subtypes using whole genome expression profiles and cranial base morphometrics. BMC Med Genomics 2014;7:39.

27. Lock EF, Soldano KL, Garrett ME, et al. Joint eQTL assessment of whole blood and dura mater tissue from individuals with Chiari type I malformation. BMC Genomics 2015;16:11.

28. Loukas M, Shayota BJ, Oelhafen K, et al. Associated disorders of Chiari Type I malformations: a review. Neurosurg Focus 2011;31(3):E3.

29. Meadows J, Kraut M, Guarnieri M, et al. Asymptomatic Chiari Type I malformations identified on magnetic resonance imaging. J Neurosurg 2000;92(6): 920–6.

30. Provenzano A, La Barbera A, Scagnet M, et al. Chiari 1 malformation and exome sequencing in 51 trios: the emerging role of rare missense variants in chromatin-remodeling genes. Hum Genet 2021; 140(4):625–47.

31. Martinez-Gil N, Mellibovsky L, Manzano-Lopez Gonzalez D, et al. On the association between Chiari malformation type 1, bone mineral density and bone related genes. Bone Rep 2022;16:101181.

Chiari I Malformations and the Heritable Disorders of Connective Tissue

Meghan Ellington, Clair A. Francomano, MD*

KEYWORDS

- Chiari I malformation • Heritable disorders of connective tissue • Ehlers-Danlos syndrome
- Marfan syndrome • Complex Chiari

KEY POINTS

- There are more than 450 distinct heritable disorders of connective tissue (HDCTs).
- The underlying genes causing most of the HDCT have been identified, and in most cases, the diagnosis can be made by genetic testing.
- The most common type of Ehlers-Danlos syndrome, the hypermobile type, is the exception as the gene(s) underlying hEDS have not been identified. Diagnosis of hEDS depends on clinical criteria.
- Chiari I malformation has been associated with many of the HDCTs.
- Chiari I malformation is more likely to be complex in the setting of an HDCT.
- Recognition of an HDCT in a patient with Chiari has prognostic and therapeutic implications.

HERITABLE DISORDERS OF CONNECTIVE TISSUE

The term "connective tissue" is used to describe the ubiquitous and diverse tissue that serves to support and give structure to other tissues and organs in the body. Different types of connective tissue vary in the type of cells, which constitute the tissue, and in their cellularity, which may be loose or dense. Specialized connective tissues include ligaments, tendons, cartilage, and adipose tissue. Connective tissues play an important role in virtually every organ system in the body, including the vascular tree, the gastrointestinal system, the musculoskeletal system, and the neuraxis. Recent understanding of the role of connective tissue throughout the body has informed our understanding of the wide range of signs and symptoms that may be seen in patients who are living with HDCTs.

The term "heritable disorder of connective tissue" was coined by Dr Victor McKusick, who first wrote about the concept in the 1955 article, "The Cardiovascular Aspects of Marfan's Syndrome: A Heritable Disorder of Connective Tissue."[1] The first edition of McKusick's *Heritable Disorders of Connective Tissue* was published in 1956[2] and included discussion of Marfan syndrome, osteogenesis imperfecta, EDS, pseudoxanthoma elasticum, and Morquio syndrome. Since the first edition of *Heritable Disorders of Connective Tissue* was published, the concept of HDCTs has become well accepted in the practice of medicine. In 2002, Royce and Steinmann edited a volume entitled *Connective Tissue and Its Heritable Disorders*, which includes 26 chapters.[3] Many of these chapters cover multiple distinct diagnoses (eg, there is a single chapter on the skeletal dysplasias, of which there are now more than 450 well-described forms.[4] A search of Online Mendelian Inheritance in Man (OMIM) in June, 2022, for "joint hypermobility" yielded 1694 distinct entries.[5]

Two of the most common HDCTs are the Ehlers-Danlos Syndromes (EDS) and Marfan syndrome. The EDS are a heterogenous group of HDCTs that have in common joint hypermobility, skin hyperextensibility, and tissue fragility. There are

Department of Medical and Molecular Genetics, Indiana University School of Medicine, 975 W. Walnut Street, IB 130, Indianapolis, IN 46202, USA
* Corresponding author.
E-mail address: cfrancom@iu.edu

Neurosurg Clin N Am 34 (2023) 61–65
https://doi.org/10.1016/j.nec.2022.09.001
1042-3680/23/© 2022 Elsevier Inc. All rights reserved.

Abbreviations	
CM1	Chiari I Malformation
EDS	Ehlers-Danlos Syndrome(s)
HDCT	Heritable Disorders of
	Connective Tissue
LDS	Loeys-Dietz Syndrome
PCFV	Posterior Cranial Fossa Volume
SGS	Shprintzen-Goldberg
	Syndrome
hEDS	hypermobile Ehlers-Danlos
	Syndrome

13 different types of EDS currently recognized, which were put forth in the 2017 international classification.[6] The current nosology is a clinical classification, with descriptive names that have been widely used in the medical and scientific community.

Of the 13 types of EDS, the molecular basis for 12 is known. The remaining type, called the hypermobile type, is the most common of the 13. The classic type (cEDS), characterized by extremely stretchy, fragile skin and severe scarring, is caused by pathogenic variants in COL5A1 or COL5A2, which encode type V collagen.[7] The vascular type, or vEDS, causes aneurysms of the medium-sized arteries and rupture of hollow organs such as the bowel and uterus, and is caused by pathogenic variants in COL3A1, encoding type III collagen.[7] **Table 1** lists the full range of EDS types and the genetic basis for each.[6]

Because the molecular cause of hEDS is unknown, diagnosis depends on a set of clinical criteria that were published in 2017 along with the current classification.[8] The diagnostic criteria for hEDS can be found at the Ehlers-Danlos Society webpage through this QR code:[9]

Marfan syndrome is another well-recognized heritable disorder of connective tissue, caused by pathogenic variants in the gene FBN1, which encodes the protein fibrillin.[10] Presenting signs of Marfan syndrome include tall stature with unusually long arms and legs, pectus deformity, aortic aneurysm, and dislocation of the ocular lenses. Dural ectasia is a common feature, and there have been several case reports describing CM1 in the setting of Marfan syndrome.[11–13]

A more recently described syndrome, Loeys-Dietz Syndrome (LDS), has cardiovascular manifestations similar to those seen in Marfan syndrome, with dilation of the aortic root and predisposition to aortic dissection.[14] However, the aorta in LDS is more vulnerable to dissection at a smaller diameter and surgery is usually recommended earlier for the patients. Arterial aneurysms and tortuosity may be seen throughout the arterial tree, with tortuosity most prominent in the vessels of the head and neck. In addition, patients with LDS may have craniofacial features such as hypertelorism, craniosynostosis, and a bifid uvula or cleft palate that are not seen in Marfan syndrome.[15] LDS is genetically heterogeneous, with pathogenic variants identified in TGFBR2, TGFBR1, SMAD3, TGFB2, SMAD2, and TGFB3.[14] Suarez and colleagues[16] described a case with LDS and CM1. Of 25 patients with LDS reported by Rodrigues and colleagues,[17] 2 had CM1.

Shprintzen-Goldberg syndrome (SGS), a rare heritable disorder of connective tissue caused by pathogenic variants in SKI, is characterized by craniosynostosis, craniofacial and skeleletal anomalies, marfanoid habitus, cardiac anomalies, and intellectual disability.[18] SGS may also present with CM1. Of 15 cases reported by Greally and colleagues in 1998, one had CM1.[19]

CHIARI I MALFORMATIONS AND THE HERITABLE DISORDERS OF CONNECTIVE TISSUE

In the late 1990s to early 2000s, there were a series of case reports describing patients with joint hypermobility or specific HDCTs and CM1. Braca and colleagues[11] described a 39-year old man with Marfan syndrome who presented with hemifacial spasm and was found to have a CM1. Jacome reported on 18 patients with EDS and chronic headache; one of these had a CM1.[20] Of 4 patients with blepharoclonus and CM1 reported in 2001, 2 had joint hypermobility and other

Table 1
Ehlers-Danlos syndrome types, inheritance pattern, and genetic basis

EDS Type	Abbreviation	IP	Genetic Basis	Affected Protein
Classic	cEDS	AD	*COL5A1, COL5A2*	Type V collagen
Classic-like	clEDS	AR	*TNXB*	Tenascin XB
Cardiac-valvular	cvEDS	AR	*COL1A2*	Type I collagen
Vascular	vEDS	AD	*COL3A1*	Type III collagen
Hypermobile	hEDS	AD	Unknown	Unknown
Arthrochalasia	aEDS	AD	*COL1A1, COL1A2*	Type I collagen
Dermatosporaxis	dEDS	AR	*ADAMTS2*	ADAMTS-2
Kyphoscoliotic	kEDS	AR	*PLOD1* *FKBP14*	LH1 FKBP22
Brittle Cornea syndrome	BCS	AR	*ZNF469* *PRDM5*	ZNF469 PRDM5
Spondylodysplastic	spEDS	AR	*B4GALT7* *B3GALT6* *SLC39A13*	β4GalT7 β3FalT6 ZIP13
Musculocontractural	mcEDS	AR	*CHST14* *DSE*	D4ST1 DSE
Myopathic	mEDS	AD or AR	*COL12A1*	Type XII collagen
Periodontal	pEDS	AD	*C1R* *C1S*	C1r C1s

Abbreviations: IP, inheritance pattern; AD, autosomal dominant; AR, autosomal recessive.
Modified from Malfait et al.[6]

features suggestive of an underlying HDCT.[21] Puget and colleagues[12] and Dickman and Klani[13] published 2 additional cases of Marfan syndrome with CM1.

Martin and Neilson[21] published a review of HDCT and headache and discussed mechanisms through which HDCT might confer increased risk for headache disorders. They cite Milhorat and colleagues[22] who reported on a prospectively collected cohort of 2813 patients with CM1, of whom 357 (12.1%) were found to have signs and symptoms suggestive of a heritable disorder of connective tissue. Another case series finding that EDS may be associated with CM1 was reported by Castori and colleagues.[23]

CM1 is conventionally thought to be secondary to a failure of the occipital enchondrium, which constitutes the mesodermal element of the occipital bone, to develop fully, leading to a small posterior cranial fossa. The hindbrain, which emerges from neuroectoderm, develops normally and there is a resulting mismatch between the hindbrain and the posterior cranial fossa in which it sits.[24]

Milhorat and colleagues[25] discussed possible mechanisms of cerebellar tonsil herniation in patients with Chiari malformation. They studied 741 patients with CM1 and 11 patients with CM2. In each case, the size of the occipital enchondrium

and volume of the posterior cranial fossa (PCFV) were measured and compared with those seen in 80 age-matched and sex-matched control persons. They found significant reductions of PCF size and volume were present in 388 patients with classic CM1, 11 patients with CM2 and 5 patients with CM1 and craniosynostosis. However, occipital bone size and PCFV were normal in 225 patients with CM1 and occipitoatlantoaxial joint instability (OAAJI), 55 patients with CM1 and a tethered cord syndrome, 30 patients with CM1 and intracranial mass lesions, and 28 patients with CM1 and lumboperitoneal shunts. They suggested that 5 different causal mechanisms could result in CM1: cranial constriction, cranial settling, spinal cord tethering, OAAJI, and intraspinal hypotension. In their population, CM1 was seen in the setting OAAJI and cranial settling in 173 patients with a range of hereditary disorders of connective tissue, including EDS, Marfan syndrome, Mitral, Aorta, Skin and Skeleton (MASS) phenotype, and undiagnosed HDCTs with phenotypes overlapping several different recognized conditions. In 4 out of 4 patients with achondroplasia (the most common skeletal dysplasia), reductions of occipital bone size, PCFV and foramen size and area were seen, whereas in 3 out of 3 patients with osteogenesis imperfecta, these measurements were within 1 SD of normal.

Milhorat and colleagues[25] propose that the primary mechanism of cerebellar tonsillar herniation in patients with OAAJI is cranial settling. They note that evidence of descent of the cerebellar tonsils due to gravity may be provided by upright MRI. Pathologic enlargement of the foramen magnum was seen in patients with CM2 and in patients with CM1 occurring in the setting of a tethered spinal cord, suggesting that the foramen magnum may be impacted by tonsillar pressure early in development, before closure of the foraminal sutures.

Brockmeyer[26] has written about the "complex Chiari" in which the cerebellar tonsil herniation defining a CM1 is accompanied by brainstem herniation through the foramen magnum, retroflexed odontoid, kinking of the medulla, a kyphotic clivo-axial angle, basilar invagination, occipitalization of the atlas, syringomyelia, or scoliosis. Brockmeyer[26] proposes that patients presenting with a "complex Chiari" are more likely to require more complex operative intervention than a typical suboccipital decompression, which may include odontoid resection or craniocervical fusion. By the nature of their underlying connective tissue defects, patients with HDCTs are more likely to present with a complex Chiari.

Henderson and colleagues[27] reported on surgical outcomes for a series of 20 patients with hereditary disorders of connective tissue and cranio-cervical instability, of whom 18 (90%) also had Chiari malformation or cerebellar ectopia. In this series, 11 patients had CM1 as defined by descent of the cerebellar tonsils of 5 mm or more below the foramen magnum. One patient had a Chiari 0, and 6 subjects had low-lying cerebellar tonsils with cerebellar ectopia of less than 5 mm descent.

A case report[12] described a 12-year-old girl with Marfan syndrome, sacral dural ectasia, and tonsillar herniation who underwent surgical decompression of the foramen magnum. She developed spontaneous intracranial hypotension after surgery as evidenced by a CSF leak at the level of the dural ectasia. A blood patch at the level of the leak was successful in alleviating the headache. This case is illustrative of the fragility of the dura, which is common among persons with HDCT and may complicate recovery from surgery. In the case reported by Dickman and Kalani,[13] severe basilar invagination secondary to a retroflexed odontoid and CM1 were observed on imaging, with circumferential compression at the foramen magnum of the medulla and upper cervical spine. A large syrinx was present from C3 to C7. This patient was treated by transoral traspalatal odontoidectomy to decompress the ventral medulla and spinal cord, followed by posterior occiput through C6 fixation and fusion. The cervical syrinx resolved after 3 months.

Sadler and colleagues[28] reported on the prevalence and implications of underlying diagnosis in a retrospective chart review of 612 patients with CM1. They found that a significant number of patients reported either self-identified joint hypermobility or a diagnosed hereditary disorder of connective tissue, consistent with the observations of Milhorat and colleagues.[25]

SUMMARY

CM1 is seen in a wide range of heritable disorders of connective tissue. It is likely that the lax tendons and ligaments characterizing these conditions contribute to the development of symptomatic Chiari I through several different mechanisms, namely: cranial settling, instability of the craniocervical junction, and the development of tethered cord. Clinicians are encouraged to screen for the presence of HDCTs in patients with CM1. This can be easily done through the use of the Beighton score to assess for generalized joint hypermobility,[8] echocardiogram to look for aortic root dilatation, and assessment of morphometric measurements to look for evidence of dolichostenomelia. The recognition of an HDCT in a patient with CM1 may have important implications for prognosis and management.

DISCLOSURES

Dr Francomano has served as a consultant for Acer Therapeutics. Meghan Ellington has nothing to disclose.

ACKNOWLEDGMENTS

This work was supported in part by the Ehlers-Danlos Society, the Bruhn-Morris Family Foundation and the Indiana University Health Foundation.

REFERENCES

1. McKusick VA. The cardiovascular aspects of Marfan's syndrome: a heritable disorder of connective tissue. Circulation 1955;11(3):321–42. https://doi.org/10.1161/01.cir.11.3.321.
2. McKusick VA. Heritable disorders of connective tissue. 1st edition. St. Louis, MO: CV Mosby co; 1956.
3. Royce PM, Steinmann B. Connective tissue and its heritable disorders: molecular, genetic, and medical Aspects. 2nd edition. New York: Wiley; 2002.
4. Mortier GR, Cohn DH, Cormier-Daire V, et al. Nosology and classification of genetic skeletal disorders: 2019 revision. Am J Med Genet A 2019;

179(12):2393–419. https://doi.org/10.1002/ajmg.a.61366.

5. Online Mendelian Inheritance in Man (OMIM®). Available at. http://www.omim.org. Accessed June 22, 2022.

6. Malfait F, Francomano C, Byers P, et al. The 2017 international classification of the Ehlers-Danlos syndromes. Am J Med Genet C Semin Med Genet 2017;175(1):8–26. https://doi.org/10.1002/ajmg.c.31552.

7. Symoens S, Syx D, Malfait F, et al. Comprehensive molecular analysis demonstrates type V collagen mutations in over 90% of patients with classic EDS and allows to refine diagnostic criteria. Hum Mutat 2012;33(10):1485–93. https://doi.org/10.1002/humu.22137.

8. Tinkle B, Castori M, Berglund B, et al. Hypermobile Ehlers-Danlos syndrome (a.k.a. Ehlers-Danlos syndrome Type III and Ehlers-Danlos syndrome hypermobility type): Clinical description and natural history. Am J Med Genet C Semin Med Genet 2017;175(1):48–69. https://doi.org/10.1002/ajmg.c.31538.

9. Ehlers-Danlos Society The. Diagnostic Criteria for Hypermobile Ehlers-Danlos Syndrome (hEDS). Available at. https://www.ehlers-danlos.com/wp-content/uploads/hEDS-Dx-Criteria-checklist-1.pdf. Accessed June 23, 2022.

10. Dietz HC, Cutting GR, Pyeritz RE, et al. Marfan syndrome caused by a recurrent de novo missense mutation in the fibrillin gene. Nature 1991;352(6333):337–9. https://doi.org/10.1038/352337a0.

11. Braca J, Hornyak M, Murali R. Hemifacial spasm in a patient with Marfan syndrome and Chiari I malformation. Case report. J Neurosurg 2005;103(3):552–4. https://doi.org/10.3171/jns.2005.103.3.0552.

12. Puget S, Kondageski C, Wray A, et al. Chiari-like tonsillar herniation associated with intracranial hypotension in Marfan syndrome. Case report. J Neurosurg 2007;106(1 Suppl):48–52. https://doi.org/10.3171/ped.2007.106.1.48.

13. Dickman CA, Kalani MY. Resolution of cervical syringomyelia after transoral odontoidectomy and occipitocervical fusion in a patient with basilar invagination and Type I Chiari malformation. J Clin Neurosci 2012;19(12):1726–8. https://doi.org/10.1016/j.jocn.2012.04.006.

14. Loeys BL, Dietz HC. Loeys-Dietz Syndrome. In: Adam MP, Mirzaa GM, Pagon RA, et al, editors. GeneReviews®. Seattle (WA): University of Washington, Seattle; 2008.

15. Meester JAN, Verstraeten A, Schepers D, et al. Differences in manifestations of Marfan syndrome, Ehlers-Danlos syndrome, and Loeys-Dietz syndrome. Ann Cardiothorac Surg 2017;6(6):582–94. https://doi.org/10.21037/acs.2017.11.03.

16. Suarez B, Caldera A, Castillo M. Imaging and clinical features in a child with Loeys-Dietz syndrome. A case report. Interv Neuroradiol 2011;17(1):9–11. https://doi.org/10.1177/159101991101700102.

17. Rodrigues VJ, Elsayed S, Loeys BL, et al. Neuroradiologic manifestations of Loeys-Dietz syndrome type 1. AJNR Am J Neuroradiol 2009;30(8):1614–9. https://doi.org/10.3174/ajnr.A1651.

18. Greally MT. Shprintzen-Goldberg Syndrome. In: Adam MP, Mirzaa GM, Pagon RA, et al, editors. GeneReviews®. Seattle (WA): University of Washington, Seattle; 2006.

19. Greally MT, Carey JC, Milewicz DM, et al. Shprintzen-Goldberg syndrome: a clinical analysis. Am J Med Genet 1998;76(3):202–12.

20. Jacome DE. Headache in Ehlers-Danlos syndrome. Cephalalgia 1999;19(9):791–6. https://doi.org/10.1046/j.1468-2982.1999.1909791.x.

21. Martin VT, Neilson D. Joint hypermobility and headache: the glue that binds the two together–part 2. Headache 2014;54(8):1403–11. https://doi.org/10.1111/head.12417.

22. Milhorat TH, Bolognese PA, Nishikawa M, et al. Syndrome of occipitoatlantoaxial hypermobility, cranial settling, and chiari malformation type I in patients with hereditary disorders of connective tissue. J Neurosurg Spine 2007;7(6):601–9. https://doi.org/10.3171/SPI-.

23. Castori M, Camerota F, Celletti C, et al. Natural history and manifestations of the hypermobility type Ehlers-Danlos syndrome: a pilot study on 21 patients. Am J Med Genet A 2010;152A(3):556–64. https://doi.org/10.1002/ajmg.a.33231.

24. Nishikawa M, Sakamoto H, Hakuba A, et al. Pathogenesis of Chiari malformation: a morphometric study of the posterior cranial fossa. J Neurosurg 1997;86(1):40–7. https://doi.org/10.3171/jns.1997.86.1.0040.

25. Milhorat TH, Nishikawa M, Kula RW, et al. Mechanisms of cerebellar tonsil herniation in patients with Chiari malformations as guide to clinical management. Acta Neurochir (Wien) 2010;152(7):1117–27. https://doi.org/10.1007/s00701-010-0636-3.

26. Brockmeyer DL. The complex Chiari: issues and management strategies. Neurol Sci 2011;32(Suppl 3):S345–7. https://doi.org/10.1007/s10072-011-0690-5.

27. Henderson FC Sr, Francomano CA, Koby M, et al. Cervical medullary syndrome secondary to craniocervical instability and ventral brainstem compression in hereditary hypermobility connective tissue disorders: 5-year follow-up after craniocervical reduction, fusion, and stabilization. Neurosurg Rev 2019;42(4):915–36. https://doi.org/10.1007/s10143-018-01070-4.

28. Sadler B, Kuensting T, Strahle J, et al. Prevalence and Impact of Underlying Diagnosis and Comorbidities on Chiari 1 Malformation. Pediatr Neurol 2020;106:32–7. https://doi.org/10.1016/j.pediatrneurol.2019.12.005.

Imaging in Chiari I Malformation

Jonathan Pindrik, MD[a],*, Aaron S. McAllister, MS, MD[b], Jeremy Y. Jones, MD[b]

KEYWORDS

- Chiari I malformation • Cerebellar tonsillar descent • Brain MRI • Spine MRI • Syringomyelia
- Spinal cord syrinx • CSF flow study • Cervicomedullary cisterns

KEY POINTS

- Often found incidentally or in the context of related clinical symptoms, Chiari I Malformation entails inferior descent of the cerebellar tonsils 5 mm or greater below the foramen magnum.
- Brain MRI offers optimal visualization of the cerebellar tonsils and local anatomy, whereas spine MRI may reveal the presence of syringomyelia or scoliosis.
- Specialized imaging sequences contribute important information for evaluation including enhanced visualization of ventral and dorsal cervicomedullary cisterns and cerebrospinal fluid flow at the craniocervical junction (CCJ).
- The clinical impact of several additional imaging features related to Chiari I Malformation (eg, magnitude of inferior cerebellar tonsillar descent, effacement of ventral or dorsal cervicomedullary cisterns, decreased or absent flow at the CCJ) remains unclear.
- Radiographic measures like pBC2 and clival-axial angle may impact surgical planning and may suggest the need for additional surgical techniques (eg, posterior occipito-cervical fusion, anterior decompression) beyond standard posterior fossa decompression with or without duraplasty.

INTRODUCTION AND DEFINITIONS

The radiographic definition of Chiari I Malformation entails inferior descent of the cerebellar tonsils 5 mm or greater below the foramen magnum.[1–12]

- Defining the plane of the foramen magnum, McRae's line extends from the basion to the opisthion.

Tonsillar descent can be measured on a midline or paramedian sagittal image from McRae's line to the most inferior tonsillar tissue (**Fig. 1**A). Although the original description in 1891 did not incorporate a diagnostic threshold of tonsillar descent, present studies and clinical practices typically use 5 mm for diagnostic purposes.[13,14] However, symptoms may be associated with measures of tonsillar descent less than 5 mm.[15,16]

In many instances, imaging performed for other purposes identifies the presence of cerebellar tonsil ectopia or Chiari I Malformation as an incidental finding. The increasing use of imaging for diagnostic evaluations has resulted in greater numbers of radiographic diagnoses of Chiari I Malformation in asymptomatic patients.[5,17,18]

- The prevalence of radiographic Chiari I malformation among children within the general population undergoing brain or cervical spine imaging approximates 0.77% to 1.0%.[1,5,6,10–12]

Syringomyelia, defined as dilation of the spinal cord central canal with a diameter 3 mm or greater, may occur in conjunction with Chiari I Malformation.[12]

- The prevalence of syringomyelia within pediatric patients with Chiari I Malformation varies between 12% and 80%.[3–7,10,17,19,20]

[a] The Ohio State Department of Neurological Surgery, Division of Pediatric Neurosurgery, Nationwide Children's Hospital, Faculty Office Building, Suite 4A.2, 700 Children's Drive, Columbus, OH 43205, USA;
[b] Department of Radiology, Nationwide Children's Hospital, 700 Children's Drive, Columbus, OH 43205, USA
* Corresponding author.
E-mail address: Jonathan.pindrik@nationwidechildrens.org

Neurosurg Clin N Am 34 (2023) 67–79
https://doi.org/10.1016/j.nec.2022.08.006
1042-3680/23/© 2022 Elsevier Inc. All rights reserved.

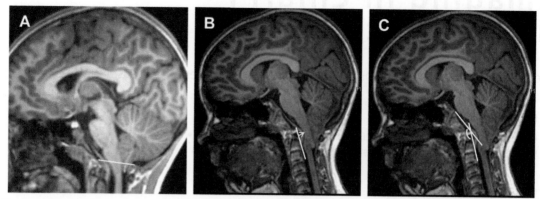

Fig. 1. Radiographic measurements related to Chiari I Malformation. T1-weighted paramedian sagittal view (*A*) demonstrates the vertical measure of cerebellar tonsil descent (*arrowed line*) below McRae's line (*horizontal bar*). Measurements of pBC2 (*B*) and clival-axial angle (CXA) (*C*) are also depicted in T1-weighted paramedian sagittal views.

Given the wide variation in reported prevalence of syringomyelia and the inability to predict the presence or future development of a syrinx based on brain MRI findings, practice patterns regarding spinal imaging in the setting of Chiari I Malformation differ. Rapid spine MRI techniques may obviate the need for sedation while screening for syringomyelia.[21]

Imaging that identifies Chiari I Malformation may include head computed tomography (CT) initially when performed in the appropriate clinical context such as trauma, acute neurological change, or concern for intracranial hemorrhage. However, further evaluation of this hindbrain anomaly requires better delineation of local and surrounding anatomy with MRI. In addition to confirming the diagnosis of Chiari I Malformation, brain and spine MRI may provide useful information impacting surgical decision-making and surgical planning. Spine MRI may also demonstrate the presence of scoliosis or tethered spinal cord which may be associated with Chiari I Malformation.[3,4]

DISCUSSION
Conventional Imaging Sequences

Multiple MRI sequences provide adequate visualization of Chiari I Malformation. At the authors' institution, T1-weighted magnetization prepared rapid gradient echo (MPRAGE) represents a standard imaging sequence for neuroanatomic structures including the cerebellar tonsils. Balanced steady-state free precession (SSFP) imaging studies (eg, balanced fast field echo [bFFE], true fast imaging with steady-state precession [True-FISP], or fast imaging employing steady-state acquisition [FIESTA]) sequences provide optimal visualization of crowding at the craniocervical

junction (CCJ) and the degree of cisternal effacement (**Fig. 2**). Sagittal sequences best demonstrate the relationship between cerebellar tonsils and McRae's line and evaluate the ventral and dorsal cervicomedullary cisterns.

Associations between the degree of tonsillar descent and symptomatology have been reported in radiological literature, with a threshold of 12 mm suggesting a higher likelihood of symptoms.[22] Additional imaging characteristics including morphology of the cerebellar tonsils (pointed vs rounded), tonsillar pistoning, syrinx formation, and cerebrospinal fluid (CSF) flow dynamics are routinely reported.[23]

Certain imaging features (when present) warrant the classification of complex Chiari I Malformation. These radiographic characteristics include brainstem herniation through the foramen magnum, dorsal medullary kink, retroflexion of the odontoid process, abnormal clival-axial angle (CXA), occipitalization of the atlas, basilar invagination, syringomyelia, and scoliosis. Some of these imaging findings may require more complex surgical management beyond standard cervicomedullary decompression, including occipito-cervical fusion.[24,25]

Radiographic measures applicable to the CCJ in complex Chiari I Malformation include the pBC2 distance measured from a line connecting the basion and posterior-inferior aspect of the C2 vertebral body to the most dorsally projecting aspect of the odontoid process and investing soft tissue (to the ventral dura) (**Fig. 1B**).[11,26] The CXA lies between intersecting lines along the clivus and the dorsal aspect of C2 (from the posterior-inferior aspect of C2 vertebral body to the posterior-superior aspect of the odontoid process) (**Fig. 1C**).[11] In addition, the magnitude of

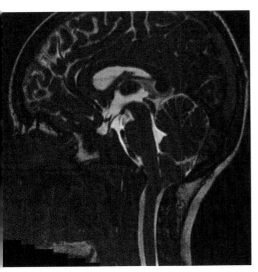

ig. 2. Midline sagittal fast imaging employing teady-state acquisition (FIESTA). Midline sagittal IESTA view highlights the enhanced visualization of entral and dorsal cervicomedullary cisterns and rowding at the craniocervical junction.

odontoid ascent above McRae's line fosters evaluation of basilar invagination.[4,11]

Designation of Chiari 1.5 indicates caudal descent of the medulla and obex (entrance into he central canal of the spinal cord) below the foramen magnum in addition to caudal descent of the cerebellar tonsils. These findings are often associated with dorsal medullary kink or spinal cord syrinx, and may impact surgical management Fig. 3).[25,27]

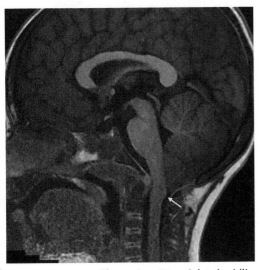

Fig. 3. Chiari 1.5 malformation. T1-weighted midline sagittal view demonstrates medullary herniation below the foramen magnum and a subtle dorsal medullary kink (*arrow*), consistent with designation of Chiari 1.5 malformation.

Box 1
Imaging characteristics of intracranial hypotension

Subdural collections

Pachymeningeal thickening and contrast enhancement

Venous engorgement and convex borders of dural venous sinuses

Pituitary gland enlargement

Cerebral sagging with decreased prominence of basal cisterns

Narrowing of the ponto-mamillary distance (<5.5 mm)

Decreased ponto-mesencephalic angle ($\leq 50°$)

Imaging should evaluate for other entities that may co-exist with or cause acquired Chiari I Malformation, including hydrocephalus, intracranial hypertension, or intracranial hypotension. Hydrocephalus may co-present in up to 10% of patients with Chiari I Malformation.[3,4] Distinguishing imaging features of intracranial hypotension have been described and are listed in **Box 1**.[16,28,29]

Intracranial hypertension may cause an acquired Chiari I Malformation in 20% of affected patients.[30] Distinguishing imaging features of intracranial hypertension are listed in **Box 2**.[31]

Following surgical decompression of Chiari I Malformation, imaging may be performed for surveillance or diagnostic purposes in the setting of persistent, new, or recurrent symptoms. Post-operative imaging should evaluate several features, including post-operative changes, pseudo-meningocele development, morphology of the cerebellar tonsils, crowding at the CCJ, compression of the ventral and dorsal cervicomedullary cisterns, and size or extent of any spinal cord syrinx (if present). Importantly, hydrocephalus may develop following surgical decompression and may require temporary or permanent CSF diversion.

Advanced Imaging Studies

Cardiac gated phase contrast CSF flow studies have been performed in the setting of Chiari I malformation for three decades, usually with a single plane midsagittal acquisition centered about the foramen magnum and/or an axial acquisition centered just below the lower tonsillar tip. These exams allow visualization of pulsatile CSF flow about the cervicomedullary junction at various phases of the cardiac cycle. Specifically, as the intracranial arterial pressure wave expands the cerebrum and extracerebral arteries during systole,

Box 2
Imaging characteristics of intracranial hypertension

Compressed dural venous sinuses with concave margins, most prominently at transverse-sigmoid sinus junction

Dilated optic nerve sheaths

Eversion of optic discs (suggesting papilledema)

Empty or partial empty sella turcica

Concave superior border of the pituitary gland

Dilated meckel's cave(s)

Small meningoceles at petrous apices

venous capacitance is transiently exceeded resulting in an approximately 1.5 mL flow of CSF across the foramen magnum. The directional flow is caudal in systole with subsequent cranial rebound in diastole. This CSF flow can be qualitatively or quantitatively assessed frame by frame cinematically during the cardiac cycle (**Fig. 4**).[32–3]

In normal individuals, relatively homogeneous CSF flow about patent cervicomedullary cisterns is appreciated in both systole and diastole. With Chiari I Malformation, cerebellar tonsils occupying the posterior cervicomedullary cistern result in alterations of CSF flow. When viewed qualitatively in the sagittal plane, there is generally decreased or obstructed flow In the dorsal cistern in the vicinity of the tonsils, and in more severe examples in the ventral cistern as well.[38] Hyperdynamic tonsillar motion, with a velocity up to 10-fold

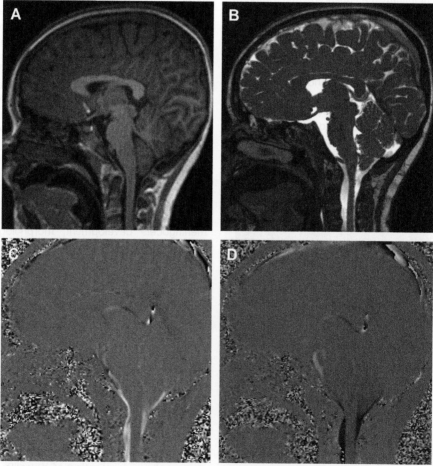

Fig. 4. Chiari I malformation in 6-year-old patient with non-exertional migraine headaches. T1-weighted paramedian sagittal image (*A*) shows 7 mm inferior cerebellar tonsil descent, whereas the sagittal balanced steady-state free precession (bSSFP) image (*B*) reveals mild effacement of the ventral and dorsal cervicomedullary cisterns. Phase contrast CSF flow study (*C, D*) demonstrates near normal flow about the cervicomedullary junction during systole and diastole.

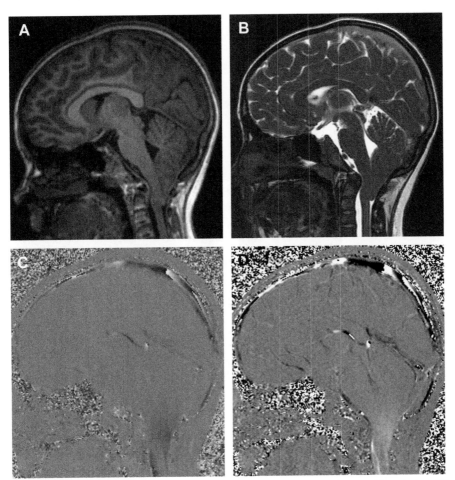

Fig. 5. Chiari I malformation in 7-year-old patient with seizures and non-exertional headaches. T1-weighted magnetization prepared rapid gradient echo (MPRAGE) sagittal view (*A*) demonstrates 16 mm inferior cerebellar tonsil descent with severe effacement of the ventral and dorsal cervicomedullary cisterns confirmed on the balanced steady state free precession (bSSFP) midline sagittal image (*B*). Phase contrast CSF flow study (*C, D*) suggests hyperdynamic tonsillar motion and absent flow about the cervicomedullary junction.

greater than normal, may also be visualized in symptomatic individuals (**Fig. 5**).[33] In the axial plane just below the foramen magnum, symptomatic patients tend to demonstrate increased CSF flow with "jets" and "bidirectional flow" in the ventrolateral aspect of the canal. These flow pattens can be followed for normalization following decompression procedures (**Fig. 6**).[39]

Yet, as an individual biomarker to distinguish those Chiari I Malformation patients with compressive symptoms or syringomyelia from those without, phase contrast CSF flow studies are probably limited. In a small cohort, radiologists evaluating qualitative CSF flow had only moderate sensitivity (75%) and less specificity (62%) in assessing for symptomatic as opposed to asymptomatic Chiari I Malformation.[38] Quantitative velocity analysis failed to add significant value in this regard.[40] With respect to syrinx, one small pediatric study reported good correlation between syrinx prevalence and abnormal qualitative CSF flow,[41] whereas other studies looking at CSF flow or tonsillar velocities have failed to show an association.[42,43] Furthermore some children with Chiari I Malformation and syrinx have normal qualitative CSF flow about the cervicomedullary junction.[44]

Despite these conflicting findings, qualitative CSF flow assessment in the sagittal plane may have surgical prognostic value. Symptom recurrence occurs long term in up to 30% of patients who undergo surgical decompression. In one series, those individuals who underwent cervicomedullary decompression in the setting of normal CSF flow had 3.4 times increased odds of having symptom recurrence at 3 years.[45] Conversely, in another series investigating children with Chiari I

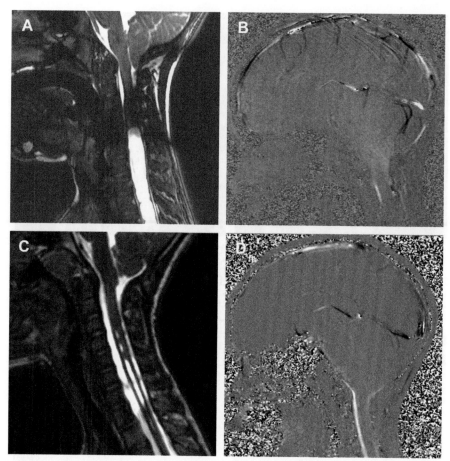

Fig. 6. Normalization of CSF flow and syrinx reduction following surgical decompression of Chiari I malformation in 7-year-old patient with syringomyelia and scoliosis. Preoperative balanced steady state free precession (bSSFP) sagittal sequences (*A*) demonstrate Chiari I malformation with 12 mm cerebellar tonsil descent below foramen magnum and a large cervico-thoracic spinal cord syrinx. The CSF flow study (*B*) shows hyperdynamic tonsillar motion and absent flow within the ventral and dorsal cervicomedullary cisterns. Postoperative bSSFP sagittal sequences (*C*) show elevation of the cerebellar tonsils, near normal caliber of cisterns at the foramen magnum, and syrinx reduction. Postoperative CSF flow study (*D*) shows restoration of normal flow ventrally and dorsally.

Malformation, those with the more severe pattern of CSF flow obstruction in both the ventral and dorsal subarachnoid spaces before decompression had a 2.6-fold reduction in the risk of symptom recurrence.[46]

Cardiac gated balanced SSFP imaging studies (eg, bFFE, TrueFISP, or FIESTA) have also been used to evaluate Chiari I Malformation. In contradistinction to phase contrast imaging which parameterizes velocity, balanced SSFP sequences provide anatomic images with high CSF and soft tissue contrast and limited CSF flow artifact (see **Figs. 4–6**). When acquired over the cardiac cycle, cine viewing allows direct visualization of tonsillar motion.[47] In normal individuals, this movement is small if apparent at all.[48,49] In study groups of Chiari I Malformation patients, there is statistically significant greater movement when compared

with normal control subjects, by measurement and visual "pulsatility." This "pulsatility" often decreases following surgical decompression. Although the range of tonsillar motion in those with Chiari I Malformation is small, approximately 0.5 to 1 mm, this anatomic information may complement phase contrast CSF flow assessment in surgical patients.[50]

Other motion-sensitive MRI techniques, including pencil beam imaging, time-spatial labeling inversion pulse (TIME-SLIP), and cine displacement encoding with stimulated echoes (DENSE), have been performed in the setting of Chiari I Malformation but are not used by these authors and are beyond the scope of this review.[51–53] Another cardiac gated three-dimensional phase contrast technique, 4D flow imaging, may provide further insight into the complex fluid and tissue

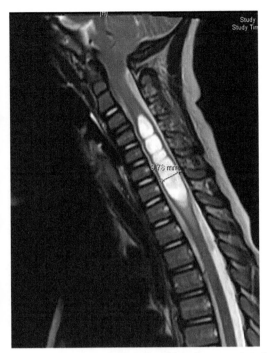

Fig. 7. Cervicothoracic spinal cord syrinx associated with Chiari I malformation. T2-weighted midline sagittal cervical and upper thoracic spine MRI demonstrates a multi-septated spinal cord syrinx extending from the C3 to T1 levels, associated with Chiari I Malformation.

dynamics of the cervicomedullary junction in Chiari I Malformation but is not widely used.[54,55]

Clinical Relevance and Considerations

Several imaging characteristics may impact surgical decision-making and surgical planning for the management of Chiari I Malformation. Although consideration of surgery typically relies upon clinical and radiographic markers, the presence of certain imaging findings may strengthen support for operative intervention even within asymptomatic patients.

- The presence of a Chiari I Malformation and spinal cord syrinx typically favors surgical intervention among most pediatric neurosurgeons.[1,2,4,6,8,10,11,17,19,56]
- The co-presentation of scoliosis with Chiari I Malformation and spinal cord syrinx typically warrants initial surgical decompression of the Chiari malformation.[2,10,17,18]

Varying in spinal cord distribution, Chiari-associated syrinx preferentially involves the cervical, cervicothoracic, or thoracic spinal cord in 55% of patients, but may present as holocord syrinx in up to 39% of patients (**Fig. 7**).[4]

- Syringomyelia typically responds well to surgical decompression of Chiari I Malformation, with syrinx reduction or resolution in 65% to 100% of affected patients (**Fig. 8**).[3–6,8,10,11,17,18]

Retrospective studies have also reported spontaneous reduction or resolution of spinal cord syringes without surgical intervention.[12,56] Although visualization of a "pre-syrinx" (T2 signal abnormality within the brainstem or spinal cord parenchyma) and its role in surgical decision-making remain controversial, this imaging finding often prompts greater precaution with routine surveillance imaging given the risk for syringomyelia development (**Fig. 9**).

Scoliosis occurs in 13%–50% of patients with Chiari I Malformation, often associated with syringomyelia (up to 82% of patients with scoliosis and Chiari I Malformation).[4,8,17] Scoliosis also may develop in patients with Chiari I Malformation without syringomyelia (up to 10% of patients).[57] However, a large retrospective analysis did not show an independent association between Chiari I Malformation and scoliosis when controlling for the presence of a syrinx (among other variables).[58] Nevertheless, radiographic evaluation of Chiari I Malformation may include full spine MRI and standing spinal radiographs to assess global alignment depending on clinician preference.

- Surgical decompression of Chiari I Malformation may impact scoliotic curvature with reported favorable outcomes (curvature stability or improvement) ranging between 32% and 100%.[8,18,57]

A meta-analysis investigating Chiari I Malformation-related scoliosis reported a success rate of 55% (37% curvature improvement, 18% curvature stability) following surgical decompression.[8] Associations between the magnitude of curvature deformity and correction following Chiari decompression have been reported, with curvatures less than 20° or 40° suggesting a higher likelihood of improvement.[4,17,18]

The significance of other imaging characteristics including diminished or absent CSF flow at the CCJ remains controversial. Retrospective studies have demonstrated the unclear impact of specialized imaging sequences (eg, phase-contrast cine MRI) on surgical decision-making.[1,56] For instance, a retrospective natural history study identified a subset of subjects with worsening CSF flow at the foramen magnum over time, all without change in clinical symptoms, development of spinal cord syrinx, nor decisions for surgical decompression over prolonged follow-up.[56] In

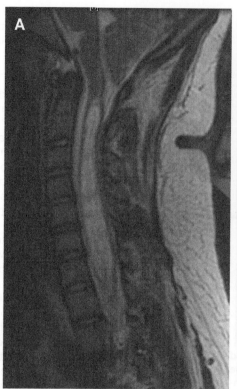
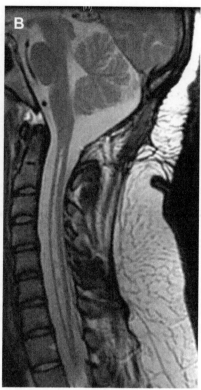

Fig. 8. Holocord syrinx reduction following surgical decompression of Chiari I malformation. T2-weighted midline sagittal cervical spine MRI views demonstrate preoperative holocord syrinx (*A*) with substantial reduction in size following posterior fossa decompression and duraplasty (*B*).

contrast, another retrospective study used a modified propensity score modeling approach with multivariate logistic regression to create a surgical decision-making tool, which incorporated abnormal cine CSF flow as a minor criterion.[2] Despite indeterminate clinical impact, abnormal CSF dynamics at the foramen magnum may explain the pathophysiology of symptom and syringomyelia development, and justify continued follow-up.[1,4,6,8,19,20]

Additional imaging characteristics often receive attention in radiologic interpretations but have an uncertain impact on clinical presentation and management (**Fig. 10, Box 3**).

In several retrospective cohort studies, the above characteristics (including degree of cerebellar tonsillar descent) and other radiographic measures did not predict clinical symptoms, likelihood for surgical intervention, or surgical outcomes.[4,5,9,10,12,56] Several retrospective studies have reported the mean (11.4 $\pm$ 4.86 mm,[1] 9.53 mm,[6] 9.1 mm[2], 11.6 mm[7]) or median (7 mm, interquartile range 6–9 mm)[5] extent of cerebellar tonsil descent without demonstrating clinical import of these measurements. Prospective long-term natural history studies have demonstrated quantitative changes in yearly surveillance radiographic examinations without impact on clinical symptoms or surgical decision-making.[12]

- The extent of cerebellar tonsil descent may vary over time (remaining stable in approximately 50%, reducing in 31% to 38%, or increasing in 4% to 12%),[12,56] without impacting clinical symptoms, neurological examination findings, or surgical management.

However, reduction in cerebellar tonsil descent may alter the diagnosis of Chiari I Malformation when cerebellar tonsil descent decreases below 5 mm (occurring in up to 12% of asymptomatic patients) (**Fig. 11**).[12] Given the unclear impact on management and surgical decision-making, routine surveillance imaging in asymptomatic patients with Chiari I Malformation has been questioned.

Other imaging features of Chiari I Malformation may influence surgical planning after the decision to proceed with operative intervention. Osseous abnormalities may occur in 23-88% of patients

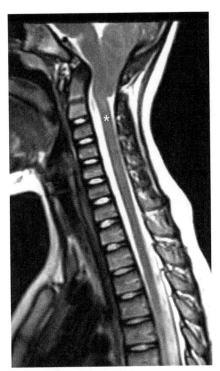

Fig. 9. Pre-syrinx in Chiari malformation. T2-weighted midline sagittal cervical spine MRI sequence demonstrates abnormal T2 hyperintensity at the cervicomedullary junction (above the *asterisk*) in a patient with Chiari (1.5) malformation.

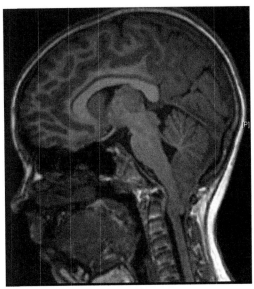

Fig. 10. Additional imaging features in Chiari I malformation. T1-weighed paramedian sagittal view shows complex Chiari I malformation with pointed cerebellar tonsils, dorsal cervicomedullary hump or kink, retroflexion of the odontoid, and effacement of the cervicomedullary cisterns. These imaging features represented incidental findings in an asymptomatic 8-year-old patient with previous history of focal epilepsy and normal overnight polysomnography (sleep study).

with Chiari I Malformation and may increase the complexity or risk assessment of surgical approaches (**Box 4**).[1] For instance, basilar invagination and retroflexion of the odontoid process may occur in up to 3% and 24% of Chiari I Malformation patients, respectively (see **Fig. 10**).[4]

Evaluation of abnormal movement or structure at the CCJ may require pre-operative cervical spine flexion-extension radiographs or CT.[2,4]

Some of the osseous anomalies associated with Chiari I Malformation may require consideration of adjunctive surgical techniques including anterior decompression or posterior occipito-cervical instrumented fixation and fusion. Radiographic measures may contribute substantively to these critical surgical decisions:

- pBC2 distance ≥ 9 mm may indicate the need for ventral brainstem decompression before posterior fossa decompression[11,26]
- CXA < 125° may indicate the need for posterior occipito-cervical fusion[11]
- Projection of the odontoid process (typically located 5 mm below McRae's line) through the foramen magnum may suggest the need for posterior occipito-cervical fusion[11]

Abnormal growth at the CCJ in patients with Chiari I Malformation and concomitant genetic syndromes (eg, syndromic craniosynostosis, achondroplasia, Paget's disease, Goldenhaar syndrome) may warrant consideration of osseous-only decompression as opposed to posterior fossa decompression with duraplasty.[7,17]

Intraoperative ultrasonography represents an additional imaging modality useful in surgical

---

Box 3
Imaging characteristics of Chiari I malformation with indeterminate clinical impact[1,4,5,19,56]

Magnitude of cerebellar tonsillar descent

Abnormal CSF flow at the foramen magnum

Cerebellar tonsil morphology

   Pointed appearance with varying severity

   Peg-like appearance

Presence of retro-cerebellar CSF collection

Angulation of the cervicomedullary junction (medullary kink)

Volume of posterior fossa

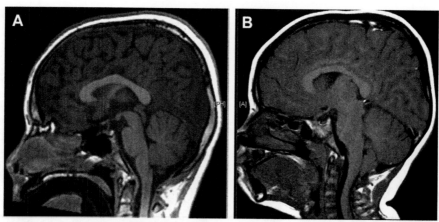

Fig. 11. Spontaneous resolution of Chiari I malformation over time. T1-weighted sagittal views demonstrate resolution of Chiari I Malformation between serial surveillance imaging studies separated by 7 years (*A*, later; *B*, earlier). Updated imaging (*A*) shows normalization of cerebellar tonsil position and normal appearance of the cervicomedullary junction.

management of Chiari I Malformation. This imaging technique may help determine adequacy of surgical decompression and contribute to decision-making regarding intradural exploration with duraplasty (**Fig. 12**).[3,17,19] Evaluation of CSF posterior to the cerebellar tonsils and physiologic pulsation patterns of the cerebellar tonsils may help determine the necessity for dural opening with duraplasty.[3]

SUMMARY

Chiari I Malformation represents a hindbrain anomaly often found incidentally (for evaluation of other symptoms or indications) or in the context of typical clinical signs or symptoms. Brain and spine MRI provide optimal anatomic detail of cerebellar tonsillar descent below the foramen magnum and may reveal additional imaging features including ventriculomegaly (potentially leading to the diagnosis of hydrocephalus), characteristics of intracranial hypertension or hypotension, spinal

cord syrinx, scoliosis, and/or tethered spinal cord. Identification of these additional imaging features may help guide initial management. Specialized imaging sequences (eg, FIESTA sagittal sequences, phase contrast CSF flow studies)

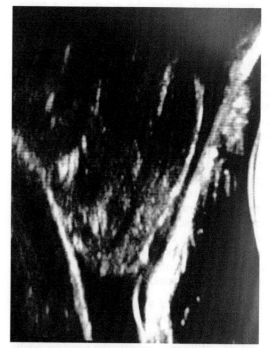

Fig. 12. Intraoperative ultrasonography in surgical Decompression of Chiari I malformation. Intraoperative ultrasound can be used to investigate adequacy of osseous decompression of Chiari I malformation when deciding upon incorporation of dural opening and duraplasty.

Box 4
Potential osseous abnormalities in Chiari I malformation[1–4]

Scoliosis

Retroflexion of the odontoid process

Basilar impression or invagination

Platybasia

Cervical spine segmentation (fusion) anomalies

Abnormal motion at the CCJ

provide enhanced visualization of ventral and dorsal cervicomedullary cisterns and CSF flow at the CCJ. Although these studies contribute critical information for evaluation, their impact on surgical decision-making remains uncertain. Additional radiographic measures (eg, pBC2, CXA) may impact surgical planning and risk assessment and may suggest the need for additional surgical techniques (eg, posterior occipito-cervical fusion, anterior decompression) beyond standard posterior fossa decompression with or without duraplasty.

CLINICS CARE POINTS

- The prevalence of radiographic Chiari I malformation among children within the general population undergoing brain or cervical spine imaging approximates 0.77% to 1.0%.[1,5,6,10-12]

- Hydrocephalus may co-present in up to 10% of patients with Chiari I Malformation.[3,4]

- The presence of a Chiari I Malformation and spinal cord syrinx typically favors surgical intervention among most pediatric neurosurgeons.[1,2,4,6,8,10,11,17,19,56]

- The co-presentation of scoliosis with Chiari I Malformation and spinal cord syrinx typically warrants initial surgical decompression of the Chiari Malformation.[2,10,17,18]

- Syringomyelia typically responds well to surgical decompression of Chiari I Malformation, with radiographic syrinx reduction or resolution in 65% to 100% of affected patients.[3-6,8,10,11,17,18]

- Surgical decompression of Chiari I Malformation may impact scoliotic curvature with reported favorable outcomes (curvature stability or improvement) ranging between 32% and 100%.[8,18,57]

- The extent of cerebellar tonsil descent may vary over time, remaining stable in approximately 50%, reducing in 31% to 38%, or increasing in 4% to 12% of patients.[12,56]

- A pBC2 distance $\geq$ 9 mm may indicate the need for ventral brainstem decompression before posterior fossa decompression.[11,26]

- Kyphosis at the CCJ reflected by CXA < 125° or projection of the odontoid process through the foramen magnum may indicate the need for posterior occipito-cervical fusion.[11]

DISCLOSURE

The authors have no commercial or financial conflicts of interest to report regarding the completion of this article. The authors have no relevant funding sources to report regarding the material presented in this article.

REFERENCES

1. Meadows J, Kraut M, Guarnieri M, et al. Asymptomatic Chiari Type I malformations identified on magnetic resonance imaging. J Neurosurg 2000;92(6):920–6.
2. Low SYY, Ng LP, Tan AJL, et al. The Seow Operative Score (SOS) as a decision-making adjunct for paediatric Chiari I malformation: a preliminary study. Child's Nervous Syst 2019;35(10):1777–83.
3. Balestrino A, Consales A, Pavanello M, et al. Management: opinions from different centers-the Istituto Giannina Gaslini experience. Child's Nervous Syst 2019;35(10):1905–9.
4. Tubbs RS, Beckman J, Naftel RP, et al. Institutional experience with 500 cases of surgically treated pediatric Chiari malformation Type I. J Neurosurg Pediatr 2011;7(3):248–56.
5. Aitken LA, Lindan CE, Sidney S, et al. Chiari type I malformation in a pediatric population. Pediatr Neurol 2009;40(6):449–54.
6. Arnautovic A, Splavski B, Boop FA, et al. Pediatric and adult Chiari malformation Type I surgical series 1965-2013: a review of demographics, operative treatment, and outcomes. J Neurosurg Pediatr 2015;15(2):161–77.
7. Speer MC, Enterline DS, Mehltretter L, et al. Review article: chiari Type I malformation with or without syringomyelia: prevalence and Genetics. J Genet Couns 2003;12(4):297–311.
8. Hwang SW, Samdani AF, Jea A, et al. Outcomes of Chiari I-associated scoliosis after intervention: a meta-analysis of the pediatric literature. Child's Nervous Syst 2012;28(8):1213–9.
9. Khalsa SSS, Geh N, Martin BA, et al. Morphometric and volumetric comparison of 102 children with symptomatic and asymptomatic Chiari malformation Type I. J Neurosurg Pediatr 2018;21(1):65–71.
10. Jussila MP, Nissilä J, Vakkuri M, et al. Preoperative measurements on MRI in Chiari 1 patients fail to predict outcome after decompressive surgery. Acta Neurochir 2021;163(7):2005–14.
11. Ho WSC, Brockmeyer DL. Complex Chiari malformation: using craniovertebral junction metrics to guide treatment. Child's Nervous Syst 2019;35(10):1847–51.
12. Whitson WJ, Lane JR, Bauer DF, et al. A prospective natural history study of nonoperatively managed Chiari I malformation: does follow-up MRI

surveillance alter surgical decision making? J Neurosurg Pediatr 2015;16(2):159–66.

13. Barkovich AJ, Wippold FJ, Sherman JL, et al. Significance of cerebellar tonsillar position on MR. AJNR Am J Neuroradiol 1986;7(5):795–9.

14. Chiari H. Ueber Veränderungen des Kleinhirns infolge von Hydrocephalie des Grosshirns. Deutsche Medizinische Wochenschrift 1891;17(42).

15. Milhorat TH, Chou MW, Trinidad EM, et al. Chiari I malformation redefined: clinical and radiographic findings for 364 symptomatic patients. Neurosurgery 1999;44(5):1005–17.

16. Farb RI, Forghani R, Lee SK, et al. The venous distension sign: a diagnostic sign of intracranial hypotension at MR imaging of the brain. AJNR Am J Neuroradiol 2007;28(8):1489–93.

17. Hersh DS, Groves ML, Boop FA. Management of Chiari malformations: opinions from different centers-a review. Child's Nervous Syst 2019; 35(10):1869–73.

18. Krieger MD, Falkinstein Y, Bowen IE, et al. Scoliosis and Chiari malformation Type I in children. J Neurosurg Pediatr 2011;7(1):25–9.

19. Gernsback J, Tomita T. Management of Chiari I malformation in children: personal opinions. Child's Nervous Syst 2019;35(10):1921–3.

20. Vinchon M. Surgery for Chiari 1 malformation: the Lille experience. Child's Nervous Syst 2019;35(10): 1875–80.

21. Ryan ME, Jaju A, Rychlik K, et al. Feasibility of rapid spine magnetic resonance evaluation for spinal cord syrinx in the pediatric population. Neuroradiology 2022;64(9):1879–85.

22. Elster AD, Chen MY. Chiari I malformations: clinical and radiologic reappraisal. Radiology 1992;183(2): 347–53.

23. Strahle J, Muraszko KM, Kapurch J, et al. Chiari malformation Type I and syrinx in children undergoing magnetic resonance imaging. J Neurosurg Pediatr 2011;8(2):205–13.

24. Brockmeyer DL, Spader HS. Complex chiari malformations in children: diagnosis and management. Neurosurg Clin N Am 2015;26(4):555–60.

25. Papachristou MD, Ward RE, Agarwal V, et al. Complex chiari malformation: what the neurosurgeon needs to know. Neurographics 2022;12(1):35–42.

26. Grabb PA, Mapstone TB, Oakes WJ. Ventral brain stem compression in pediatric and young adult patients with Chiari I malformations. Neurosurgery 1999;44(3):520–7 [discussion: 527-528].

27. Tubbs RS, Iskandar BJ, Bartolucci AA, et al. A critical analysis of the Chiari 1.5 malformation. J Neurosurg 2004;101(2 Suppl):179–83.

28. Shah LM, McLean LA, Heilbrun ME, et al. Intracranial hypotension: improved MRI detection with diagnostic intracranial angles. AJR Am J Roentgenol 2013;200(2):400–7.

29. Michali-Stolarska M, Bladowska J, Stolarski M, et al. Diagnostic imaging and clinical features of intracranial hypotension - review of literature. Pol J Radiol 2017;82:842–9.

30. Aiken AH, Hoots JA, Saindane AM, et al. Incidence of cerebellar tonsillar ectopia in idiopathic intracranial hypertension: a mimic of the Chiari I malformation. AJNR Am J Neuroradiol 2012;33(10):1901–6.

31. Sarrami AH, Bass DI, Rutman AM, et al. Idiopathic intracranial hypertension imaging approaches and the implications in patient management. Br J Radiol 2022;95(1136):20220136.

32. Bhadelia RA, Bogdan AR, Wolpert SM, et al. Cerebrospinal fluid flow waveforms: analysis in patients with Chiari I malformation by means of gated phase-contrast MR imaging velocity measurements. Radiology 1995;196(1):195–202.

33. Wolpert SM, Bhadelia RA, Bogdan AR, et al. Chiari I malformations: assessment with phase-contrast velocity MR. AJNR Am J Neuroradiol 1994;15(7): 1299–308.

34. Pujol J, Roig C, Capdevila A, et al. Motion of the cerebellar tonsils in Chiari type I malformation studied by cine phase-contrast MRI. Neurology 1995; 45(9):1746–53.

35. Pinna G, Alessandrini F, Alfieri A, et al. Cerebrospinal fluid flow dynamics study in Chiari I malformation: implications for syrinx formation. Neurosurg Focus 2000;8(3):E3.

36. Shah S, Haughton V, del Río AM. CSF flow through the upper cervical spinal canal in Chiari I malformation. AJNR Am J Neuroradiol 2011;32(6): 1149–53.

37. Haughton V, Mardal KA. Spinal fluid biomechanics and imaging: an update for neuroradiologists. AJNR Am J Neuroradiol 2014;35(10):1864–9.

38. Hofkes SK, Iskandar BJ, Turski PA, et al. Differentiation between symptomatic Chiari I malformation and asymptomatic tonsilar ectopia by using cerebrospinal fluid flow imaging: initial estimate of imaging accuracy. Radiology 2007;245(2):532–40.

39. Iskandar BJ, Quigley M, Haughton VM. Foramen magnum cerebrospinal fluid flow characteristics in children with Chiari I malformation before and after craniocervical decompression. J Neurosurg 2004; 101(2 Suppl):169–78.

40. Krueger KD, Haughton VM, Hetzel S. Peak CSF velocities in patients with symptomatic and asymptomatic Chiari I malformation. AJNR Am J Neuroradiol 2010;31(10):1837–41.

41. Ventureyra EC, Aziz HA, Vassilyadi M. The role of cine flow MRI in children with Chiari I malformation. Childs Nerv Syst 2003;19(2):109–13.

42. Gad KA, Yousem DM. Syringohydromyelia in Patients with Chiari I Malformation: a retrospective analysis. AJNR Am J Neuroradiol 2017;38(9): 1833–8.

43. Leung V, Magnussen JS, Stoodley MA, et al. Cerebellar and hindbrain motion in Chiari malformation with and without syringomyelia. J Neurosurg Spine 2016;24(4):546–55.

44. Godzik J, Kelly MP, Radmanesh A, et al. Relationship of syrinx size and tonsillar descent to spinal deformity in Chiari malformation Type I with associated syringomyelia. J Neurosurg Pediatr 2014; 13(4):368–74.

45. McGirt MJ, Nimjee SM, Fuchs HE, et al. Relationship of cine phase-contrast mri to outcome after decompression for chiari I malformation. Neurosurgery 2006;59(1):140–6.

46. McGirt MJ, Atiba A, Attenello FJ, et al. Correlation of hindbrain CSF flow and outcome after surgical decompression for Chiari I malformation. Childs Nerv Syst 2008;24(7):833–40.

47. Li AE, Wilkinson MD, McGrillen KM, et al. Clinical applications of cine balanced steady-state free precession MRI for the evaluation of the subarachnoid spaces. Clin Neuroradiol 2015;25(4):349–60.

48. Sharma A, Parsons MS, Pilgram TK. Balanced steady-state free-precession MR imaging for measuring pulsatile motion of cerebellar tonsils during the cardiac cycle: a reliability study. Neuroradiology 2012;54(2):133–8.

49. Cousins J, Haughton V. Motion of the cerebellar tonsils in the foramen magnum during the cardiac cycle. AJNR Am J Neuroradiol 2009;30(8):1587–8.

50. Radmanesh A, Greenberg JK, Chatterjee A, et al. Tonsillar pulsatility before and after surgical decompression for children with Chiari malformation type 1: an application for true fast imaging with steady state precession. Neuroradiology 2015;57(4):387–93.

51. Bhadelia RA, Patz S, Heilman C, et al. Cough-associated changes in CSF flow in chiari i malformation evaluated by real-time MRI. AJNR Am J Neuroradiol 2016;37(5):825–30.

52. Ohtonari T, Nishihara N, Ota S, et al. Novel assessment of cerebrospinal fluid dynamics by time-spatial labeling inversion pulse magnetic resonance imaging in patients with chiari malformation Type I. World Neurosurg 2018;112:e165–71.

53. Eppelheimer MS, Nwotchouang BST, Heidari Pahlavian S, et al. Cerebellar and brainstem displacement measured with DENSE MRI in chiari malformation following posterior fossa decompression surgery. Radiology 2021;301(1):187–94.

54. Bunck AC, Kroeger JR, Juettner A, et al. Magnetic resonance 4D flow analysis of cerebrospinal fluid dynamics in Chiari I malformation with and without syringomyelia. Eur Radiol 2012;22(9):1860–70.

55. Williams G, Thyagaraj S, Fu A, et al. In vitro evaluation of cerebrospinal fluid velocity measurement in type I Chiari malformation: repeatability, reproducibility, and agreement using 2D phase contrast and 4D flow MRI. Fluids Barriers CNS 2021;18(1):12.

56. Strahle J, Muraszko KM, Kapurch J, et al. Natural history of Chiari malformation Type I following decision for conservative treatment. J Neurosurg Pediatr 2011;8(2):214–21.

57. Tubbs RS, Doyle S, Conklin M, et al. Scoliosis in a child with Chiari I malformation and the absence of syringomyelia: case report and a review of the literature. Child's Nervous Syst 2006;22(10):1351–4.

58. Strahle J, Smith BW, Martinez M, et al. The association between Chiari malformation Type I, spinal syrinx, and scoliosis. J Neurosurg Pediatr 2015;15(6):607–11.

Cerebrospinal Fluid Hydrodynamics in Chiari I Malformation and Syringomyelia: Modeling Pathophysiology

John D. Heiss, MD

KEYWORDS

- Chiari I malformation • Syringomyelia • Hydrocephalus • Cerebrospinal fluid dynamics
- Pathophysiology • Glymphatic system • Aquaporin 4 • Foramen magnum decompression

KEY POINTS

- The Chiari I malformation narrows Cerebrospinal fluid (CSF) flow pathways at the foramen magnum.
- Chiari I malformation patients with critically obstructed CSF flow develop cervical syringomyelia.
- Operative decompression of the Chiari I malformation usually relieves the obstruction of the CSF pathways at the foramen magnum and resolves syringomyelia.
- Syringomyelia persistence after decompressive surgery indicates that the CSF pathways remain obstructed at the foramen magnum.
- Pulsatile movement of the Chiari I malformation produces tonsillar gliosis and other hindbrain manifestations.

INTRODUCTION

The pathophysiology linking Chiari I malformation to syringomyelia development and progression remains controversial. Neurosurgeons and scientists generally agree that obstruction of the normal circulation of cerebrospinal (CSF) flow in and around the foramen magnum is a critical component of Chiari I-associated syringomyelia pathogenesis. This article reviews the experimental and clinical observations about Chiari I malformation-associated syringomyelia and scientific investigations providing insights into how obstruction of normal CSF flow at the foramen magnum could, by a hydrodynamic mechanism, lead to syringomyelia development and progression.

HISTORY

In 1891, Hans Chiari originally described his type I malformation as involving tonsillar ectopia and hydrocephalus, but not syringomyelia.[1] Earlier, the German pathologist Theodor Langhans published a case of cerebellar tonsillar extension inferior to the foramen magnum associated with an intramedullary cystic fluid collection in the cervical spinal cord. The title of his 1881 article, *Über Höhlenbildung im Rückenmark als Folge Blutstauung* (translated as "Regarding cavity creation in the spinal cord as a consequence of obstruction to blood flow"), implied an ischemic etiology for syringomyelia. However, the text noted cerebrospinal (CSF) flow obstruction as another factor in syrinx formation, "The increase in pressure in the cerebellar cavity will hinder or greatly impede the outflow of blood and cerebral spinal fluid."[2] Later, neurosurgeons recognized that syringomyelia resolved after decompressing the Chiari I malformation at the foramen magnum and reestablishing normal CSF flow there.[3,4] Classic theories of syringomyelia pathogenesis associated with Chiari I

Clinical Unit, Surgical Neurology Branch, National Institute of Neurological Diseases and Stroke, National Institutes of Health, 10 Center Drive, Room 3D20, MSC-1414, Bethesda, MD 20892, USA
E-mail address: heissj@ninds.nih.gov

Neurosurg Clin N Am 34 (2023) 81–90
https://doi.org/10.1016/j.nec.2022.08.007
1042-3680/23/Published by Elsevier Inc.

malformation included Gardner's Theory, in which the fourth ventricle created a "water-hammer" pulse wave during cardiac systole. The pulse wave passed through the obex to the central canal of the spinal cord, which progressively expanded into a syrinx.[3] Williams believed that pressure differentials created between the intracranial cavity and spinal canal during coughing and straining (Valsalva) drive CSF from the fourth ventricle to the spinal cord central canal, forming a syrinx.[4] Both theories require the presence of a patent central canal of the spinal cord between the fourth ventricle and syrinx. However, pathologic and radiographic studies showed that the central canal is rarely patent and usually obstructed at several spinal segments in adults with or without syringomyelia.[5,6]

More recently, investigators demonstrated various factors associated with syringomyelia in Chiari I malformation patients. One factor was the extent to which the cerebellar tonsillar ectopia obstructed the normal flow of cerebrospinal fluid at the foramen magnum as evaluated by phase-contrast cine MRI. Caudal location of the medulla also significantly heightened the risk of syringomyelia. Syringomyelia was three times likelier in Chiari I malformation patients with a low-obex position (54%) than a normal position (18%).[7] Other factors were the reduced volume of the entire posterior fossa or its inferior part around the foramen magnum and abnormal tapering of the width of the adjacent upper cervical spinal canal.[8–10] Syringomyelia also accompanied intradural adhesions and arachnoidopathy, which narrow the CSF pathways at the foramen magnum.[11] Narrowing of the foramen of Magendie also impeded CSF flow.[12,13] Basilar invagination, if present, can compress the anterior subarachnoid CSF pathway across the craniospinal junction in patients with Chiari I malformation. In short, Chiari I malformation patients with syringomyelia have severely narrowed CSF pathways in and around the foramen magnum.

DEFINITIONS

Syringomyelia is an intramedullary fluid-filled cavity that distends the spinal cord and is longer than one spinal segment. Communicating syringomyelia is an enlargement of the spinal cord central canal communicating with an enlarged fourth ventricle.[14] Hydromyelia is communicating syringomyelia that may be associated with hydrocephalus. Noncommunicating syringomyelia is an enlargement of the spinal cord central canal that does not communicate with an enlarged fourth ventricle.[14] Extracanalicular syringomyelia is an intramedullary fluid-filled cavity within the spinal cord parenchyma that does not communicate with the fourth ventricle or spinal cord central canal. Atrophic syringomyelia is an intramedullary fluid-filled cavity associated with myelomalacia. Tumor-related syringomyelia is an intramedullary fluid collection often communicating with the spinal cord central canal and consisting of plasma ultrafiltrate of permeable tumor capillaries. A neoplastic cyst is a local intramedullary tumor cyst.[14] The obex is a thin triangular gray matter membrane located 1 to 2 mm posterior to the apertura canalis centralis, the ostia of the central canal in the inferior fourth ventricle.[15] On MRI the location of the apertura canalis centralis is referred to as the obex. Medical personnel often refer to the apertura canalis centralis as the obex.

BACKGROUND

Hydrodynamics is the branch of physics exploring the motion and forces of fluids on adjacent solid bodies.[16] In spinal hydrodynamics, the subarachnoid space and the central canal of the spinal cord are the fluid sites, and the solid body is the spinal cord parenchyma. Neurosurgeons and engineers have long been intrigued by the possibility of a hydrodynamic link between the Chiari I malformation and syringomyelia. The Chiari I malformation consists of hindbrain herniation, a process in which the cerebellar tonsils and medulla extend inferior to their normal anatomic position. Hindbrain herniation into the foramen magnum reduces the area for CSF flow across the foramen magnum. A severe reduction of CSF flow area (A) within and around the foramen magnum is associated with syringomyelia. Syringes resolve after surgical procedures that expand the CSF flow area. Reduced CSF flow area is a critical hydrodynamic factor in syringomyelia development and progression.[17–19]

A central formula in hydrodynamics is the Hagen–Poiseuille equation: $\Delta P = 8\mu \, LQ/\pi r^4$, in which ΔP is the difference in pressure between the ends of a circular pipe of a certain length (L), radius (r), volumetric laminar flow rate (Q), and dynamic viscosity (μ).[20] The formula for cross-sectional area of a circle is $A = \pi r^2$ so $\Delta P = 8\mu LQ/\pi r^4$ can also be stated $\Delta P = 8\mu LQ\pi/\pi^2 r^4$ or $\Delta P = 8\mu LQ\pi/A^2$. The Hagen–Poiseuille equation is better suited to predicting blood flow in a cylindrical artery than in the CSF pathway at the foramen magnum, where a CSF layer surrounds the neural elements. However, the Hagen–Poiseuille equation can be modified to predict flow in annular pathways.[21] The Hagen–Poiseuille equation does not consider non-laminar CSF flow (turbulent flow), wall stress, friction, and irregular flow areas that reduce fora-men magnum CSF flow. CSF flow at the foramen magnum varies from tubular laminar flow even further because the CSF flow across the foramen magnum is oscillatory, with ΔP changing from positive to negative and CSF flow (Q) changing in direction during every cardiac cycle, unlike an ar-tery in which ΔP is always positive and flow (Q) al-ways moves in the same direction (away from the heart).[21] To further complicate the modeling of CSF flow across the foramen magnum, the neural elements move within the foramen magnum during the cardiac cycle, although less than the surround-ing CSF.[22] Nonetheless, the Hagen–Poiseuille equation is a guide for estimating the effect of the Chiari I malformation in narrowing the CSF pathways. We can simplify the Hagen–Poiseuille equation to $\Delta P = KQ/A^2$ by considering 8 $\mu L\pi$ a constant, K. Using that formula, a one-half reduc-tion of the cross-sectional area at the foramen magnum (A) would require four times the pressure differential (ΔP) to displace the normal amount of CSF across the foramen magnum during the sys-tolic and diastolic phases of the cardiac cycle.[17]

The Chiari I malformation's reduction of the cross-sectional area (A) for CSF flow at the foramen magnum prevents dampening of the intracranial pressure pulse wave afforded by normal CSF outflow from the intracranial cavity to the spinal subarachnoid space in cardiac systole. Reduced CSF flow across the foramen magnum heightens the pressure change (ΔP) across the foramen mag-num because the intracranial cavity has reduced compliance in patients with Chiari I and syringomy-elia (**Fig. 1**). The high-pressure differential (ΔP) across the foramen magnum causes the hindbrain (cerebellar tonsils and medulla) to descend in car-diac systole and ascend in cardiac diastole in a pul-satile motion as seen on intraoperative ultrasonography after craniectomy[17] (**Fig. 2**A). Dur-ing cardiac systole, the hindbrain and CSF descend and transfer the enlarged intracranial pulse pres-sure (ΔP) to the partially enclosed spinal subarach-noid space (**Fig. 2**B).[17] Craniocervical decompression, the operative treatment of Chiari I malformation, relieves dorsal compression on the cerebellar tonsils and cisterna magna. The cisterna magnum capacity expands as it fills with CSF after this procedure. The cross-sectional area (A) for CSF flow at the foramen magnum increases, and the pressure differential required for normal CSF flow across the foramen magnum during the cardiac cy-cle decreases. In addition, craniocervical decom-pression removes the rigid bony dorsal covering of the foramen magnum, replacing it with compliant soft tissue that can dampen CSF pressure waves across it.[17]

OBSERVATIONS

Hydrocephalus resembles syringomyelia in many ways. For example, hydrocephalus enlarges the cerebral ventricles, the ependyma-lined internal CSF spaces of the brain, and syringomyelia en-larges the central canal, the ependyma-lined inte-rior CSF space of the spinal cord. Hydrocephalus and syringomyelia can be communicating, obstructive, post-traumatic, chemically induced, and post-hemorrhagic. Obstructed CSF flow in the lateral ventricles or cranial subarachnoid space and impaired CSF absorption cause hydro-cephalus. Analogously, obstruction of CSF flow at the craniovertebral junction and impaired syrinx fluid absorption may cause syringomyelia. Hydro-cephalus and syringomyelia distend surrounding central nervous system (CNS) structures and create neurologic deficits. Hydrocephalus can be associated with syringomyelia in patients with Chiari I malformation.[23]

Hydrocephalus and syringomyelia differ in several ways, primarily in the CNS structure involved. Obstructing the ventricular system causes hydrocephalus, but the spinal cord central canal is blocked in over 90% of normal adults and does not cause syringomyelia.[5] In the brain, gray matter nuclei and white matter surround the epen-dyma of the ventricles. In the spinal cord, the cen-tral gray matter surrounds the ependyma of the central canal. The choroid plexus produces roughly one-half to two-thirds of intracranial CSF in the brain, and extrachoroidal locations make the rest. The production of CSF in the spinal cord is extrachoroidal, although CSF can enter the spinal cord from the spinal subarachnoid space.

Treatment of hydrocephalus associated with Chiari I malformation is recommended before cra-niocervical decompression because reducing ven-tricular volume may reduce hindbrain herniation and syrinx size.[24] Compression of the hindbrain within the foramen magnum narrows the foramen of Magendie, bows the dorsal wall of the fourth ventricle, and impairs fourth ventricular drainage. Hydrocephalic enlargement of the fourth ventricle within the neural elements further narrows the sur-rounding cisterna magna and basal cisterns. It can increase the cardiac cycle-related intracranial pressure pulses transmitted to the spinal canal.

The central canal of the spinal cord expands in syringomyelia. The normal central canal is lined by ependymal cells and surrounded by a layer of tanycytes within the center of the spinal cord gray matter. The ependyma and tanycytes regu-late water movement between the central canal and extracellular compartment.[25] The mature

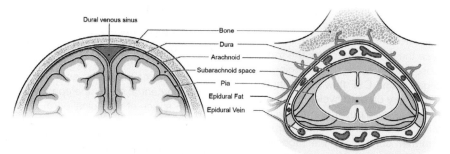

Fig. 1. The rigid skull surrounds the intracranial cavity (*left*), which is much less compliant than the spinal intradural space (*right*). The spinal dura (right) can expand into the epidural space during cardiac systole because of the surrounding compressible fat and veins and the ligamentum flavum covering the interlaminar spaces. CSF is normally driven across from the incompliant intracranial cavity to the more compliant spinal subarachnoid space to compensate for the volumetric expansion of intracranial arteries during cardiac systole.

ependyma is a barrier protecting neural tissue from potentially harmful substances.[26] In embryonic life, the central canal extends from the apertura canalis centralis near the fourth ventricular obex to the conus medullaris. The typical adult central canal is less than 1 mm in diameter, and its lumen is obstructed at one or several locations, preventing communication with the apertura canalis centralis of the fourth ventricle.[5] Milhorat

and colleagues, in an autopsy study of children and adults dying from "various causes," found that the spinal cord central canal was stenotic in 3% of infants, 18% of children, 88% of adolescents and young adults, and 90% of middle-aged adults. Stenosis of the central canal was most prominent in the thoracic spinal cord.[5] They thought that the location of the spinal cord segments affected by syringomyelia was related to

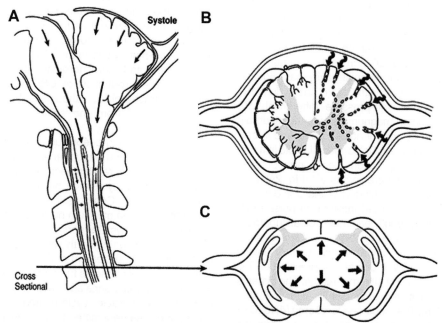

Fig. 2. During cardiac systole, the Chiari I malformation obstructs typical CSF displacement from the intracranial cavity to the spinal subarachnoid space. In place of CSF, the cerebellar tonsils and medulla are displaced inferiorly, creating an enlarged cervical subarachnoid pressure wave (*A*). The pressure wave propels syrinx fluid motion that elongates the syrinx (*A*). The pressure wave also drives CSF into the perivascular spaces of the spinal cord. It may oppose spinal cord interstitial fluid egress through the glymphatic system and into the spinal subarachnoid space (*B*). The distending force within the syrinx that expands the syrinx radially may arise from increased resistance to fluid outflow from the spinal cord central canal, syrinx, and spinal cord interstitial spaces to the spinal subarachnoid space (*C*).

the period of life in which the syrinx began, with central–holocord syringes arising in childhood and central focal and paracentral syringes arising later in life. The presumed cause of central canal occlusion was intermittent inflammatory events. The central canal can be as wide as 2 to 5 mm in patients without present or future myelopathy symptoms.[27] This normal variant contrasts with syringes associated with neurologic deficit, typically of larger diameter, distending the spinal cord, and associated with signs and symptoms of central myelopathy.

RESEARCH

Phase-contrast cine MRI shows the CSF pathway size, velocity, and flow (Q = velocity $\times$ A) in an individual patient with Chiari I malformation and syringomyelia. Physical models can simulate the anatomy of the Chiari I malformation and surrounding structures and the physiologic effects of cardiac pulsation and Valsalva. These models demonstrate the Chiari I malformation's complex and myriad effects on CSF flow and physical stress on the hindbrain and spinal cord tissue.[28]

Phase-contrast cine MRI showed that patients with Chiari I malformation had greater cerebellar tonsillar movement than controls.[29] However, the amount of tonsillar movement in that study could not distinguish between Chiari I malformation patients with and without syringomyelia.[29] Another study showed that 150 microns of cardiac-related tissue motion during 70 ms of the cardiac cycle increased diastolic velocity by 60% and pressure by 20% at the craniocervical junction.[22] The tonsils and hindbrain oscillate in response to cardiac-cycle-related intracranial volume changes and pressure differentials across the foramen magnum. Accentuated hindbrain and CSF motion across the foramen magnum creates high cervical subarachnoid pulse pressure waves in the partially enclosed spinal subarachnoid space.[17] The subarachnoid pressure waves act on the outer surface of the cervical spinal cord to drive syrinx fluid motion. The pulsatile movement of the hindbrain could also oscillate fluid between obstructing septa in the central canal fluid, expand the central canal, and begin syrinx development. In phase-contrast cine MRI CSF flow studies, syrinx fluid oscillates superiorly and inferiorly during the cardiac cycle in response to cerebral and cerebellar tonsillar pulsation.

The origin of syrinx fluid in patients with Chiari I malformation-related syringomyelia remains controversial. Syrinx fluid has the same appearance and protein concentration as spinal cord interstitial fluid and CSF.[30] Fluorescently labeled tracers injected into the cisterna magna of normal mice were distributed to the entire cross-section of the C5 level of the spinal cord within 70 minutes. They were primarily concentrated in the gray matter. The fluorescent tracer entered the spinal parenchyma through the perivascular spaces and across the pial surface. The aquaporin-4 (AQP4)-specific inhibitor, TGN-020, significantly reduced the tracer uptake.[31] This study confirmed that it was normal for cerebrospinal fluid to enter the spinal cord from the subarachnoid space and that AQP4 mediated this process.

AQP4 is highly expressed along the entire spinal cord in the rat spinal cord, labeling astrocytic fiber bundles protruding from the gray matter to the glia limitans adjacent to the pia mater.[32] AQP4 label also encircles neurovascular units. In contrast, AQP1 labeling occurs in the dorsal gray matter's unmyelinated neuronal fibers and endothelial cells.[32] Astrocytes around syrinx cavities expressed AQP4 in an excitotoxic model of post-traumatic syringomyelia.[33] Hypoxia-inducible factor 1-alpha accompanied increased AQP4 expression in areas of CNS injury.[34] Water retention in the murine brain occurs after knockout of subpial astrocytic AQP4 but not after knockout of perivascular astrocytic AQP4 or ependymal AQP4.[35]

The spinal cord central canal is a sink attracting intramedullary interstitial fluid.[36] The spinal cord interstitial fluid drains into small lymphatic-like perivascular spaces and empties into the surrounding spinal subarachnoid space.[37] Intramedullary edema develops when intramedullary fluid production exceeds interstitial fluid drainage. Syringes form when this excess interstitial fluid enters the central canal or adjacent central gray matter, creating a cyst distending those anatomic structures (**Fig. 3**).[38] The development of a symptomatic syrinx associated with Chiari I malformation may be preceded by spinal cord edema or a smaller syrinx.[38,39]

Arterial pulsations can drive CSF through the perivascular spaces and into the extracellular space of the brain and spinal cord.[40] Obstruction of CSF egress from the interstitial spaces of the CNS can also lead to fluid accumulation and hydrocephalus.[41] In patients with Chiari I malformation and syringomyelia, increased cervical subarachnoid pressure waves can increase CSF movement from the subarachnoid space to the perivascular spaces and into the spinal cord interstitial space.[17]

The mechanism of syrinx distension is contentious (**Fig. 2**C). Extrachoroidal CSF produced in the spinal cord could join subarachnoid CSF as a source of syrinx fluid. The spinal cord constantly makes extrachoroidal CSF that maintains its

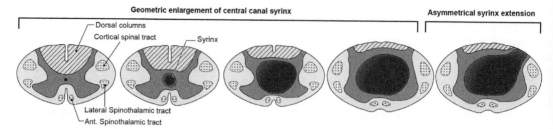

Fig. 3. Syrinx enlargement is a slow process that proceeds from the central canal and surrounding gray matter of the spinal cord. The growing syrinx initially stretches gray matter structures and the spinothalamic crossing tracts. Syrinx pressure can injure the central spinal cord structures irreversibly.

functional milieu.[42] A unidirectional ion pump in the capillary wall moves water from plasma to the CNS interstitial (extracellular) space and creates extrachoroidal CSF. The capillary is impermeable to transcapillary back diffusion of ions from the extracellular space and extrachoroidal CSF reuptake. Immunohistochemical techniques that preserve the meninges show that AQP1 and Na+/K+/2Cl cotransporter-1 are present in leptomeningeal vascular endothelia of the spinal cord.[43] The Chiari I malformation could promote syrinx formation by preventing normal spinal cord absorption of extrachoroidal CSF or increasing extrachoroidal CSF production. The constant output of intramedullary extrachoroidal CSF without compensatory syrinx drainage could contribute to the development of syrinx pressure and distension. Increased spinal subarachnoid CSF pressure waves could also prevent normal absorption of CSF from the spinal cord.

Extrachoroidal CSF fluid retention could be a reason Chiari I malformation-related syringes do not form immediately adjacent to the site of CSF blockage at the foramen magnum but lower in the cervical spinal cord. Gray matter comprises a more significant percentage of the cross-sectional area of the spinal cord in lower than the upper cervical spinal cord. Extrachoroidal CSF production predominates in gray compared with white matter.[44] Therefore, the lower cervical spinal cord produces more extrachoroidal CSF per spinal segment than the upper cervical spinal cord. Individual variation in the pattern of central canal occlusion also influences syrinx location.[5] Aquaporin levels influence the distensibility of the ventricular ependyma and may also affect the distensibility of the central canal.[45] Finally, in some patients with Chiari I malformation and syringomyelia, syrinx formation may occur inferior to narrowing of the upper cervical spinal canal that accompanies hypoplasia of the posterior fossa.[8]

CSF obstruction at the foramen magnum could slow CSF drainage from the spinal subarachnoid space and the exit of interstitial fluid from the syrinx and spinal cord. After surgically expanding the CSF pathways at the foramen magnum, it usually takes 3 to 6 months before the syrinx diameter becomes less than one-half its preoperative diameter.[46] In rare cases, syringes regress spontaneously, presumably because of anatomic changes that improve CSF flow at the foramen magnum.[47] Syrinx collapse, on the other hand, occurs immediately with syrinx shunting.[48] These observations suggest that in patients with Chiari I malformation and syringomyelia, the syrinx's pressure and distension resolve slowly after craniocervical decompression because of slow syrinx drainage through tiny interstitial pathways to the subarachnoid space.

Other observations also support that efflux of syrinx fluid from the spinal cord is a slow process. Subarachnoid space and syrinx puncture through the dura show that Chiari I-related syringes and the spinal subarachnoid space have similar mean and pulse pressures.[17] After opening the dura, Chiari I-related syringes remain expanded and maintain a pressure greater than the atmospheric pressure in the spinal subarachnoid space.[49] Computed tomography (CT) myelography also shows that syrinx drainage is slow. The bulk flow of water-soluble myelogram dye out of syringes is much slower than the clearance of dye from the subarachnoid space, leading to the target sign on CT, in which dye is retained in the syrinx after being absorbed in the surrounding subarachnoid space. Another finding in CT myelography is that syringes associated with Chiari I malformation or spinal subarachnoid space obstructions accumulate higher concentrations of myelogram dye than tumor-related syringes, suggesting bulk flow into the syrinx from the subarachnoid space occurs in obstruction-related syringes.[50] In Chiari I malformation patients, increased bulk flow of CSF into the syrinx from the spinal subarachnoid space and slow syrinx fluid outflow favor the syrinx' development and maintenance.[50]

Pathophysiology of Different Syringomyelia Types

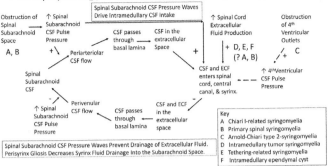

Fig. 4. Syringes arise from diverse mechanisms that share the feature that they create a net increase in the intramedullary fluid. ECF, extracellular fluid.

Despite its slow drainage rate, syrinx fluid associated with Chiari I malformation typically has a normal protein level as assessed by laboratory measures.[30] Syrinx fluid associated with conditions causing CSF obstruction typically has the same MRI signal as CSF. Fluid-attenuated inversion recovery (FLAIR) MRI sequences can detect protein in the CSF at levels as low as 95 mg/dL, somewhat above the normal CSF protein range of 20 to 50 mg/dL.[51]

Usually, intramedullary fluid production and absorption are balanced, and syringes do not form. The cause of intramedullary fluid accumulation appears straightforward in some types of syringomyelia unassociated with Chiari I malformation. For example, there is a case report of syringomyelia associated with choroid plexus within the central canal of the spinal cord. In this case, intramedullary CSF accumulation and a syrinx appear related to intramedullary CSF produced by the choroid plexus remnant that exceeded intramedullary absorption capabilities.[52] In syringes related to intramedullary tumors, plasma ultrafiltrate escapes the tumor interstitium under pressure, enters the central canal, exceeds absorption capabilities, and creates a syrinx.[50] These cases highlight the spinal cord's limited capacity to drain excess interstitial fluid (**Fig. 4**).

Syrinx distension requires a distending force. The process of syrinx expansion must produce enough pressure to expand the central canal's diameter until fluid production and absorption come into balance. Syringes come in various sizes, and as syringes enlarge, the spinal cord diameter increases and the spinal cord parenchyma stretches around the syrinx fluid (see **Fig. 3**). The viscoelastic stretching of the spinal cord elements around the syrinx requires energy from the syrinx fluid transmitted by pressure, usually over a long time, to the wall of the syrinx.

The development of a syrinx associated with Chiari I malformation may be preceded by spinal cord edema.[38,39] Alternatively, the syrinx may progressively enlarge over time from a net increase of fluid within the central canal due to increased interstitial CSF production or reduced absorption of extracellular fluid from the central canal. The central canal in histologic cross-sections is usually not round but irregular, with multiple fluid-filled protrusions from its center into the medial spinal cord. This shape has a larger perimeter than a circle, allowing the central canal to expand initially into a cylindrical shape without stretching its ependymal lining.[53] The syrinx size will enlarge or remain stable until the obstruction at the craniocervical junction is relieved. Radial enlargement of the syrinx stretches and displaces tanycytes, neurons, astrocytes, oligodendrocytes, veins, and capillaries and softens the surrounding tissue. A gliotic capsule forms around the syrinx. The spinal cord adjusts to the syrinx, loses its inherent stiffness, and its fluid distends the spinal cord. Gravitation-related hydrostatic forces distend the syrinx's inferior component and narrow the syrinx's superior part, leading to phenomena known as the "collapsing cord sign" in response to raising the head of the table during myelography.[30,54,55] The pia and arachnoid maters provide much of the inherent stiffness to the spinal cord.[56,57] A loss of this stiffness demonstrates that syringomyelia weakened the pia and arachnoid. The spinal cord diameter increases with the enclosed syrinx. A permanent loss of central spinal cord structures occurs if the obstruction to CSF flow is not relieved. Improving the CSF flow at the foramen magnum reduces the size of the syrinx and arrests the neurologic progression.

CURRENT EVIDENCE

The Chiari I malformation obstructs CSF flow at the foramen magnum and results in cervical subarachnoid CSF pressure waves. These pressure waves increase the volume of cerebrospinal fluid entering the cervical spinal cord through the perivascular space. They could also impede spinal cord extrachoroidal CSF transport from the spinal cord's central canal and extracellular space to the spinal subarachnoid space, contributing to syrinx fluid accumulation. Extrachoroidal CSF is a potential pressure source for a growing syrinx because active transcapillary ionic gradients make it inexorably. Syringes may not form immediately adjacent to the site of CSF blockage, the foramen magnum because extrachoroidal CSF production predominates in the gray matter compared with the white matter.[44] Gray matter forms a more significant percentage of the cross-sectional area of the spinal cord in the lower cervical spinal cord, where the gray matter is larger to support upper extremity motor and sensory function. More fluid per spinal segment may be made in the lower cervical spinal cord than at higher levels. Another consideration influencing syrinx location is individual variation in the central canal occlusion pattern.[5] Finally, in some patients with Chiari I malformation and syringomyelia, narrowing the upper cervical spinal canal may favor syrinx formation in the lower spinal canal.

CLINICAL RELEVANCE

Syringomyelia arises because the Chiari I malformation obstructs the CSF pathway at the foramen magnum. Craniocervical decompression relieves this obstruction and restores normal CSF flow across the foramen magnum. Syringomyelia persisting or expanding after craniocervical decompression signifies that the operative procedure did not relieve the Chiari I malformation's obstruction to CSF flow. In those cases, reoperation can usually restore CSF flow at the foramen magnum and resolve syringomyelia, except in cases of severe arachnoiditis.[18] In those cases, shunting syrinx fluid can collapse the syrinx and stabilize syrinx-related central myelopathy. Further understanding of Chiari I pathophysiology and the mechanism of syrinx enlargement may lead to pharmacotherapeutic approaches for patients with syringomyelia that cannot be remediated successfully with operative therapy.[58,59]

SUMMARY

Syringomyelia develops in association with Chiari I malformation because the hindbrain is ectopic and partially obstructs the CSF pathways at the foramen magnum. Fluid accumulates within the central canal or the adjacent gray matter and forms a syrinx. The force pressurizing the syrinx fluid arises from spinal subarachnoid pressure waves generated by brain artery expansion during cardiac systole. Gliosis forming around the syrinx impairs syrinx fluid absorption. The distending force of expanding syrinx fluid compresses and injures the central gray matter and crossing fibers of the anterior spinothalamic tract and expands the spinal cord diameter. The syrinx eventually compresses the long tracts of the spinal cord, leading to long tract signs. The syrinx transforms the spinal cord slowly, usually over months to years, from a solid, viscoelastic structure to a flaccid structure whose walls are inflated by the syrinx fluid. Surgical relief of the CSF obstruction at the foramen magnum results in syrinx resolution, defined as more than a 50% decrease in syrinx diameter.[46]

CLINICS CARE POINTS

- Syringomyelia associated with the Chiari I malformation arises because the Chiari I malformation obstructs normal CSF flow across the foramen magnum during the cardiac cycle.
- Syringomyelia resolves after an operative procedure relieves the obstruction to normal CSF flow at the foramen magnum.
- Syringomyelia persisting after an operative procedure indicates that the operation was unsuccessful in establishing normal CSF flow at the foramen magnum.

DISCLOSURE

The author has nothing to disclose.

FUNDING

The Intramural Research Program of the National Institute of Neurological Diseases and Stroke supported this research.

REFERENCES

1. Chiari H. Concerning alterations in the cerebellum resulting from cerebral hydrocephalus. 1891. Pediatr Neurosci 1987;13(1):3–8.
2. Mortazavi MM, Tubbs RS, Brockerhoff MA, et al. The first description of Chiari I malformation with intuitive correlation between tonsillar ectopia and syringomyelia. J Neurosurg Pediatr 2011;7(3):257–60.
3. Gardner WJ, Angel J. The mechanism of syringomyelia and its surgical correction. Clin Neurosurg 1958; 6:131–40.

4. Williams B. The distending force in the production of "communicating syringomyelia. Lancet 1969; 2(7613):189–93.

5. Milhorat TH, Kotzen RM, Anzil AP. Stenosis of central canal of spinal cord in man: incidence and pathological findings in 232 autopsy cases. J Neurosurg 1994;80(4):716–22.

6. Williams B. Syringomyelia. Neurosurg Clin N Am 1990;1(3):653–85.

7. Haller G, Sadler B, Kuensting T, et al. Obex position is associated with syringomyelia and use of posterior fossa decompression among patients with Chiari I malformation. J Neurosurg Pediatr 2020;26(1): 45–52.

8. Hirano M, Haughton V, Munoz del Rio A. Tapering of the cervical spinal canal in patients with Chiari I malformations. AJNR Am J Neuroradiol 2012;33(7): 1326–30.

9. Nishikawa M, Sakamoto H, Hakuba A, et al. Pathogenesis of Chiari malformation: a morphometric study of the posterior cranial fossa. J Neurosurg 1997;86(1):40–7.

10. Noudel R, Jovenin N, Eap C, et al. Incidence of basioccipital hypoplasia in Chiari malformation type I: comparative morphometric study of the posterior cranial fossa. Clinical article. J Neurosurg 2009; 111(5):1046–52.

11. Dlouhy BJ, Dawson JD, Menezes AH. Intradural pathology and pathophysiology associated with Chiari I malformation in children and adults with and without syringomyelia. J Neurosurg Pediatr 2017; 20(6):526–41.

12. Guan J, Yuan C, Zhang C, et al. Intradural Pathology Causing Cerebrospinal Fluid Obstruction in Syringomyelia and Effectiveness of Foramen Magnum and Foramen of Magendie Dredging Treatment. World Neurosurg 2020;144:e178–88.

13. Orakdogen M, Emon ST, Erdogan B, et al. Fourth Ventriculostomy in Occlusion of the Foramen of Magendie Associated with Chiari Malformation and Syringomyelia. NMC Case Rep J 2015;2(2):72–5.

14. Milhorat TH. Classification of syringomyelia. Neurosurg Focus 2000;8(3):E1.

15. Longatti P, Fiorindi A, Marton E, et al. Where the central canal begins: endoscopic in vivo description. J Neurosurg 2022;136(3):895–904.

16. Merriam-Webster.com. Hydrodynamics. 2022. https://www.merriam-webster.com. [Accessed 16 May 2022].

17. Heiss JD, Patronas N, DeVroom HL, et al. Elucidating the pathophysiology of syringomyelia. J Neurosurg 1999;91(4):553–62.

18. Heiss JD, Suffredini G, Smith R, et al. Pathophysiology of persistent syringomyelia after decompressive craniocervical surgery. Clin article. *J Neurosurg Spine* 2010;13(6):729–42.

19. Oldfield EH, Muraszko K, Shawker TH, et al. Pathophysiology of syringomyelia associated with Chiari I malformation of the cerebellar tonsils. Implications for diagnosis and treatment. J Neurosurg 1994; 80(1):3–15.

20. Srivastava A, Sood A, Joy SP, et al. Principles of physics in surgery: the laws of flow dynamics physics for surgeons - Part 1. Indian J Surg 2009;71(4):182–7.

21. Loth F, Yardimci MA, Alperin N. Hydrodynamic modeling of cerebrospinal fluid motion within the spinal cavity. J Biomech Eng 2001;123(1):71–9.

22. Pahlavian SH, Loth F, Luciano M, et al. Neural Tissue Motion Impacts Cerebrospinal Fluid Dynamics at the Cervical Medullary Junction: A Patient-Specific Moving-Boundary Computational Model. Ann Biomed Eng 2015;43(12):2911–23.

23. Williams B, Sgouros S, Nenji E. Cerebrospinal fluid drainage for syringomyelia. Eur J Pediatr Surg 1995;5(Suppl 1):27–30.

24. Muthukumar N. Syringomyelia as a presenting feature of shunt dysfunction: Implications for the pathogenesis of syringomyelia. J Craniovertebr Junction Spine 2012;3(1):26–31.

25. Del Bigio MR. The ependyma: a protective barrier between brain and cerebrospinal fluid. Glia 1995; 14(1):1–13.

26. Bruni JE. Ependymal development, proliferation, and functions: a review. Microsc Res Tech 1998; 41(1):2–13.

27. Holly LT, Batzdorf U. Slitlike syrinx cavities: a persistent central canal. J Neurosurg 2002;97(2 Suppl): 161–5.

28. Thyagaraj S, Pahlavian SH, Sass LR, et al. An MRI-Compatible Hydrodynamic Simulator of Cerebrospinal Fluid Motion in the Cervical Spine. IEEE Trans Biomed Eng 2018;65(7):1516–23.

29. Leung V, Magnussen JS, Stoodley MA, et al. Cerebellar and hindbrain motion in Chiari malformation with and without syringomyelia. J Neurosurg Spine 2016;24(4):546–55.

30. Ellertsson AB. Syringomyelia and other cystic spinal cord lesions. Acta Neurol Scand 1969;45(4):403–17.

31. Wei F, Zhang C, Xue R, et al. The pathway of subarachnoid CSF moving into the spinal parenchyma and the role of astrocytic aquaporin-4 in this process. Life Sci 2017;182:29–40.

32. Oklinski MK, Lim JS, Choi HJ, et al. Immunolocalization of Water Channel Proteins AQP1 and AQP4 in Rat Spinal Cord. J Histochem Cytochem 2014; 62(8):598–611.

33. Hemley SJ, Bilston LE, Cheng S, et al. Aquaporin-4 expression in post-traumatic syringomyelia. J Neurotrauma 2013;30(16):1457–67.

34. Xiong A, Li J, Xiong R, et al. Inhibition of HIF-1α-AQP4 axis ameliorates brain edema and neurological functional deficits in a rat controlled cortical injury (CCI) model. Sci Rep 2022;12(1):2701.

35. Vindedal GF, Thoren AE, Jensen V, et al. Removal of aquaporin-4 from glial and ependymal membranes causes brain water accumulation. Mol Cell Neurosci 2016;77:47–52.

36. Storer KP, Toh J, Stoodley MA, et al. The central canal of the human spinal cord: a computerised 3-D study. J Anat 1998;192(Pt 4):565–72.

37. Koh L, Zakharov A, Johnston M. Integration of the subarachnoid space and lymphatics: is it time to embrace a new concept of cerebrospinal fluid absorption? Cerebrospinal Fluid Res 2005;2:6.

38. Levy EI, Heiss JD, Kent MS, et al. Spinal cord swelling preceding syrinx development. Case Report J Neurosurg 2000;92(1 Suppl):93–7.

39. Takamura Y, Kawasaki T, Takahashi A, et al. A craniocervical injury-induced syringomyelia caused by central canal dilation secondary to acquired tonsillar herniation. Case Report J Neurosurg 2001;95(1 Suppl):122–7.

40. Kedarasetti RT, Drew PJ, Costanzo F. Arterial vasodilation drives convective fluid flow in the brain: a poroelastic model. Fluids Barriers CNS 2022;19(1):34.

41. Rasmussen MK, Mestre H, Nedergaard M. Fluid transport in the brain. Physiol Rev 2022;102(2):1025–151.

42. Hammock MK, Milhorat TH. The cerebrospinal fluid: current concepts of its formation. Ann Clin Lab Sci 1976;6(1):22–6.

43. Li Q, Aalling NN, Förstera B, et al. Aquaporin 1 and the Na(+)/K(+)/2Cl(-) cotransporter 1 are present in the leptomeningeal vasculature of the adult rodent central nervous system. Fluids Barriers CNS 2020;17(1):15.

44. Milhorat TH, Hammock MK, Fenstermacher JD, et al. Cerebrospinal fluid production by the choroid plexus and brain. Science 1971;173(3994):330–2.

45. Trillo-Contreras JL, Toledo-Aral JJ, Echevarría M, et al. AQP1 and AQP4 Contribution to Cerebrospinal Fluid Homeostasis. Cells 2019;8(2). https://doi.org/10.3390/cells8020197.

46. Wetjen NM, Heiss JD, Oldfield EH. Time course of syringomyelia resolution following decompression of Chiari malformation Type I. J Neurosurg Pediatr 2008;1(2):118–23.

47. Vaquero J, Ferreira E, Parajón A. Spontaneous resolution of syrinx: report of two cases in adults with Chiari malformation. Neurol Sci 2012;33(2):339–41.

48. Rhoton ALJ. Microsurgery of syringomyelia and syringomyelic cord syndrome. In: Schmidek HH, Sweet WH, editors. Operative neurosurgical techniques. Philadelphia, PA: WB Saunders; 1988. p 1307–26.

49. Milhorat TH, Capocelli AL Jr, Kotzen RM, et al. Intramedullary pressure in syringomyelia: clinical and pathophysiological correlates of syrinx distension. Neurosurgery 1997;41(5):1102–10.

50. Heiss JD, Jarvis K, Smith RK, et al. Origin of Syrinx Fluid in Syringomyelia: A Physiological Study. Neurosurgery 2019;84(2):457–68.

51. Melhem ER, Jara H, Eustace S. Fluid-attenuated inversion recovery MR imaging: identification of protein concentration thresholds for CSF hyperintensity. AJR Am J Roentgenol 1997;169(3):859–62.

52. Shtaya A, Sadek AR, Nicoll JAR, et al. Choroid Plexus in the Central Canal of the Spinal Cord Causing Recurrent Syringomyelia. World Neurosurg 2018;111:275–8.

53. Moore SA. The Spinal Ependymal Layer in Health and Disease. Vet Pathol 2016;53(4):746–53.

54. Merriam-webster.com. Hydrostatics. 2022. https://www.merriam-webster.com. [Accessed 16 May 2022].

55. Schlesinger EB, Antunes JL, Michelsen WJ, et al. Hydromyelia: clinical presentation and comparison of modalities of treatment. Neurosurgery 1981;9(4):356–65.

56. Ramo NL, Troyer KL, Puttlitz CM. Viscoelasticity of spinal cord and meningeal tissues. Acta Biomater 2018;75:253–62.

57. Bilston LE, Thibault LE. The mechanical properties of the human cervical spinal cord in vitro. Ann Biomed Eng 1996;24(1):67–74.

58. Itoh T, Nishimura R, Matsunaga S, et al. Syringomyelia and hydrocephalus in a dog. J Am Vet Med Assoc 1996;209(5):934–6.

59. Plessas IN, Rusbridge C, Driver CJ, et al. Long-term outcome of Cavalier King Charles spaniel dogs with clinical signs associated with Chiari-like malformation and syringomyelia. Vet Rec 2012;171(20):501.

Adult Chiari Malformation Type I
Surgical Anatomy, Microsurgical Technique, and Patient Outcomes

Alisa Arnautovic, BS[a], Mirza Pojskić, MD[b,c], Kenan I. Arnautović, MD, PhD[d,*]

KEYWORDS

- Adult Chiari malformation • 270° decompression • Suboccipital ligament

KEY POINTS

- Increased body mass index is an independent risk factor associated with symptomatic Chiari malformation in adults, which has shown not only positive correlation to symptomatic syrinx formation but also a certain influence to increased length and width of the syrinx; our research group proposed a hypothesis with possible explanation of the underlying pathophysiological mechanism.
- The suboccipital ligament is an important structure at the craniocervical junction whose identification, proper dissection, and resection play an important part in the surgical management of the adult Chiari malformation type I (CM-I).
- The 270° circumferential decompression of foramen magnum includes suboccipital craniectomy, C-1 laminectomy, resection of the suboccipital ligament, lateral decompression with drilling of the 1/5 of the occipital condyles, dural opening, arachnoid dissection, and lateral decompression and opening of the foramina of Luschka and opening of the fourth ventricle.
- Clinical results of this operative technique have shown almost uniform resolution or substantial improvement of suboccipital headaches and neurologic symptoms with good neuroradiological outcome in resolution or substantial decrease of syrinx.
- The placement technique of an abdominal fat graft to obliterate postoperative suboccipital "dead space" is a further technical addition to eliminate and prevent most common complication of CM-I decompression—cerebrospinal fluid leak and/or pseudomeningocele.

 Video content accompanies this article at http://www.neurosurgery.theclinics.com.

INTRODUCTION

Chiari malformation type I (CM-I), first described by an Austrian pathologist Hans Chiari in 1891, is a hindbrain disorder that occurs in pediatric and adult populations and is mainly characterized by elongation and descent of the cerebellar tonsils of more than 5 mm below the foramen magnum into the spinal canal (Video 1).[1–3] Altered cerebrospinal fluid (CSF) flow at the level of foramen magnum is the key element in its pathophysiology and development of syringomyelia.[4] Further subtypes include CM-II, characterized by downward displacement of the medulla, fourth ventricle, and cerebellum into the cervical spinal canal,

a George Washington University School of Medicine and Health Sciences, Washington, DC, USA; b Department of Neurosurgery, University of Marburg, Marburg, Germany; c Faculty of Medicine, Josip Juraj Strossmayer University, Osijek, Croatia; d Department of Neurosurgery, Semmes Murphey Neurologic & Spine Institute, University of Tennessee Health Science Center, 6325 Humphreys Boulevard, Memphis, TN 38120, USA
* Corresponding author.
E-mail address: kenanarnaut@yahoo.com

Neurosurg Clin N Am 34 (2023) 91–104
https://doi.org/10.1016/j.nec.2022.09.004
1042-3680/23/© 2022 Elsevier Inc. All rights reserved.

which occurs almost exclusively with myelomeningocele.[5] Type III is a form of dysraphism with occipital encephalocele and has a high mortality in infancy,[6] whereas type IV encompasses cerebellar hypoplasia or anaplasia and is usually fatal during infancy. Secondary CM may be associated with hydrocephalus, idiopathic intracranial hypertension, pseudotumor cerebri, idiopathic intracranial hypotension, and intracranial mass lesion, and the treatment includes the treatment of the underlying condition. Complex CMs are associated with platybasia, basilar invagination, retroflexed odontoid, and/or craniospinal instability with predominantly ventral neural compression, and these conditions are predominantly treated with ventral decompression and craniocervical fusion.

Surgical treatment of CM type I that resolves or at least stabilizes the symptoms in most of the patients includes decompression of the foramen magnum and reestablishment of the CSF flow across the craniocervical junction, which leads to resolution of the syrinx.[3,7] Conservative treatment includes prescriptive medications, physical therapy, and swimming and is reserved for selected adult patients without severe symptoms or neurologic deficits.[8] Differences in surgical treatment between pediatric and adult population have been described.[3] Although posterior fossa and foramen magnum decompression with duraplasty are the treatment of choice in most of the pediatric, adult, and combined series, opening of the arachnoid membrane and intra-arachnoid dissection were reported in 72% and 70% of the combined and adult series, respectively, but only 47% of the pediatric series.[3] Arachnoidal preservation following duraplasty in pediatric patients is believed to prevent CSF leak, pseudomeningocoele, and meningitis, which are the probable reasons for this difference.[3,9] Further variations to the acknowledged surgical technique include posterior fossa decompression without dural opening, posterior fossa decompression with resection of tonsils as well as filum terminale sectioning, syringosubarachnoid shunting, and syringoperitoneal shunting in CM-I, all of which have shown no evidence over any posterior fossa decompression techniques.[10] Up to 15% of pediatric patients in recent literature review underwent posterior fossa decompression without dural opening[11]; however, in comparison, techniques using dural opening were associated with better symptom improvement, syrinx reduction, and reduced revision rate.[11] Atlantoaxial fixation has been proposed as an alternative technique to decompression surgery, under viewpoint that atlantoaxial instability lies in the core of pathogenesis of Chiari.[12] Although this technique leads indirectly to enlargement of posterior fossa through distraction of dens and ventral stem decompression, current evidence remains limited, and C1-C2 fixation is not recommended in patients with CM without atlantoaxial instability.[13]

In this study, we summarize the current knowledge on epidemiology, demographics, risk factors, and prognostic factors that influence outcome in patients with adult CM-I ("simple CM-I") who undergo posterior fossa decompression surgery. Furthermore, we describe the relevant surgical anatomy and surgical technique of 270° microsurgical decompression, report on common complications in the literature, and describe techniques for prevention of complications. Lastly, we present several illustrative cases to demonstrate the current concept of treatment and how outcomes are affected.

CHIARI I MALFORMATION DEFINITIONS

Simple CM-I is a hindbrain disorder associated with underdeveloped (small) posterior cranial fossa and descent of cerebellar tonsils below the level of foramen magnum greater than 5 mm, alteration of the CSF flow at the craniocervical junction, frequent association of brain stem/spinal cord syrinx, and compression of the brainstem and/or spinal cord. Proper diagnostics includes ruling out spinal instability (extremely rare in simple CM-I). Symptomatic patients are treated with suboccipital craniectomy, dural opening (almost all patients, adult and pediatric), arachnoid opening (almost all adult and about 50% of pediatric patients), and with tonsillar coagulation and sporadically resection. *Secondary CM-I* may be associated with hydrocephalus, idiopathic intracranial hypertension, pseudotumor cerebri, idiopathic intracranial hypotension, and intracranial mass lesion.

The treatment consists of resolving underlying condition. *Complex CM-I* are associated with platybasia, basilar invagination, retroflexed odontoid, and other craniocervical developmental abnormalities and/or variants. It is associated with craniospinal instability with predominantly ventral neural compression. It is treated predominantly with ventral decompression and craniocervical fusion.

EPIDEMIOLOGY AND DEMOGRAPHICS

More than 50 surgical adult CM series have been published in the time period 2013 to 2022 in the English literature. In the studies with adult patients, the mean duration was 8 years (range 2–30 years)[3] and most of the studies were published in the United States and Europe. In adult series, there is a predominance of women (57% vs 43%), with 2 age peaks of 41 and 46 years[3]; 69% of all patients in the literature present with syringomyelia.[3]

RISK FACTORS

A direct comparison among the age groups revealed a negative age effect on surgical decompression outcomes in patients with CM-I.[14] Age of the patients also did not show correlation to syrinx formation.[15] Literature shows a female predominance in patients with adult CM-I. One reason for this predominance might be that adult women present more commonly with headache syndrome, which may prompt more frequent MRI diagnostics.[3]

Body mass index (BMI) is described as an independent risk factor for syringomyelia in patients with adult CM-I, and a reduction in body weight should be recommended for all overweight and obese patients with CM-I.[15] Increased BMI has shown correlation not only to syrinx but also to increased length and width of the syrinx.[15]

CM-I is the leading cause of syringomyelia.[2] Increased intracranial pressure is associated with pseudotumor cerebri and CM-I in children.[16] The creation and enlargement of a syrinx may contribute to the transformation of asymptomatic to symptomatic CM-I.[3] Syringomyelia is more common in adult than in pediatric population, with the rates of association of syringomyelia with CM-I of 69% in adult patients.[3]

The hypothesis that was raised by our group is that in patients with adult CM-I with increased BMI, the pressure transmission that normally exists between the intrathoracic/intraabdominal and vertebral valveless venous compartments is exaggerated because of the increased BMI, which worsens the pressure gradient between the cranial and spinal compartments and their possibility of equalization, both of which are already altered by the CM-I syndrome. In turn, this phenomenon could precipitate the symptomatic presentation of a CM-I.[15] Because most of the published studies are from the United States and Europe, we speculate that these findings may have a regional or uniform character.

In the cohort of 60 patients with adult CM-I, in the syringomyelia subgroup, we identified 2 patients who had de novo formation of a syrinx on a significant increase in their BMI.[15] De novo CM-I in patients following decompression surgery after follow-up of 2 years have been firstly described by the senior author.[17] The hypothesis is that with obstruction of the rapid to-and-fro movement of CSF in the subarachnoid spaces across the foramen magnum during systole and diastole, the cerebellar tonsils, which plug subarachnoid spaces posteriorly, move down with each systolic pulse and act as a piston on the partially isolated spinal CSF compartment.[18,19] "This movement then produces a systolic pressure wave in the spinal CSF that acts on the surface of the spinal cord, causing a progression of the syrinx from the pulsatile pressure waves forcing CSF into the cord through the perivascular and interstitial spaces; this is aggravated in patients with increased BMI."[15]

"Future directions for the treatment of Chiari anomalies and syringomyelia include the application of advanced imaging techniques, more widespread use of genetic evaluation, large-scale outcome studies, and the further refinement of surgical technique."[20]

SURGICAL ANATOMY IN PATIENTS WITH CHIARI MALFORMATION TYPE I

Several differences in the anatomy of the craniocervical junction exist in patients with CM-I compared with healthy subjects. Patients with CM-I are more often reported to have a shorter clivus, shorter posterior fossa height and steeper tentorial angle, shorter McRae line, flatter atlantooccipital joints, as well as increased cerebellar descent length.[21] Recent MRI study on patients with CM-I compared with healthy controls has shown that the length of transverse ligament and alar ligament in the normal population was significantly longer than in patients with CM-I.[22] However, morphologic parameters of posterior fossa failed to predict the response to decompression in patients with CM-I[23] and also have shown not be reflective of CM-I disease severity as indicated by the Chiari Severity Index (CSI).[24] Neuroradiological workup for patients to exclude craniocervical instability is advised.[17]

The suboccipital ligament is a structure of paramount importance for surgery of craniocervical region and posterior decompression in patients with CM-I in particular, firstly described by research group of the senior author.[25] Although the posterior suboccipital membrane is located between the occipital bone and C-1 lamina (ventral) the rectus capitis posterior major and minor (dorsal), the suboccipital ligament extends horizontally between the bilateral occipital condyles and superior rims of the C-1 laminae with two separate branches: the condyle (superior) branch and the C-1 or atlantal (inferior) branch, which both form a ligament with horizontally oriented fibers.[25] In its middle third, the ligament is loosely attached to the dura, and in this portion, it can be easily resected and detached from dura. Toward the lateral third, it becomes more densely attached to the dura. Interestingly, this ligament did not show signs of hypertrophy in patients with CM-I but structural differences in form of the presence of hyaline nodules and an altered fiber orientation in patients with CM-I.[25] Dissection and controlled resection of this ligament enables clean dural incision and facilitates the preservation of the arachnoid membrane as well as dural graft suturing to dura due to preservation of an even thickness of dural edges above, below, and at the level of the ligament.[25] Resection of suboccipital ligament is one important surgical step in the technique of 270° decompression.

MICROSURGICAL TECHNIQUE

Principle goals of surgery for CM type I were defined as resolving craniospinal pressure dissociation, restoration of subarachnoid spaces and the cisterna magna, syrinx reduction and elimination, relieving compression of the brainstem, and improvement or elimination of symptoms and signs of CM-I.[26] Ninety-nine percent of the studies in the literature report posterior fossa decompression as a surgical technique, with 92% of studies that advocate dural opening.[3] A recent study on failure to resolve syringomyelia following CM decompression emphasized adequate lateral bony decompression and opening of the fourth ventricle as paramount in the resolution of syrinx.[27] The so-called all-factors surgery, which includes posterior fossa decompression, enlarged cranioplasty, duraplasty, cerebellar tonsil partial resection, and adhesion release, has been advocated to improve symptoms, reduce syrinx, and reduce the complication rate.[28] Recently it has been advocated that the surgery can be safely performed without intraoperative neuromonitoring.[29]

Our surgical technique named the 270° circumferential microsurgical decompression of the foramen magnum has been published by the senior author and shows improved clinical patient reported outcomes, reduction of syrinx, and low complication rate.[17] Following harvest of abdominal fat pad in supine position, patient is positioned prone, with head fixed in a 3-point Mayfield head rest. Following incision from the external occipital protuberance (EOP) to the C2 spinous process, nuchal ligament and paraspinal muscles are separated from the squama of the suboccipital bone and C1 lamina with retractors. Following C1 laminectomy, a high-speed drill is used to create an oval-shaped sulcus in the suboccipital bone with the base toward C1 extending halfway between the rim of foramen magnum and the EOP. The posterior medial 1/5 of the occipital condyle is drilled

using a 3-mm coarse diamond. The lateral decompression is more important than the vertical extent of bone removal. The craniectomy itself is about 2 cm (around 1 inch) high to avoid any possibility of cerebellar ptosis. Following this, the suboccipital ligament is dissected and resected in its medial portion as described previously. The dura is opened in a shape of letter "Y" and tacked to surrounding soft tissues with 4-0 Nurolon stitches. The arachnoid membrane is opened in the midline and then in the bilateral cerebellomedullary cisterns, releasing CSF and decompressing both Luschka foramina; 270° arachnoid dissection (enabled by limited condyle drilling) facilitates a more complete release of arachnoid adhesions obstructing the CSF flow. "Enlarging the cisterna magna is based on the premise that CSF pulsations in an enlarged cisterna magna will promote ascent of the cerebellar tonsils, as well as aid in the propagation of CSF pulsations into the spinal subarachnoid space. Reducing the size of the cerebellar tonsils contributes to the enlargement of the cisterna magna and initiates ascent of the tonsils."[17] Following division of arachnoid adhesions, previous drilling of parts of posterolateral condyles enables visualization of bilateral vertebral arteries and posterior inferior cerebellar artery origin. The entrance in the fourth ventricle is opened by releasing arachnoid adhesions, and the tips of the cerebellar tonsils are coagulated. Closure is done with a triangular piece of bovine pericardium allograft (Durepair, Medtronic, Minneapolis, MN, USA) using 4-0 Nurolon sutures. Duraplasty affects intracranial compliance and seems to be associated with a lower risk of reoperation.[20] Valsalva maneuver ensures a watertight closure, whereas the previously harvested abdominal fat is now placed on top of the dura along with fibrin glue to eliminate the "dead space" created by bone removal and to prevent CSF leak, with special care not to "overpack" the space.[17] Coagulating tonsillar tips and dural patch grafting maintain a wide craniocervical decompression simultaneously, which ensures resolution of syringomyelia.[17] Details of our microsurgical technique can be seen in our Video 1. Operative video (Supplemental material).

PATIENT OUTCOMES

Improvement of suboccipital headaches and neurologic deficits as well as reduction of syrinx remain the mainstay of the outcome assessment in patients with adult CM-I. There were several attempts to identify prognostic and surgery factors for CM-I.[30,31] Aliaga and colleagues developed Chicago Chiari Outcome Scale (CCOS), which graded 4 postoperative outcome categories (pain, nonpain symptoms, functionality, and complications) with a maximum of 16 points.[31] This scoring system was externally validated, although functionality and nonpain symptoms were found to be less reliable.[32] CSI was described in 2015 by Greenberg and colleagues[33] in order to identify the prognostic predictors of outcome following surgery. CSI has found its application foremost in pediatric patients and differentiates 3 severity grades of patients with CM-I: grade I (classic poorly localized Chiari headache, best prognosis), grade II (no headache or frontotemporal headache), and grade III (myelopathic symptoms, worse prognosis). A recent study of 149 adult patients with CM-I, with 39 patients (26%) with syrinx, has shown poor ability of CSI in identifying improved patients and urged for future model and more practical scoring system.[30] Same investigators proposed a novel risk calculator for likelihood of reoperation and discharge other than home, based on age, sex, BMI, presence of diabetes, and American Society of Anesthesiologists (ASA) score of 2 and more,[34] which still awaits its validation.

The relationship of increased BMI to CM is complex. Our research group in a consecutive series of 60 patients described that the extension of the vertical syrinx was greater in overweight patients than in those with a normal body weight.[15] Gaining weight may influence the de novo creation of a syrinx in adults who previously had minimally symptomatic or asymptomatic CM-I, and reducing weight can improve a syrinx after unsuccessful surgical decompression.[15] However, in a series of 1310 patients undergoing MRI for any reason, there was no relationship between BMI and the level of the cerebellar tonsils or the diagnosis of CM-I on imaging.[35] Increased BMI was recognized as a risk factor for cerebrospinal fluid disturbance with postoperative hydrocephalus following posterior fossa decompression requiring CSF diversion.[36] In pediatric series, up to 42% of patients were obese or overweight, whereas younger obese patients presented the highest incidence of Chiari-related headache symptoms and older obese patients, the highest incidence of findings other than headache.[37]

Posterior fossa decompression is assumed to normalize intracranial pressure (ICP) and craniospinal pressure dissociation; however, a study on 11 patients where ICP was monitored following decompression has shown that anatomic restoration of cerebrospinal fluid pathways does not lead to immediate normalization of preoperatively altered pulsatile and static ICP in patients with CM, which can explain persistent symptoms

during the early period.[38] Comparable and elevated pulsatile ICP, which indicates impaired intracranial compliance, in both CM-I and idiopathic intracranial hypertension (IIH) cohorts was described, whereas static ICP was higher in the IIH cohort in an analysis of 107 patients who underwent ICP monitoring due to CM or IHH.[39] MRI-based volumetric measurements imply that PF alterations may be partly responsible for the development of IIH and CM-I.[40]

Fourth ventricular drainage is thought to be essential for syrinx resolution, and persistence or progression of the syrinx after decompression is an indication for reoperation with shunting, albeit associated with high failure rates.[27] In revisions to treat progressive syringomyelia after failed decompression, following adequate bony decompression, lysis of adhesions around cisterna magna, and opening of the fourth ventricle, insertion of a shunt from the fourth ventricle to cervical subarachnoid space has been advocated.[41] Shunting procedures have been proposed in case of extensive arachnoiditis or repeated failures in a recent study of Knafo and colleagues, whereas revision of duraplasty at the level of foramen magnum is the first-line treatment.[42] Syrinx to subarachnoid shunting[41] as well as syringo-subarachnoid-peritoneal shunt was also described as an option in patients who have not responded to the primary treatment.[41]

The correlation between hydrocephalus and CM-I has been debated since the first descriptions.[43] In a series of 297 patients who underwent posterior decompression, 22 patients required long-term postoperative CSF diversion.[44] Age less than 6 years, higher intraoperative blood loss, and the presence of a fourth ventricular web were significantly associated with the need for long-term CSF diversion after decompressive surgery.[44] Endoscopic third ventriculostomy without the need for shunting has been advocated in a case series of 10 patients with hydrocephalus and Chiari, where 80% of the patients were reported to have resolved hydrocephalus following this intervention.[43] Opposite to this, secondary cranial vault thickening and development of CM-I has been described as a late complication of supratentorial shunting.[45]

Posterior decompression triggers dynamic process that can lead to significant modifications of intracranial venous drainage.[46] The dura mater at the craniovertebral junction in cadaver studies had a well-developed vascular network consisted of veins or the venous sinus and were mainly located around the interface between the inner layer of the cranial dura mater and the rectus capitis posterior minor muscle layer.[47] Assessment of the venous drainage pattern using magnetic resonance venography has been recently advocated for safe surgical treatment in patients with CM-I. In case of persistent patent occipital sinus (OS), the sinus is usually obliterated and divided; however, in patients with prominent OS, more thorough presurgical preparation should be performed. Instead of performing Y-shaped dural incision and duraplasty, surgical procedures can be modified depending on the types of the oblique unilateral OS to preserve their venous drainage routes.[48]

Feghali and colleagues and Labuda and colleagues also identified depression as independently associated with poor outcome in patients with adult CM-1, even with pain and functionality improvement.[49,50] The SHORE score is one further predictive model for patient outcome in adult Chiari I, which identified headache with Valsalva, nonwhite race, absence of visual symptoms), syrinx absence, and increased odontoid retroflexion, as predictive of clinical improvement following decompression surgery.[51] Thakar and colleagues reported the presence of gait imbalance, and motor deficits independently predict worse clinical and radiological outcomes after decompressive surgery for CM-I.[52] Assessment of visuospatial and visuo-constructional performance as well as cognitive and psychological functioning have been the subject of interest and has shown no significant impairment or improvement following decompressive surgery.[53] Hereditary CM-I may present a subset of patients with poorer outcomes.[50] Motor deficits, syrinx, and C1-C2 facet malalignment were found to have significant negative associations with the CCOS score.[54] A recent algorithm for precise management of CM-I, including the preoperative multimodality neuroimaging and individual surgical therapy, has been published, adding to the growing body of literature on treatment modalities and prognosis outcomes in patients with adult CM-I.[55] Headache improvement reached statistical significance when comparing pediatric and adult series in favor of pediatric group, whereas neurologic improvement was higher in pediatric group but without statistical significance.[3]

European Myelopathy Score has been used for the first time by our group to validate the neurologic improvement of patients with adult CM-I.[17] Our patients were generally slightly younger than the reported literature median age (38 vs 41 years), with female predominance and less syrinx (35 vs 65%) and male predominance in patients with syringomyelia.[17] Eighty-eight percent of patients were overweight or obese, which confirmed previously proven correlation of increased BMI and Chiari that was published by our group.[15,17]

In our series of 130 patients with adult CM-I who were surgically treated with the described surgical technique, all patients had neurologic improvement and 98% of patients experienced headache improvement.[17] Studies published from 2000 to 2019 have shown a mean headache improvement rate of 79% and mean neurologic improvement rate of 77%.[17] Mean reported headache improvement in adult series published in 1965 to 2013 was even lower with 73%.[3] Of 1126 patients in the adult series published in the period 1965 to 2013, neurologic improvement/resolution was noted in 823 patients (73%), no change in 225 (20%), and worsening in 78 (7%).[3] Application of our surgical technique and treatment concept has increased the headache improvement rate by 21% and neurologic improvement by 23% compared with the literature.

Complete syrinx resolution occurred in 81% of our patients (35/43), with 19% of patients (8) with significant improvement. Median time to resolving/improving syrinx was 4 months.[17] In studies published from 2000 to 2019, mean syrinx improvement rate was only 74%.[17] Our technique resulted in 7% increase of syrinx resolution compared with current literature. Resolution of symptoms despite insufficient resolution of syrinx has been reported following posterior fossa decompression for Chiari.[56] The reported ranges for adult CM-I regarding syrinx resolution were 38% to 100% improvement/resolution, 11% to 64% no change, and 2% to 40% worsening.[3] Insertion of a shunt from the fourth ventricle to the cervical subarachnoid space as well as bipolar coagulation of the lateral tonsillar pia to ensure the CSF flow has been advocated as one of the techniques for syrinx resolution,[27] although according to international consensus agreement only as a reserve option following causative treatment.[57] Grading system consisting of 4 grades has been proposed by our group for simplification of the assessment of syrinx size and syringomyelia severity and preoperative and postoperative comparison.[15]

COMPLICATIONS

Three patients in our series of 130 patients with adult CM developed pseudomeningocele/CSF leak after surgery (1 man, 2 women) and needed reoperation. After adoption of the fat graft technique, there were no further complications of this kind.[17] Superficial wound infection occurred in 4/130 patients with 3 patients who underwent wound revision surgery.[17] Complication rates in the literature have been reported between 4% and 5%; however, only 41% of the studies reported any complications.[3] The most common complications were pseudomeningocele, aseptic meningitis, CSF leak, meningitis, and neurologic deficits.[3] Mortality was reported in only 11% of the studies (2% in adult and 3% in the combined), with the most common causes being pneumonia, sepsis, postoperative bleeding, and sleep apnea.[3] Recent literature review suggested that posterior fossa decompression with duraplasty and arachnoid dissection had a greater prevalence of total complications and CSF-related complications compared with arachnoid preservation, with 25 times greater risk of reoperation.[9] However, this review did not report on neurologic outcome and reduction of syringomyelia in these patients. One further analysis showed that the more aggressive is the surgery, the longer is the operating time, the higher are the complication rates (the CSF leakage–related ones for posterior fossa decompression with duraplasty and neurologic symptoms for posterior fossa decompression with duraplasty and tonsillar resection), but the higher the efficacy of surgery on symptoms and even more on syrinx resolution.[57] Obesity is a recognized risk for readmission and reoperation, with overall readmission rate of 9.3% and return-to-operating-room rate of 6.8% in analysis of 672 patients with adult CM-I.[58]

Nearly two-thirds of reoperations occur due to CSF leak, which account for 2.5% of complications in the adult series.[3,58] Our strategy of prevention of CSF leaks include harvest of abdominal fat graft, which is then placed on top of the dura along with fibrin glue to eliminate the "dead space" created by bone removal with the enforcement of suture with a fat autograft as necessary.[17] Utility of autologous fat graft has been previously shown for CSF leak prevention in intradural spinal tumor surgery.[59] This technique reduced the complication rate, that is, CSF leak and pseudomeningocoele occurrence significantly compared with the current literature. Recent international consensus document on treatment of CM-I identified the main causes of surgical failures.[57] Three-dimensional computed tomography can help diagnose the incomplete foraminal decompression, needing bone erosion widening; furthermore, constructive interference in steady-state (CISS) and flow MRI can help detect posterior fossa arachnoiditis, needing adhesiolysis and possibly tonsil resection (88.5%); these factors were identified as the most frequent cause of failure.[60]

In pediatric and adult Chiari cohorts, autologous fascia or pericranium for expansile duraplasty has been advocated, as the use of nonautologous materials may cause excessive scarring.[27] Possible complications of placement of abdominal fat graft

is the morbidity of the abdominal wound such as infection. Although we did not account any infections of the donor site, a special care of the abdominal wound needs to be taken care of. Autograft was the dural graft material that most frequently had the lowest rate of complications as shown in the meta-analysis by Yahanda and colleagues and was associated with significantly lower rates of pseudomeningocele compared with collagen-based graft, allograft, and nonautologous graft materials, although autografts and nonautologous grafts yielded similar outcomes for revision surgery, symptoms, and syrinx size.[61]

Ratio for implementation of 270° decompression, that is, limited condyle drilling, lies in the fact that it enables more aggressive 270° arachnoid dissection (enabled by limited condyle drilling) and facilitates a more complete release of arachnoid adhesions obstructing the CSF flow and decompression of the lateral cerebellomedullary cisterns and Luschka foramina bilaterally. CSF evacuation from the fourth ventricle as well as vertical CSF flow across the craniospinal junction circumferentially are facilitated. Coagulating tonsillar tips shriveling them up and dural patch grafting maintains a wide craniocervical decompression simultaneously, which ensures resolution of syringomyelia.[17] None of the patients in our series showed any clinical or radiological signs of instability during the course of lengthy follow-up, which averaged almost 4.5 years; however, only patients without instability ruled out by extensive preoperative neuroradiological workup were included in the study using this operative treatment.[17] Goel and colleagues published their experience with patients with CM-I with complex malformations and craniocervical instability with satisfactory postoperative results with fusion as a predominant treatment option.[12] Analyses of data from the Park-Reeves Syringomyelia Research Consortium have shown that although posterior decompression alone is adequate for treating most of the patients with CM-I, occipitocervical fusion and ventral decompression can be occasionally used.[62] In pediatric cohorts, neurologic examination deficits of gait instability and weak neck rotation, with prior history of basilar invagination, were associated with occipitocervical fusion.[62] Henderson and colleagues suggest that fusion may be considered in patients with clinical symptoms, Chiari 1 or 0, and a clivo-axial angle (CXA) less than 135°.[63] Bollo and colleagues introduced the term "complex Chiari malformations" and identified a set of radiological features to use as guide in choosing the most appropriate surgical treatment (ie, decompression with or without fusion) in pediatric patients.[64] C1/2 fusion technique and

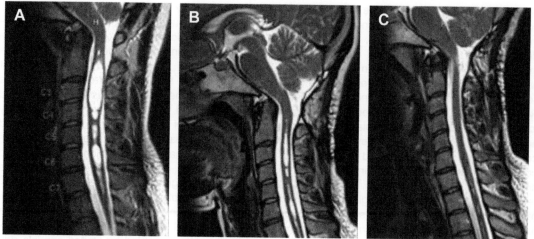

Fig. 1. 20-year-old female patient. Complete resolution of symptoms and significant reduction of syringomyelia following decompression. (*A*) Preoperative sagittal T1-weighted MRI of the cervical spine. (*B*) Postoperative sagittal T1-weighted MRI of the cervical spine at 1-year follow-up. (*C*) Postoperative sagittal T1 MRI of the cervical spine 3 years following surgery.

proposed hypothesis of CM being seen as a result of craniocervical junction instability as proposed by Goel[12,65,66] and advocated by Salunke and colleagues[67] has sparked a controversy on role of instability and fusion technique in treatment of Chiari, although most of the surgical series use a posterior fossa decompression with possible additional fusion in cases of apparent instability. However, in adult series, recent analysis of C1/2 facet configurations as well as CXAs revealed that for adult CM without basilar invagination, C1/2 facet configurations and CXA are irrelevant and that posterior decompression alone provides excellent long-term outcomes.[68] In CM-I with

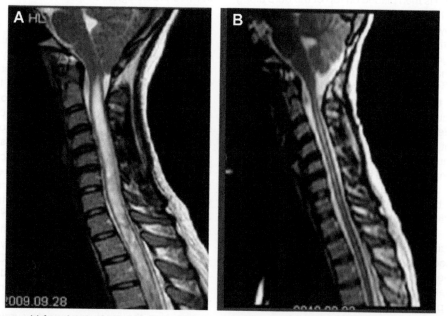

Fig. 2. 43-year-old female patient. Complete resolution of symptoms and significant reduction of syringomyelia following decompression. (*A*) Preoperative sagittal T1-weighted MRI of the cervical spine. (*B*) Postoperative sagittal T1-weighted MRI of the cervical spine.

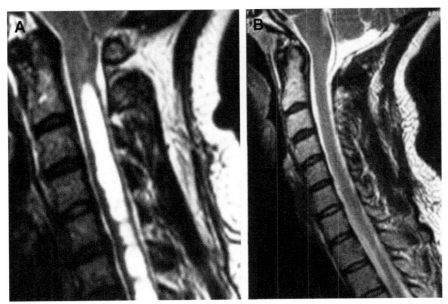

Fig. 3. 23-year-old female patient. Complete resolution of symptoms and significant reduction of syringomyelia following decompression. (*A*) Preoperative sagittal T1-weighted MRI of the cervical spine. (*B*) Postoperative sagittal T1-weighted MRI of the cervical spine.

basilar invagination, anterior C1 facet displacements indicate C1/2 instability and require posterior fusion in patients with ventral compression or C1/2 instability.[68] Risk of postoperative complications is higher in patients with fusion and with increased number of instrumented levels, compared with patients who underwent decompression alone.[69] However, treatment of recurrent cases of CM with syringomyelia in which posterior fossa decompression has failed has been advocated with C1/2 fusion.[70] The definitions of atlantoaxial instability itself vary throughout literature as do the treatment guidelines; however, commonly, lateral radiographs of the craniovertebral junction demonstrating an atlantodental interval of at least 3 mm in adults and 5 mm in children indicate instability, whereas newer investigations by computed tomography set the cutoff at 2 mm for adults.[71,72] CM may be associated with craniovertebral junction deformities.[71] The simultaneous

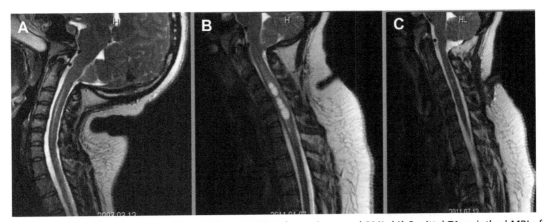

Fig. 4. 36-year-old female patient. Case of de novo CM-I due to increased BMI. (*A*) Sagittal T1-weigthed MRI of the cervical spine with syringomyelia; BMI of the patient 28.5. (*B*) Sagittal T1-weighted MRI of the cervical spine; BMI of the patient increased to 41, with subsequent development of CM-I with syrinx progression. (*C*) Sagittal T1-weighted MRI of the cervical spine following decompression with resolution of syrinx and improvement of symptoms. Note also the fat graft in position.

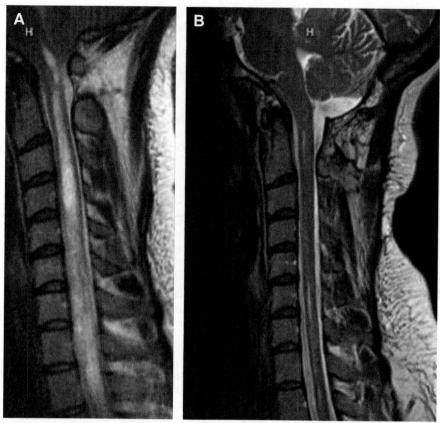

Fig. 5. 34-year-old female patient. Complete resolution of symptoms and significant reduction of syringomyelia following decompression. (*A*) Preoperative sagittal T1-weighted MRI of the cervical spine. (*B*) Postoperative sagittal T1-weighted MRI of the cervical spine.

presence of craniocervical instability and the need for a proper preoperative work-up has been widely accepted.[71] Initially, instability was mainly noted after suboccipital decompression and laminectomy.[73] The reported association of CM-I and atlantoaxial subluxation is around 30% in pediatric cohorts[74]

ILLUSTRATIVE CASES

All illustrative cases are treated with 270° decompression microsurgical technique (**Figs. 1–5**).

SUMMARY

In this article, we have summarized the impact of our research group on knowledge of adult CM-I. We have described for the first time the association of increased BMI and influence of an increasing BMI on the de novo formation of a spinal cord syrinx in adults. The suboccipital ligament is an important structure on the craniocervical junction whose identification and proper

dissection and resection play an important role in surgical management of the adult CM-I. The 270° circumferential decompression of foramen magnum including resection of suboccipital ligament, wide lateral decompression with limited drilling of the posterior 1/5 of the occipital condyles, arachnoid dissection, lateral release, and opening of foramina Luschka and the fourth ventricle has shown excellent clinical results in terms of improvement of headache and neurologic symptoms as well as neuroradiological outcome in resolution or elimination of syrinx. Our technique of placement of abdominal fat graft in the suboccipital epidural area to eliminate "dead space" is a further addition to improvement of adult CM-I treatment in terms of prevention of the most common complication—prevention of CSF leak and pseudomeningocele. These contributions add to a growing body of literature in treatment of adult CM-I and pose a starting point for future prospective outcome studies and further refinement of diagnostic, preoperative evaluation and surgical technique.

CLINICS CARE POINTS

- Principle goals of surgery for CM type I were defined as resolving craniospinal pressure dissociation, restoration of subarachnoid spaces and the cisterna magna, syrinx reduction and elimination, relieving compression of the brainstem, and improvement or elimination of symptoms and signs of CM-I

- Surgical technique named the 270° circumferential microsurgical decompression of the foramen magnum has been published by the senior author and shows improved clinical patient reported outcomes, reduction of syrinx, and low complication rate

- Fourth ventricular drainage and opening is thought to be essential for syrinx resolution

- The most common complications are pseudomeningocele, aseptic meningitis, CSF leak, meningitis, and neurologic deficits

- Strategy of prevention of CSF leaks include harvest of abdominal fat graft, which is then placed on top of the dura along with fibrin glue to eliminate the "dead space" created by bone removal with the enforcement of suture with a fat autograft as necessary

SUPPLEMENTARY DATA

Supplementary data related to this article can be found online at https://doi.org/10.1016/j.nec.2022.09.004.

REFERENCES

1. Vanaclocha V, Saiz-Sapena N, Garcia-Casasola MC. Surgical technique for cranio-cervical decompression in syringomyelia associated with Chiari type I malformation. Acta Neurochir (Wien) 1997;139(6): 529–39 [discussion: 539–40].

2. Milhorat TH, Chou MW, Trinidad EM, et al. Chiari I malformation redefined: clinical and radiographic findings for 364 symptomatic patients. Neurosurgery 1999;44(5):1005–17.

3. Arnautovic A, Splavski B, Boop FA, et al. Pediatric and adult Chiari malformation Type I surgical series 1965-2013: a review of demographics, operative treatment, and outcomes. J Neurosurg Pediatr 2015;15(2):161–77.

4. Alfieri A, Pinna G. Long-term results after posterior fossa decompression in syringomyelia with adult Chiari Type I malformation. J Neurosurg Spine 2012; 17(5):381–7.

5. Zhou Q, Song C, Huang Q, et al. Evaluating craniovertebral stability in Chiari malformation coexisting with Type II basilar invagination: an observational study based on kinematic computed tomography and its clinical application. World Neurosurg 2022. https://doi.org/10.1016/j.wneu.2022.05.045.

6. Elbaroody M, Mostafa HE, Alsawy MFM, et al. Outcomes of Chiari Malformation III: A Review of Literature. J Pediatr Neurosci 2020;15(4):358–64.

7. Mugge L, Caras A, Henkel N, et al. Headache and Other Symptoms in Chiari Malformation Type I Are Associated with Cerebrospinal Fluid Flow Improvement After Decompression: A Two-Institutional Study. World Neurosurg 2022. https://doi.org/10.1016/j.wneu.2022.03.108.

8. Abdallah A, Rakip U. Conservative Treatment of Chiari Malformation Type I Based on the Phase-Contrast Magnetic Resonance Imaging: A Retrospective Study. World Neurosurg 2022. https://doi.org/10.1016/j.wneu.2022.03.126.

9. Osborne-Grinter M, Arora M, Kaliaperumal C, et al. Posterior Fossa Decompression and Duraplasty with and without Arachnoid Preservation for the Treatment of Adult Chiari Malformation Type 1: A Systematic Review and Meta-Analysis. World Neurosurg 2021;151:e579–98.

10. Antkowiak L, Tabakow P. Comparative Assessment of Three Posterior Fossa Decompression Techniques and Evaluation of the Evidence Supporting the Efficacy of Syrinx Shunting and Filum Terminale Sectioning in Chiari Malformation Type I. A Systematic Review and Network Meta-Analysis. World Neurosurg 2021;152:31–43.

11. Akbari SHA, Yahanda AT, Ackerman LL, et al. Complications and outcomes of posterior fossa decompression with duraplasty versus without duraplasty for pediatric patients with Chiari malformation type I and syringomyelia: a study from the Park-Reeves Syringomyelia Research Consortium. J Neurosurg Pediatr 2022;15:1–13.

12. Goel A, Jadhav D, Shah A, et al. Chiari 1 Formation Redefined-Clinical and Radiographic Observations in 388 Surgically Treated Patients. World Neurosurg 2020;141:e921–34.

13. Salunke P, Karthigeyan M, Malik P, et al. Changing Perception but Unaltered Reality: How Effective Is C1-C2 Fixation for Chiari Malformations without Instability? World Neurosurg 2020;136:e234–44.

14. Gilmer HS, Xi M, Young SH. Surgical Decompression for Chiari Malformation Type I: An Age-Based Outcomes Study Based on the Chicago Chiari Outcome Scale. World Neurosurg 2017;107:285–90.

15. Arnautovic KI, Muzevic D, Splavski B, et al. Association of increased body mass index with Chiari malformation Type I and syrinx formation in adults. J Neurosurg 2013;119(4):1058–67.

16. Kurschel S, Maier R, Gellner V, et al. Chiari I malformation and intra-cranial hypertension:a case-based review. Childs Nerv Syst 2007;23(8):901–5.

17. Arnautovic KI, Qaladize BF, Pojskic M, et al. The 270° Circumferential Microsurgical Decompression of the Foramen Magnum in Adult Chiari Malformation Type I: Single Surgeon Series of 130 Patients with Syringomyelia, Neurologic, and Headache Outcomes. World Neurosurg 2021;146:e1103–17.

18. Heiss JD, Patronas N, DeVroom HL, et al. Elucidating the pathophysiology of syringomyelia. J Neurosurg 1999;91(4):553–62.

19. Oldfield EH, Muraszko K, Shawker TH, et al. Pathophysiology of syringomyelia associated with Chiari I malformation of the cerebellar tonsils. Implications for diagnosis and treatment. J Neurosurg 1994;80(1):3–15.

20. Holly LT, Batzdorf U. Chiari malformation and syringomyelia. J Neurosurg Spine 2019;31(5):619–28.

21. Shuman WH, DiRisio A, Carrasquilla A, et al. Is there a morphometric cause of Chiari malformation type I? Analysis of existing literature. Neurosurg Rev 2022;45(1):263–73.

22. Karaaslan B, Börcek A, Uçar M, et al. Can the Etiopathogenesis of Chiari Malformation Be Craniocervical Junction Stabilization Difference? Morphometric Analysis of Craniocervical Junction Ligaments. World Neurosurg 2019;128:e1096–101.

23. Liu Z, Hao Z, Hu S, et al. Predictive value of posterior cranial fossa morphology in the decompression of Chiari malformation type I: A retrospective observational study. Medicine (Baltimore) 2019;98(19):e15533.

24. Thakar S, Kanneganti V, Talla Nwotchouang BS, et al. Are Two-Dimensional Morphometric Measures Reflective of Disease Severity in Adult Chiari I Malformation? World Neurosurg 2022;157:e497–505.

25. Alabaster K, Fred Bugg M, Splavski B, et al. The suboccipital ligament. J Neurosurg 2018;128(1):165–73.

26. Batzdorf U, McArthur DL, Bentson JR. Surgical treatment of Chiari malformation with and without syringomyelia: experience with 177 adult patients. J Neurosurg 2013;118(2):232–42.

27. Emerson SN, Scott RM, Al-Mefty O. Resolution of Primary or Recalcitrant Chiari-Associated Syringomyelia Requires Adequate Cerebrospinal Fluid Egress from the Fourth Ventricle. World Neurosurg 2022;163:24.

28. Chu W, Chen X, Xue X, et al. Treatment of symptomatic Chiari I malformation by "all-factors-surgery": a report of 194 cases. Eur Spine J 2021;30(6):1615–22.

29. Schaefer J, Atallah E, Tecce E, et al. Utility of intraoperative neuromonitoring for decompression of Chiari type I malformation in 93 adult patients. J Neurosurg 2022;1–6. https://doi.org/10.3171/2022.3.JNS22127.

30. Feghali J, Xie Y, Chen Y, et al. External validation of current prediction systems of improvement after decompression surgery in Chiari malformation type I patients: can we do better? J Neurosurg 2020;134(5):1466–71.

31. Aliaga L, Hekman KE, Yassari R, et al. A novel scoring system for assessing Chiari malformation type I treatment outcomes. Neurosurgery 2012;70(3):656–64 [discussion: 664–5].

32. Yarbrough CK, Greenberg JK, Smyth MD, et al. External validation of the Chicago Chiari Outcome Scale. J Neurosurg Pediatr 2014;13(6):679–84.

33. Greenberg JK, Yarbrough CK, Radmanesh A, et al. The Chiari Severity Index: a preoperative grading system for Chiari malformation type 1. Neurosurgery 2015;76(3):279–85 [discussion: 285].

34. Feghali J, Marinaro E, Lubelski D, et al. Novel Risk Calculator for Suboccipital Decompression for Adult Chiari Malformation. World Neurosurg 2020;139:526–34.

35. Smith BW, Strahle J, Kazarian E, et al. Impact of body mass index on cerebellar tonsil position in healthy subjects and patients with Chiari malformation. J Neurosurg 2015;123(1):226–31.

36. Almotairi FS, Tisell M. Cerebrospinal fluid disturbance in overweight women after occipitocervical decompression in Chiari malformation type I. Acta Neurochir (Wien) 2016;158(3):589–94 [discussion: 594].

37. Lam S, Auffinger B, Tormenti M, et al. The relationship between obesity and symptomatic Chiari I malformation in the pediatric population. J Pediatr Neurosci 2015;10(4):321–5.

38. Frič R, Eide PK. Perioperative monitoring of pulsatile and static intracranial pressure in patients with Chiari malformation type 1 undergoing foramen magnum decompression. Acta Neurochir (Wien) 2016;158(2):341–7 [discussion: 346–7].

39. Frič R, Eide PK. Comparative observational study on the clinical presentation, intracranial volume measurements, and intracranial pressure scores in patients with either Chiari malformation Type I or idiopathic intracranial hypertension. J Neurosurg 2017;126(4):1312–22.

40. Milarachi EN, Gourishetti SC, Ciriello J, et al. Posterior fossa volume in idiopathic intracranial hypertension: a magnetic resonance imaging-based study. Acta Radiol 2021. https://doi.org/10.1177/028418512110665 64. 2841851211066564.

41. Soleman J, Roth J, Bartoli A, et al. Syringo-Subarachnoid Shunt for the Treatment of Persistent Syringomyelia Following Decompression for Chiari Type I Malformation: Surgical Results. World Neurosurg 2017;108:836–43.

42. Knafo S, Malcoci M, Morar S, et al. Surgical Management after Chiari Decompression Failure: Craniovertebral Junction Revision versus Shunting Strategies. J Clin Med 2022;11(12). https://doi.org/10.3390/jcm11123334.

43. Wu Y, Li C, Zong X, et al. Application of endoscopic third ventriculostomy for treating hydrocephalus-correlated Chiari type I malformation in a single

Chinese neurosurgery centre. Neurosurg Rev 2018; 41(1):249–54.

44. Guan J, Riva-Cambrin J, Brockmeyer DL. Chiari-related hydrocephalus: assessment of clinical risk factors in a cohort of 297 consecutive patients. Neurosurg Focus 2016;41(5):E2.

45. Caldarelli M, Novegno F, Di Rocco C. A late complication of CSF shunting: acquired Chiari I malformation. Childs Nerv Syst 2009;25(4):443–52.

46. Cinalli G, Russo C, Vitulli F, et al. Changes in venous drainage after posterior cranial vault distraction and foramen magnum decompression in syndromic craniosynostosis. J Neurosurg Pediatr 2022;1–12. https://doi.org/10.3171/2022.6.PEDS22171.

47. Ito K, Yamada M, Horiuchi T, et al. Microanatomy of the dura mater at the craniovertebral junction and spinal region for safe and effective surgical treatment. J Neurosurg Spine 2020;1–7. https://doi.org/10.3171/2020.1.SPINE191424.

48. Tochigi S, Isoshima A, Ohashi H, et al. Preoperative assessment of dominant occipital sinus in patients with Chiari malformation type I: anatomical variations and implications for preventing potentially life-threatening surgical complications. J Neurosurg 2022;1–10. https://doi.org/10.3171/2022.5.JNS212973.

49. Feghali J, Chen Y, Xie Y, et al. The impact of depression on surgical outcome in Chiari malformation type I: an assessment based on the Chicago Chiari Outcome Scale. J Neurosurg Spine 2020;1–8. https://doi.org/10.3171/2020.2.SPINE2069.

50. Labuda R, Loth D, Allen PA, et al. Factors Associated With Patient-Reported Postsurgical Symptom Improvement in Adult Females with Chiari Malformation Type I: A Report from the Chiari1000 Dataset. World Neurosurg 2022;161:e682–7.

51. Feghali J, Xie Y, Chen Y, et al. The SHORE Score: A Novel Predictive Tool for Improvement After Decompression Surgery in Adult Chiari Malformation Type I. World Neurosurg 2020;142:e195–202.

52. Thakar S, Sivaraju L, Jacob KS, et al. A points-based algorithm for prognosticating clinical outcome of Chiari malformation Type I with syringomyelia: results from a predictive model analysis of 82 surgically managed adult patients. J Neurosurg Spine 2018;28(1):23–32.

53. Seaman SC, Deifelt Streese C, Manzel K, et al. Cognitive and Psychological Functioning in Chiari Malformation Type I Before and After Surgical Decompression - A Prospective Cohort Study. Neurosurgery 2021;89(6):1087–96.

54. Loe ML, Vivas-Buitrago T, Domingo RA, et al. Prognostic significance of C1-C2 facet malalignment after surgical decompression in adult Chiari malformation type I: a pilot study based on the Chicago Chiari Outcome Scale. J Neurosurg Spine 2020;1–7. https://doi.org/10.3171/2020.6.SPINE20544.

55. Guo F, Turgut M. Precise Management of Chiari Malformation with Type I. Front Surg 2022;9:850879.

56. Tosi U, Lara-Reyna J, Chae J, et al. Persistent Syringomyelia After Posterior Fossa Decompression for Chiari Malformation. World Neurosurg 2020;136:454–61.e1.

57. Ciaramitaro P, Massimi L, Bertuccio A, et al. Diagnosis and treatment of Chiari malformation and syringomyelia in adults: international consensus document. Neurol Sci 2022;43(2):1327–42.

58. Bhimani AD, Esfahani DR, Denyer S, et al. Adult Chiari I Malformations: An Analysis of Surgical Risk Factors and Complications Using an International Database. World Neurosurg 2018;115:e490–500.

59. Arnautovic KI, Kovacevic M. CSF-Related Complications After Intradural Spinal Tumor Surgery: Utility of an Autologous Fat Graft. Med Arch 2016;70(6):460–5.

60. Silva A, Thanabalasundaram G, Wilkinson B, et al. Experience with revision craniovertebral decompression in adult patients with Chiari malformation type 1, with or without syringomyelia. Br J Neurosurg 2020;23:1–6.

61. Yahanda AT, Simon LE, Limbrick DD. Outcomes for various dural graft materials after posterior fossa decompression with duraplasty for Chiari malformation type I: a systematic review and meta-analysis. J Neurosurg 2021;1–14. https://doi.org/10.3171/2020.9.JNS202641.

62. CreveCoeur TS, Yahanda AT, Maher CO, et al. Occipital-Cervical Fusion and Ventral Decompression in the Surgical Management of Chiari-1 Malformation and Syringomyelia: Analysis of Data From the Park-Reeves Syringomyelia Research Consortium. Neurosurgery 2021;88(2):332–41.

63. Henderson FC, Wilson WA, Mark AS, et al. Utility of the clivo-axial angle in assessing brainstem deformity: pilot study and literature review. Neurosurg Rev 2018;41(1):149–63.

64. Bollo RJ, Riva-Cambrin J, Brockmeyer MM, et al. Complex Chiari malformations in children: an analysis of preoperative risk factors for occipitocervical fusion. J Neurosurg Pediatr 2012;10(2):134–41.

65. Goel A, Sathe P, Shah A. Atlantoaxial Fixation for Basilar Invagination without Obvious Atlantoaxial Instability (Group B Basilar Invagination): Outcome Analysis of 63 Surgically Treated Cases. World Neurosurg 2017;99:164–70.

66. Goel A, Kaswa A, Shah A. Atlantoaxial Fixation for Treatment of Chiari Formation and Syringomyelia with No Craniovertebral Bone Anomaly: Report of an Experience with 57 Cases. Acta Neurochir Suppl 2019;125:101–10.

67. Salunke P, Karthigeyan M, Malik P. Foramen magnum decompression without bone removal: C1-C2 posterior fixation for Chiari with congenital atlantoaxial dislocation/basilar invagination. Surg Neurol Int 2019;10:38.

68. Klekamp J. Relevance of C1/2 Facet Configurations and Clivus-Canal-Angles for Adult Patients with Chiari I Malformation with and without Basilar Invagination. World Neurosurg 2022;162:e156–67.

69. Passias PG, Naessig S, Para A, et al. Complication rates following Chiari malformation surgical management for Arnold-Chiari type I based on surgical variables: A national perspective. J Craniovertebr Junction Spine 2020;11(3):169–72.

70. İştemen İ, Harman F, Arslan A, et al. Is C1-C2 Reduction and Fixation A Good Choice in the Treatment of Recurrent Chiari-Like Symptoms With Syringomyelia? World Neurosurg 2021;146:e837–47.

71. Meyer B, Wagner A, Grassner L, et al. Chiari malformation type I and basilar invagination originating from atlantoaxial instability: a literature review and critical analysis. Acta Neurochir (Wien) 2020; 162(11):2925.

72. Wagner A, Grassner L, Kögl N, et al. Chiari malformation type I and basilar invagination originating from atlantoaxial instability: a literature review and critical analysis. Acta Neurochir (Wien) 2020; 162(7):1553–63.

73. Aronson DD, Kahn RH, Canady A, et al. Instability of the cervical spine after decompression in patients who have Arnold-Chiari malformation. J Bone Joint Surg Am 1991;73(6):898–906.

74. Chatterjee S, Shivhare P, Verma SG. Chiari malformation and atlantoaxial instability: problems of coexistence. Childs Nerv Syst 2019;35(10):1755–61.

Posterior Fossa Decompression with or Without Duraplasty for Chiari I Malformation

Alexander T. Yahanda, MD, MPHS[a,*], David D. Limbrick Jr, MD, PhD[a,b]

KEYWORDS

- Chiari I malformation • Dural augmentation • Dural graft • Duraplasty
- Posterior fossa decompression • Syringomyelia

KEY POINTS

- Posterior fossa decompression with duraplasty (PFDD) or posterior fossa decompression without duraplasty (PFD) duraplasty remains the mainstay of surgical treatment of symptomatic Chiari I malformation.
- PFDD is a more invasive procedure than PFD that, although associated with longer hospitalizations and greater complication rates, may provide better symptomatic relief and syrinx reduction with a lower risk of revision surgery.
- Further studies are needed to establish the ideal type of dural graft for PFDD.
- Additional surgical procedures may be employed in addition to PFD/PFDD given complex craniovertebral anatomy or symptoms.

INTRODUCTION

Chiari malformation type I (CM-1) is a common congenital anomaly resulting in herniation of the cerebellar tonsils through the foramen magnum. It is estimated that CM-1 may be present in up to 4% of children.[1] Though CM-1 can remain asymptomatic, patients can present with a myriad of symptoms, including (but not limited to) headaches, cranial nerve dysfunction, ataxia, paresthesias, motor deficits, and apnea.[2] Moreover, CM-1 is often accompanied by syringomyelia (SM), which may yield additional symptoms. Surgery remains the most definitive treatment of symptomatic CM-1. The goal of surgery is to sufficiently decompress the cerebellar tonsils to reduce the effects of herniation through the foramen magnum and restore normal flow of cerebrospinal fluid (CSF) across the craniovertebral junction (CVJ).

Broadly, the standard of care operation for symptomatic CM-1 is referred to as posterior fossa decompression. This decompression may involve occipital craniectomy (often with C1 laminectomy and removal of the atalanto-occipital membrane) and remain extradural (herein referred to as posterior fossa decompression, or PFD), or it can include dural augmentation in addition to osseous decompression (posterior fossa decompression with duraplasty, or PFDD). There are additional surgical techniques that may be used as adjuncts to PFD or PFDD given certain patient presentations or anatomical findings. This article provides a comprehensive overview of literature on PFD and PFDD as well as nuances of operative techniques.

[a] Department of Neurological Surgery, Washington University School of Medicine, 660 South Euclid Avenue, St Louis, MO 63110, USA; [b] Department of Pediatrics, Washington University School of Medicine, 660 South Euclid Avenue, St Louis, MO 63110, USA
* Corresponding author. Department of Neurosurgery, Washington University School of Medicine, 660 South Euclid Avenue, CB 8057, St Louis, MO 63110.
E-mail address: ayahanda@wustl.edu

Neurosurg Clin N Am 34 (2023) 105–111
https://doi.org/10.1016/j.nec.2022.08.008
1042-3680/23/© 2022 Elsevier Inc. All rights reserved.

DIFFERENCES IN OPERATIVE TECHNIQUE
Posterior Fossa Decompression Without Duraplasty

PFD involves suboccipital craniectomy, often with C1 laminectomy or more depending on the extent of tonsillar ectopia, to alleviate compression upon the cerebellar tonsils and restore normal CSF flow. For this surgery, the patient is positioned prone on the operating table. A midline posterior incision is made, which allows for exposure from the inion to the upper cervical spine. A subperiosteal dissection is used to expose the occipital bone and posterior cervical spine. A suboccipital craniectomy is performed to decompress the foramen magnum. Laminectomy of C1 is subsequently performed for additional decompression. In some instances, the surgeon may elect to score the dura, lyse epidural adhesions, remove the atalanto-occipital membrane, or split the outer dural membrane.[3] As no duraplasty is employed, the entire procedure remains extradural.

Posterior Fossa Decompression with Duraplasty

PFDD largely follows the same initial steps as PFD, including the incision, exposure, osseous decompression, and laminectomy of C1. The primary difference is that PFDD also requires opening of the dura with subsequent dural augmentation. The rationale behind PFDD is that extradural decompression alone may be insufficient as the dura surrounding the cerebellar tonsils (or intradural sources of flow restriction such as arachnoid adhesions or veils) may also be providing a degree of constriction. Typically, the dura is incised in a Y-shaped manner and a dural graft is sewed over the opening to yield additional intradural space. This dural graft may be of several different origins, either autologous or nonautologous.

The goals for any dural graft material are to be easily manipulated during surgery, enable a watertight dural seal, avoid generating an immunological or inflammatory reaction, and lead to minimal scarring. Ultimately, the graft should serve as a scaffold over which the patient's native dura may grow. Common autologous grafts that have been used for PFDD include pericranium, nuchal ligament, or fascia lata. The main benefits of autologous grafts are that they are derived from the patient's own tissues and thus theoretically minimize the chances of an immunological reaction to the graft. They furthermore negate the financial burden of nonautologous grafts. These grafts may be harvested as part of the PFDD procedure. Pericranium, perhaps the most commonly used autologous graft,[4] is often harvested through a separate

incision or by elongation of the initial posterior fossa incision to include a greater region of the posterior skull from which the pericranium may be harvested. Similarly, nuchal ligament is harvested at a point along its midline course from the posterior skull to the upper cervical spine. Fascia lata harvest, which perhaps incurs the most additional morbidity to the patient, is achieved thorough a separate incision on the patient's lateral thigh.

There is a wide range of potential nonautologous grafts that may be used, each with a unique commercial moniker. Regarding specific types of materials, these grafts may be broken down into a few categories: bovine or other animal-based grafts, synthetic grafts, and nonautologous human-derived grafts. Animal-based grafts typically are comprised of the acellular remnants of connective tissue—for instance, pericardium or collagen matrix. Rare reports in the literature highlight the use of porcine small intestine as a possible dural graft.[5] Synthetic grafts consist of waterproof materials such as expanded polytetrafluoroethylene (PTFE) or similar polymers. Nonautologous human-derived graft may include cadaveric dura or acellular dermal matrices. Each type of graft—either autologous or nonautologous—no doubt has its own risks and benefits as well as a characteristic side effect profile, though, as will be discussed later in this article, the literature comparing various dural grafts is of poor quality overall and lacks the ability to discern potentially important distinctions among graft types.

OUTCOMES AFTER POSTERIOR FOSSA DECOMPRESSION WITHOUT DURAPLASTY OR POSTERIOR FOSSA DECOMPRESSION WITH DURAPLASTY

Improvement in Chari-related symptoms is often achieved after decompression with or without duraplasty. One meta-analysis placed the overall rate of postoperative symptomatic improvement between 61% and 93%.[6] This is in large part due to normalization of CSF flow dynamics after adequate decompression.[7] Indeed, patients with *normal* preoperative CSF dynamics have been found to derive significantly less benefit from PFD than those with abnormal CSF dynamics.[8] Radiographically, it has been found that patients frequently experience improvements in CSF flow after PFD.[9–11] For patients with SM, improved CSF flow around the CVJ can also lead to decreased CSF pulsatility within the syrinx. Significant improvements in syrinx size have been described after either PFD or PFDD, though PFDD has been independently associated with greater syrinx reduction compared with PFD.[12] Nevertheless, it should be noted that decreased syrinx size does not necessarily yield symptomatic improvement as syrinx size and symptoms are not always directly correlated.

The overall postoperative complication rate for PFD has been found to be somewhere between 12% and 24%.[2,13–16] As no dural opening is employed for PFD, the rates of CSF leak, pseudomeningocele, or chemical or infectious meningitis appear to be very low. By comparison, the reported postoperative complication rate for PFDD ranges from 18-40%, though the exact incidence of complications for individual dural graft types is not well-established and can vary widely across studies. In any case, it is generally accepted that the postoperative complication rate is higher for PFDD than for PFD due to its more invasive nature and potential reactions to nonautologous graft materials. The most common complications for PFDD include CSF leak, pseudomeningocele, and aseptic meningitis, all of which have been found in multiple prior studies to be significantly more common than after PFD.[13,16]

Posterior Fossa Decompression Without Duraplasty Versus Posterior Fossa Decompression with Duraplasty?

The decision to pursue PFD or PFDD for the treatment of CM-1 with or without SM remains a source of some controversy. Proponents of PFD argue that this technique provides satisfactory outcomes while reducing complications and other morbidity compared with the more-invasive PFDD. In addition to postoperative complications, prior studies have shown that PFDD is associated with greater blood loss, longer OR times, and longer hospital stays compared with PFD.[2,17] On the other hand, surgeons who prefer PFDD cite literature supporting the fact that PFDD may provide greater long-term relief of symptoms, particularly for patients with SM.[12] Furthermore, patients undergoing PFDD have significantly lower rates of revision surgery when compared with PFD.[2,6,16,18]

Akbari and colleagues,[2] in the largest multicenter retrospective study examining outcomes for patients receiving PFD (*n* = 117) versus PFDD (*n* = 575) for CM-1 and SM found that PFDD was associated with higher 6-month complication rates but higher rates of symptomatic improvement, larger decreases in syrinx size, and lower rates of revision surgery compared with PFD. These findings have been echoed to varying degrees by prior meta-analyses. Durham and colleagues[13] compared 316 PFDD patients and 266 PFD patients from seven different studies.

They found that PFDD led to fewer revision surgeries but that it did not improve symptoms or syrinx sizes significantly compared with PFD. Lu and colleagues[16] compared 1963 PFD and 1492 PFDD cases from 12 studies and concluded that PFDD resulted in greater clinical improvement but was not significantly different from PFD with respect to revision surgery rate, blood loss, or syrinx improvement. Lin and colleagues[18] examined 3481 patients undergoing PFD or PFDD from 13 studies. These researchers found that PFDD yielded greater clinical improvement for patients with SM, but that PFDD and PFD were not significantly different in clinical improvement for patients without SM and did not produce significantly different improvements in imaging. PFDD was associated with significantly more complications than PFD. Sadler and colleagues[19] found that patients with CM-1, SM, and scoliosis who were treated with PFDD were less likely to experience curve progression compared with patients treated with PFD.

A forthcoming randomized clinical trial comparing outcomes for PFD versus PFDD (ClincalTrials.gov identifier: NCT02669836) will provide the most definitive evidence for outcomes between these procedures. Until then, based on existing retrospective evidence, the preoperative planning process should consider the risks of benefits of PFD versus PFDD, weighing the lower complication risks of PFD against the potential for superior long-term symptomatic relief and lower risk of revision surgery with PFDD. This discussion may be especially important for patients with concurrent SM.

Differences Among Dural Grafts for Posterior Fossa Decompression with Duraplasty

Ideally, given the many different graft types that are available for PFDD, we would have a thorough understanding of the complication profiles for commonly-used graft materials to reduce postoperative complications after PFDD. However, this is not the case. Complication rates and profiles for each type of dural graft are not well-established. Moreover, though there have been many prior studies that compare different graft types, the results have been heterogenous.[20–46] These prior studies have often used limited patient cohorts (<50 patients), examined only one or two types of grafts, and used data from single institutions, which makes comparing graft types difficult. Only a few meta-analyses have been performed on this topic.[4,47,48]

Yahanda and colleagues[49] performed the largest multicenter retrospective study examining complication rates for 5 types of dural graft materials (autograft, bovine pericardium, bovine collagen, synthetic, and allograft). This study used the Park-Reeves Syringomyelia Research Consortium (PRSRC) database, which included data for 781 patients from >30 different institutions. These authors found that nonautologous grafts were associated with higher rates of pseudomeningocele and meningitis compared with autograft. Among nonautologous grafts, allograft had the lowest complication rate. Autograft and nonautologous grafts were associated with similar improvements in syrinx size and postoperative symptoms.

Yahanda, Simon, and Limbrick also conducted the largest meta-analysis to date examining complication rates and outcomes among dural grafts for nearly 1500 patients across 27 studies.[48] The authors found that autograft was likely the most advantageous graft type, as it was associated with the lowest rates of overall complications, pseudomeningocele, revision PFDD, and aseptic meningitis, though it was also associated with increased wound complications. This meta-analysis also determined that the current literature comparing various dural graft materials is of poor quality and that large prospective studies are required to fully elucidate differences among grafts.

ADJUNCT PROCEDURES TO POSTERIOR FOSSA DECOMPRESSION WITHOUT DURAPLASTY/POSTERIOR FOSSA DECOMPRESSION WITH DURAPLASTY
Arachnoid Sparing

To decrease the rate of CSF leaks or other complications, an arachnoid sparing technique may be used for PFDD. In this approach, care is taken to not breach the arachnoid membranes before performing the duraplasty. A prior meta-analysis found that using an arachnoid sparing method produced similar outcomes compared with PFDD with arachnoid dissection while decreasing the rate of overall complications.[50] The effect on syrinx size reduction, however, may be equivalent between the two techniques.[51]

Tonsillar Reduction

Given that the symptoms of CM-1 are ultimately from cerebellar tonsillar ectopia, some surgeons may elect for adjunctive tonsillar reduction while they perform their decompression. As this requires entering the dura to approach the tonsils, these additional surgical techniques can only be performed with PFDD. Cauterization or resection of the tonsils is generally tolerated well, but prior

studies have indicated that this technique may not yield superior outcomes in symptom improvement or syrinx resolution when compared with PFD/PFDD alone.[52,53]

Occipital-Cervical Fusion ± Ventral Decompression

Certain patients who receive PFD or PFDD may require additional stabilization or decompression of the CVJ. In these cases, it may be advantageous to perform an occipital-cervical fusion (OCF) or ventral decompression (VD). OCF involves fusing the occiput to the cervical spine to reduce instability across the CVJ. This procedure, unfortunately, provides stability at the cost of reduced mobility of the head and neck, but it may be required for patients with certain symptoms or anatomical findings. Several prior studies have examined prognostic factors for necessitating OCF for CM-1.[54–57] Anatomical anomalies of the CVJ and skull base, including several factors of the "complex Chiari malformation" (clivoaxial angle <125°, basilar invagination, condylar-C2 sagittal vertical alignment ≥5 mm), increase the risk for requiring OCF, as do the presence of certain genetic abnormalities.[56,57] In rare instances, ventral brainstem impingement may require VD to alleviate symptoms, which involves decompression of ventral bony CVJ elements. The risk factors for requiring VD are similar to those for OCF.

SUMMARY

PFD with/without duraplasty is the standard surgical treatment of symptomatic CM-1. PFD may be associated with shorter operative times and hospitalizations, fewer complications, and may yield significant improvements in symptoms and syrinx sizes. PFDD may be associated with superior long-term symptomatic relief, larger syrinx reduction, and a lower need for revision decompression. Various dural graft materials may be used for PFDD, though the ideal type of graft has not been definitively established. Other adjunct surgical procedures may be added to PFD/PFDD given certain symptomatic or anatomical considerations.

CLINICS CARE POINTS

- Surgical management of Chari I malformation can yield significant improvements in symptoms and syrinx sizes.

- When deciding on PFD versus PFDD, one must consider the risks/benefits inherent to each procedure type.
- Future studies are underway to establish the choice of PFD versus PFDD, the optimal dural graft material, and adjunct surgical procedures that may augment the benefits provided by PFD/PFDD.

REFERENCES

1. Strahle J, Muraszko KM, Kapurch J, et al. Chiari malformation Type I and syrinx in children undergoing magnetic resonance imaging: clinical article. J Neurosurg Pediatr 2011;8(2):205–13.
2. Akbari SHA, Yahanda AT, Ackerman LL, et al. Complications and outcomes of posterior fossa decompression with duraplasty versus without duraplasty for pediatric patients with Chiari malformation type I and syringomyelia: a study from the Park-Reeves Syringomyelia Research Consortium. J Neurosurg Pediatr 2022;1–13. https://doi.org/10.3171/2022.2.PEDS21446.
3. Limonadi FM, Selden NR. Dura-splitting decompression of the craniocervical junction: reduced operative time, hospital stay, and cost with equivalent early outcome. J Neurosurg 2004;101(2 Suppl):184–8.
4. Abla AA, Link T, Fusco D, et al. Comparison of dural grafts in Chiari decompression surgery: Review of the literature. J Craniovertebr Junction Spine 2010;1(1):29–37.
5. Bejjani GK, Zabramski J, Durasis Study Group. Safety and efficacy of the porcine small intestinal submucosa dural substitute: results of a prospective multicenter study and literature review. J Neurosurg 2007;106(6):1028–33.
6. Xu H, Chu L, He R, et al. Posterior fossa decompression with and without duraplasty for the treatment of Chiari malformation type I—a systematic review and meta-analysis. Neurosurg Rev 2017;40(2):213–21.
7. Iskandar BJ, Quigley M, Haughton VM. Foramen magnum cerebrospinal fluid flow characteristics in children with Chiari I malformation before and after craniocervical decompression. J Neurosurg 2004;101(2 Suppl):169–78.
8. McGirt MJ, Atiba A, Attenello FJ, et al. Correlation of hindbrain CSF flow and outcome after surgical decompression for Chiari I malformation. Childs Nerv Syst 2008;24(7):833–40.
9. Luzzi S, Giotta Lucifero A, Elsawaf Y, et al. Pulsatile cerebrospinal fluid dynamics in Chiari I malformation syringomyelia: Predictive value in posterior fossa decompression and insights into the syringogenesis. J Craniovertebral Junction Spine 2021;12(1):15–25.
10. Delavari N, Wang AC, Bapuraj JR, et al. Intraoperative phase contrast MRI analysis of cerebrospinal fluid velocities during posterior fossa decompression for Chiari I malformation. J Magn Reson Imaging 2020;51(5):1463–70.
11. Quon JL, Grant RA, DiLuna ML. Multimodal evaluation of CSF dynamics following extradural decompression for Chiari malformation Type I. J Neurosurg Spine 2015;22(6):622–30.
12. Hale AT, David Adelson P, Albert GW, et al. Factors associated with syrinx size in pediatric patients treated for Chiari malformation type I and syringomyelia: a study from the Park-Reeves Syringomyelia Research Consortium. J Neurosurg Pediatr 2020;25(6):629–39.
13. Durham SR, Fjeld-Olenec K. Comparison of posterior fossa decompression with and without duraplasty for the surgical treatment of Chiari malformation Type I in pediatric patients: a meta-analysis. J Neurosurg Pediatr 2008;2(1):42–9.
14. Mozaffari K, Davidson L, Chalif E, et al. Long-term outcomes of posterior fossa decompression for Chiari malformation type 1: which patients are most prone to failure? Childs Nerv Syst 2021;37(9):2891–8.
15. Tam SKP, Brodbelt A, Bolognese PA, et al. Posterior fossa decompression with duraplasty in Chiari malformation type 1: a systematic review and meta-analysis. Acta Neurochir (Wien) 2021;163(1):229–38.
16. Lu VM, Phan K, Crowley SP, et al. The addition of duraplasty to posterior fossa decompression in the surgical treatment of pediatric Chiari malformation Type I: a systematic review and meta-analysis of surgical and performance outcomes. J Neurosurg Pediatr 2017;20(5):439–49.
17. James HE, Brant A. Treatment of the Chiari malformation with bone decompression without durotomy in children and young adults. Child's Nerv Syst 2002;18(5):202–6.
18. Lin W, Duan G, Xie J, et al. Comparison of results between posterior fossa decompression with and without duraplasty for the surgical treatment of chiari malformation type I: a systematic review and meta-analysis. World Neurosurg 2018;110:460–74.e5.
19. Sadler B, Skidmore A, Gewirtz J, et al. Extradural decompression versus duraplasty in Chiari malformation type I with syrinx: outcomes on scoliosis from the Park-Reeves Syringomyelia Research Consortium. J Neurosurg Pediatr 2021;28(2):167–75.
20. Fischer EG. Posterior fossa decompression for Chiari I deformity, including resection of the cerebellar tonsils. Child's Nerv Syst 1995;11(11):625–9.
21. Anson JA, Marchand EP. Bovine pericardium for dural grafts: Clinical results in 35 patients. Neurosurgery 1996;39(4):764–8.
22. Vanaclocha V, Saiz-Sapena N. Duraplasty with freeze-dried cadaveric dura versus occipital

pericranium for Chiari type I malformation: Comparative study. Acta Neurochir (Wien) 1997;139(2):112–9.

23. Alzate JC, Kothbauer KF, Jallo GI, et al. Treatment of Chiari I malformation in patients with and without syringomyelia: a consecutive series of 66 cases. Neurosurg Focus 2001;11(1):E3.

24. Sindou M, Chávez-Machuca J, Hashish H. Cranio-cervical decompression for Chiari type I-malformation, adding extreme lateral foramen magnum opening and expansile duroplasty with arachnoid preservation. Technique and long-term functional results in 44 consecutive adult cases – comparison with I. Acta Neurochir (Wien) 2002;144(10):1005–19.

25. Danish SF, Samdani A, Hanna A, et al. Experience with acellular human dura and bovine collagen matrix for duraplasty after posterior fossa decompression for Chiari malformations. J Neurosurg 2006;104(Suppl. 1):16–20.

26. Messing-Jünger AM, Ibáñez J, Calbucci F, et al. Effectiveness and handling characteristics of a three-layer polymer dura substitute: a prospective multicenter clinical study. J Neurosurg 2006;105(6):853–8.

27. Galarza M, Sood S, Ham S. Relevance of surgical strategies for the management of pediatric Chiari type I malformation. Childs Nerv Syst 2007;23(6):691–6.

28. Hoffman CE, Souweidane MM. Cerebrospinal fluid-related complications with autologous duraplasty and arachnoid sparing in type I Chiari malformation. Oper Neurosurg 2008;62(3 Suppl 1):156–60.

29. Attenello FJ, McGirt MJ, Garcés-Ambrossi GL, et al. Suboccipital decompression for Chiari I malformation: Outcome comparison of duraplasty with expanded polytetrafluoroethylene dural substitute versus pericranial autograft. Child's Nerv Syst 2009;25(2):183–90.

30. Parker SR, Harris P, Cummings TJ, et al. Complications following decompression of Chiari malformation Type I in children: dural graft or sealant? J Neurosurg Pediatr 2011;8(2):177–83.

31. Foreman P, Safavi-A Bbasi S, Talley MC, et al. Perioperative outcomes and complications associated with allogeneic duraplasty for the management of Chiari malformations Type i in 48 pediatric patients: Clinical article. J Neurosurg Pediatr 2012;10(2):142–9.

32. Lam FC, Kasper E. Augmented Autologous Pericranium Duraplasty in 100 Posterior Fossa Surgeries-A Retrospective Case Series. Oper Neurosurg 2012;71(suppl_2):302–7.

33. Lam FC, Penumaka A, Chen CC, et al. Fibrin sealant augmentation with autologous pericranium for duraplasty after suboccipital decompression in Chiari 1 patients: a case series. Surg Neurol Int 2013;4(1):6.

34. Williams LE, Vannemreddy PS, Watson KS, et al. The need in dural graft suturing in Chiari I malformation decompression: A prospective, single-blind, randomized trial comparing sutured and sutureless duraplasty materials. Surg Neurol Int 2013;4(1):26.

35. Chotai S, Medhkour A. Surgical outcomes after posterior fossa decompression with and without duraplasty in Chiari malformation-I. Clin Neurol Neurosurg 2014;125:182–8.

36. Bao CS, Liu L, Wang B, et al. Craniocervical decompression with duraplasty and cerebellar tonsillectomy as treatment for Chiari malformation-I complicated with syringomyelia. Genet Mol Res 2015;14(1):952–60.

37. Bowers CA, Brimley C, Cole C, et al. AlloDerm for duraplasty in Chiari malformation: superior outcomes. Acta Neurochir (Wien) 2015;157(3):507–11.

38. Alperin N, Loftus JR, Bagci AM, et al. Magnetic resonance imaging-based measures predictive of short-term surgical outcome in patients with Chiari malformation Type I: a pilot study. J Neurosurg Spine 2017;26(1):28–38.

39. Lee CK, Mokhtari T, Connolly ID, et al. Comparison of porcine and bovine collagen dural substitutes in posterior fossa decompression for Chiari I malformation in adults. World Neurosurg 2017;108:33–40.

40. Cools MJ, Quinsey CS, Elton SW. Chiari decompression outcomes using ligamentum nuchae harvest and duraplasty in pediatric patients with Chiari malformation type I. J Neurosurg Pediatr 2018;22(1):47–51.

41. Dlouhy BJ, Menezes AH. Autologous cervical fascia duraplasty in 123 children and adults with Chiari malformation type I: Surgical technique and complications. J Neurosurg Pediatr 2018;22(3):297–305.

42. Farber H, McDowell MM, Alhourani A, et al. Duraplasty type as a predictor of meningitis and shunting after chiari I decompression. World Neurosurg 2018;118:e778–83.

43. Hidalgo ET, Dastagirzada Y, Orillac C, et al. Time to resolution of symptoms after suboccipital decompression with duraplasty in children with chiari malformation type I. World Neurosurg 2018;117:e544–51.

44. Jiang E, Sha S, Yuan X, et al. Comparison of clinical and radiographic outcomes for posterior fossa decompression with and without duraplasty for treatment of pediatric Chiari I malformation: a prospective study. World Neurosurg 2018;110:e465–72.

45. Elhadji Cheikh Ndiaye SY, Troude L, Al-Falasi M, et al. Chiari malformations in adults: a single center surgical experience with special emphasis on the kinetics of clinical improvement. Neurochirurgie 2019;65(2–3):69–74.

46. Ito K, Yamada M, Horiuchi T, et al. Appropriate surgical procedures for Chiari type 1 malformation and associated syrinx based on radiological

characteristics of the craniovertebral junction. Neurosurg Rev 2019. https://doi.org/10.1007/s10143-019-01079-3.

47. Förander P, Sjåvik K, Solheim O, et al. The case for duraplasty in adults undergoing posterior fossa decompression for Chiari i malformation: a systematic review and meta-analysis of observational studies. Clin Neurol Neurosurg 2014;125:58–64.

48. Yahanda AT, Simon LE, Limbrick DD. Outcomes for various dural graft materials after posterior fossa decompression with duraplasty for Chiari malformation type I: a systematic review and meta-analysis. J Neurosurg 2021;1–14. https://doi.org/10.3171/2020.9.JNS202641.

49. Yahanda AT, David Adelson P, Hassan S, et al. Dural augmentation approaches and complication rates after posterior fossa decompression for Chiari I malformation and syringomyelia: a Park-Reeves Syringomyelia Research Consortium study. J Neurosurg Pediatr 2021;27(4):459–68.

50. Osborne-Grinter M, Arora M, Kaliaperumal C, et al. Posterior fossa decompression and duraplasty with and without arachnoid preservation for the treatment of adult chiari malformation type 1: a systematic review and meta-analysis. World Neurosurg 2021;151:e579–98.

51. Özlen F, Kucukyuruk B, Alizada O, et al. Comparison of two surgical techniques in Chiari Malformation Type 1 Patients: Duraplasty alone vs duraplasty with arachnoid dissection. Clin Neurol Neurosurg 2021;206. https://doi.org/10.1016/J.CLINEURO.2021.106686.

52. Koueik J, Sandoval-Garcia C, Kestle JRW, et al. Outcomes in children undergoing posterior fossa decompression and duraplasty with and without tonsillar reduction for Chiari malformation type I and syringomyelia: a pilot prospective multicenter cohort study. J Neurosurg Pediatr 2019;25(1):21–9.

53. Jia C, li H, Wu J, et al. Comparison decompression by duraplasty or cerebellar tonsillectomy for Chiari malformation-I complicated with syringomyelia. Clin Neurol Neurosurg 2019;176:1–7.

54. Ho WSC, Brockmeyer DL. Complex Chiari malformation: using craniovertebral junction metrics to guide treatment. Child's Nerv Syst 2019;35(10):1847–51.

55. Smith JS, Shaffrey CI, Abel MF, et al. Basilar invagination. Neurosurgery 2010;66(SUPPL. 3).

56. Crevecoeur TS, Yahanda AT, Maher CO, et al. Occipital-cervical fusion and ventral decompression in the surgical management of chiari-1 malformation and syringomyelia: analysis of data from the park-reeves syringomyelia research consortium. Neurosurgery 2021. https://doi.org/10.1093/neuros/nyaa460.

57. Ravindra VM, Iyer RR, Yahanda AT, et al. A multicenter validation of the condylar-C2 sagittal vertical alignment in Chiari malformation type I: a study using the Park-Reeves Syringomyelia Research Consortium. J Neurosurg Pediatr 2021. https://doi.org/10.3171/2020.12.PEDS20809.

Short-Term and Long-Term Complications Associated with Posterior Fossa Decompression for Chiari Malformation

Ulrich Batzdorf, MD

KEYWORDS

- Chiari malformation • Pseudomeningocele • Cerebellar ptosis • Dural ectasia • Basilar invagination
- Cranio-cervical instability • Syringomyelia

KEY POINTS

- Posterior fossa decompression can be performed safely if the usual precautions of sterility and hemostasis are observed.
- Blood in the subarachnoid space may lead to scar formation and care should be taken to minimize the amount of subarachnoid blood.
- Instability of various causes should be considered in instances of persistent pain, particularly pain associated with head and neck movement.

INTRODUCTION

Although the surgical treatment of Chiari anomalies in adults is relatively straightforward, complications and less than satisfactory outcomes can and do occur.[1] Understanding these situations is important from the point of view of correcting the problem as well as preventing the recurrence of similar problems in the future.

DIAGNOSIS

The first consideration must always be given to the diagnosis: Was the diagnosis of (primary) tonsillar descent due to a disproportionately small posterior fossa correct, or was there an underlying condition resulting in tonsillar descent, so-called secondary Chiari malformation? Thus, the importance of careful clinical evaluation and, in most patients, completes cranio-spinal imaging to rule out other processes. Clinical assessment should focus on the specific type of headache (strain-related rather than generalized or posture-related) and other established hallmark symptoms. Imaging should be performed to rule out potential sources of cerebrospinal fluid (CSF) leakage, which may occur at any level of the spine, causing CSF hypotension,[2,3] or cerebral lesions including hydrocephalus, aqueductal stenosis, space-occupying lesions, or idiopathic intracranial hypertension (pseudotumor cerebri).[4] Relying only on the measurement of tonsillar descent, often the focus of radiologists may be misleading; the shape of the descended tonsils reflecting compression is more reliable. Minor variations in sequential imaging studies are sometimes related to the patient's

Department of Neurosurgery, David Geffen School of Medicine at UCLA, 300 Stein Plaza, Wasserman 420, Los Angeles, CA 90095-6901, USA

E-mail address: ubatzdorf@mednet.ucla.edu

Neurosurg Clin N Am 34 (2023) 113–117
https://doi.org/10.1016/j.nec.2022.09.005
1042-3680/23/© 2022 Elsevier Inc. All rights reserved.

position on the scanning table, with varying degrees of neck flexion or extension. It is also important not to mistake a residual central canal of the spinal cord for true syringomyelia.[5]

Acute Problems

Acute problems include complications associated with any surgical procedure: infection and hemorrhage, as well as problems specifically associated with posterior fossa decompression, especially when the dura has been opened, either deliberately or accidentally, notably CSF leakage. The development of new neurological deficits also needs to be considered. Wound infection will not be discussed in detail here, except to note the importance of meticulous sterile technique common to all neurosurgical procedures and especially important when the dura has been opened and a wound infection can lead to meningitis. Appropriate antibiotic therapy needs to be instituted promptly. Likewise, careful hemostasis is essential. Dural sinuses can bleed significantly and must be secured. The dura itself may be vascular and it is important to recognize that most dural vessels lie between the inner and outer dural leaves. Full thickness coagulation of the dura risks dural necrosis and thereby CSF leakage. When the dura has been opened, it is important to irrigate the intradural compartment thoroughly. Blood in the subarachnoid space may lead to significant scarring.

CSF leakage from the wound is a serious problem. When it occurs, lumbar drainage may need to be instituted for several days. If fluid leakage recurs after drainage has been discontinued, wound reopening and identification and closure of the leak site need to be performed. Measures that should be taken to prevent this complication include meticulous dural closure, with the performance of a Valsalva maneuver by the anesthesiologist to identify any potential leak in every patient. It is probably reasonable to have the anesthesiologist perform this maneuver even when the dura has not been deliberately opened as inadvertent dural openings can occur. Any identified dural leak should be sutured with a fine suture incorporating a small patch of autologous tissue harvested from the wound edge. It has been our practice to cover the dural closure with a patch of collagen sponge and dural sealant.[6] It is also helpful to have the head of the patient's bed raised 45 degrees for the first few days after surgery and to have the patient avoid straining or lifting maneuvers.

Neurological deficits are rarely seen as a complication of posterior fossa decompression for Chiari anomalies. When intradural exploration is carried out, it is essential to avoid injury to prominent vessels, notably the posterior inferior cerebellar arteries. The exact location of these vessels with respect to the cerebellar tonsils varies widely and it is important to identify these structures to avoid injury, including proximity of bipolar coagulation when this is used to reduce the size of the tonsils. Should a spasm of a major vessel be seen at the time of surgery, topical application of papaverine may be helpful. It is also important to avoid injury to vessels on the opening of the dura. Careful separation of the dura from the underlying arachnoid has been our practice and should safeguard against injuring a major vessel that would be located in the subarachnoid space.

Long-Term Problems

Long-term problems can be considered from two points of view: (a) those which are related to technical issues and (b) those related to other causes.

Technically related problems

These problems generally fall into four categories: Pseudomeningoceles, a bony opening too large or too small, inadequate restoration of CSF flow, and instability.

Pseudomeningoceles

Pseudomeningoceles occur when a leak in the dural closure has occurred, often in a delayed manner[7] (**Fig. 1**). Consideration should always be given to the possibility that the leak occurred

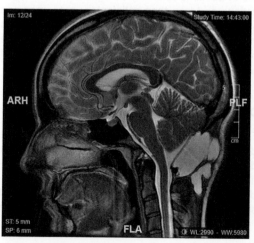

Fig. 1. Pseudomeningocele. Sagittal T2W image of a patient who had undergone an uncomplicated posterior fossa decompression for Chiari malformation approximately a year before this study. Details of the dural closure are not known. She presented with posterior cervical pain, which increased with coughing and also with neck extension.

because of unsuspected elevation in intracranial pressure, such as undiagnosed idiopathic intracranial hypertension or undiagnosed pressure issues of other etiologies. Assuming that such underlying pathology has been excluded, it is important to realize that the presence of a pseudomeningocele is not to be treated as inconsequential, and this is particularly true when the patient also has a syrinx, which may not have diminished in size as one would have expected when a pseudomeningocele is present. Pseudomeningoceles, even relatively small ones, may act as a capacitance reservoir and thereby diminish the strength of the pulsatile force propagated into the spinal subarachnoid space.[8] This is believed to be responsible for the persistence of a syrinx cavity following posterior fossa decompression when a pseudomeningocele is present. Pseudomeningoceles may also be the source of local pain, presumably the result of dural stretching. The *treatment* is reoperation with the closure of the dural defect. The specific material used for duraplasty may be of importance. Autologous pericranium has been a satisfactory material in our experience. Precautions noted above in connection with acute CSF leaks, including Valsalva maneuver, use of collagen sponge and dural sealant, as well as head elevation and, potentially, a brief period of lumbar drainage, need to be kept in mind.

Craniectomy size

Excessively large decompression, that is, a posterior fossa craniectomy that is too large can result in a delayed complication. The aim of occipital bone removal should be to expose the cerebellar tonsils and the size of the craniectomy can be estimated from the patient's imaging studies. Excessively large craniectomies may result in the descent of the cerebellar hemispheres into the decompression site, what has been termed cerebellar ptosis (**Fig. 2**), or expansion of the dural graft into the decompression site, dural ectasia (see **Fig. 4**). By stretching the surrounding dura, both of these conditions may give rise to local, that is, posterior cervical-cranial headache. Severe cerebellar ptosis may also recreate the partial obstruction of CSF flow which initially resulted from tonsillar descent. Such headaches generally develop after the patient assumes the upright position. It has been our practice to have the patient apply a sponge, held in place with an elastic bandage, to the incision area, to determine whether such counter-pressure prevents the headache from developing.[9] Dural ectasia can also result from the use of expansible material for duraplasty. In some patients, local fascia used for dural grafting,

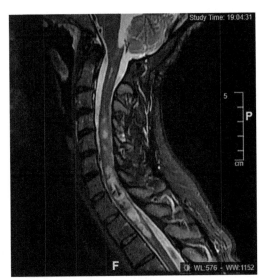

Fig. 2. Cerebellar ptosis. Sagittal T2W cervical spine MR scan of a patient who had undergone posterior fossa decompression for Chiari malformation and syringomyelia. Note descent of the cerebellar tonsils into the decompression site and narrowing of the fourth ventricle outlet, as well as persistent syringomyelia. The patient presented with recurrent headaches. T2W, T 2 weighted; MR, magnetic resonance.

can stretch considerably and thereby put tension on the posterior fossa dura to which it has been sutured. Our practice has been to line the material used for duraplasty (autologous pericranium) with a nonstretchable layer of expanded polytetrafluoroethylene (ePTFE), available as Gore-Tex.[6] *Treatment* of ptosis or ectasia consists of placing a titanium plate which reduces the size of the craniectomy[10] (**Fig. 3**). Multiperforated plates which can be secured with small screws are commercially available. In this connection, it is important to note that there are variations in posterior fossa anatomy that may give rise to the Chiari syndrome. Patients with a small posterior fossa due to a low insertion of the tentorium into the occipital bone are particularly at risk to develop cerebellar ptosis (**Fig. 4**), also known as "slump," because of the relatively small cupping support for the cerebellar hemispheres.

A craniectomy that is too small may not alleviate compression of the cerebellar tonsils and thus would also not create a more normally sized cisterna magna. It is general practice to include laminectomy of the first cervical vertebra as part of the posterior fossa decompression. Incomplete fusion of C 1 should always be kept in mind when removing this lamina. *Treatment* consists of enlarging the craniectomy and performing a duraplasty when indicated. As discussed in connection with the persistence of syringomyelia, failures may

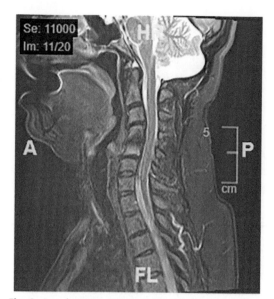

Fig. 3. Dural ectasia. Sagittal T2W image of a patient who had undergone posterior fossa decompression for Chiari malformation several years earlier. Note the large bony decompression, almost to the level of the tentorial insertion. She presented with local posterior cervical–cephalic pain which developed some months after lifting.

also occur when the outlet of the fourth ventricle is not inspected and a membrane is left intact.

Technical factors can also result in postoperative instability, although such problems are more commonly encountered in patients with certain comorbidities, as discussed in the section on other causes of long-term problems (see below). A potential source of instability is a laminectomy of the C 2 vertebra in addition to the usual C 1 laminectomy. In our experience, the C 2 lamina does not need to be removed, even in the rare situation when the tonsils have descended to the C 2 lamina

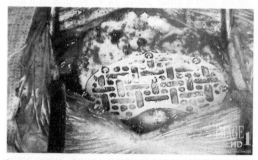

Fig. 4. Titanium plate anchored with screws to edge of prior craniectomy in a patient who developed dural ectasia following posterior fossa decompression 3 years earlier. She experienced excellent relief of headaches with sponge counter pressure, leading to a decision to perform this partial cranioplasty.

level. The cerebellar tonsils are usually sufficiently mobile to permit the tonsils to be elevated and then reduced or even resected. The large spinous process of C 2 is the site of attachment of major neck muscles and ligaments and removal thus may result in instability and kyphosis. Injury to the occiput–C1 or C1–C2 facet joints may also result in instability. *Treatment* may require an instrumented fusion of occiput to the upper cervical spine.

Other nontechnical causes of complications

Complications in this category generally fall into two distinct groups: (a) Problems related to bony structural abnormalities and (b) problems related to ligamentous abnormalities.

Problems related to bony abnormalities

Patients with Chiari anomaly should always be assessed for evidence of basilar invagination, which is associated with a greater incidence of cranio-cervical instability. Measurements of clivo-axial angle are helpful in this respect. Not all patients with basilar invagination require cranio-cervical fusion at the time of decompression, but consideration should be given to this possibility. Flexion and extension radiographs may give an indication of potential instability. Likewise, a severely retroflexed odontoid may give rise to problems. Grabb-Oakes measurements are helpful in evaluating this problem.[11] Neck flexion in this group of patients may give rise to cervical-medullary compression.

Problems related to ligamentous abnormalities

Hereditary connective tissue disorders, such as Ehlers-Danlos syndrome, have been recognized as a source of postoperative instability following posterior fossa decompression procedures.[12] Again, it is important to establish preoperatively whether there is ligamentous instability, and some patients with severe ligamentous laxity may require cranio-cervical fusion at the time of the decompression procedure.

Persistent Syringomyelia

The usual expectation is that a syrinx cavity will diminish in size following posterior fossa decompression for a Chiari abnormality. It has been our experience that the collapse of the syrinx cavity is more complete in younger patients. Presumably, tissue changes may have taken place in patients with a long-standing syrinx cavity that prevents more complete collapse. Consideration must be given to the possibility that some impediment to free CSF equilibration between the cranial and cervical compartments has occurred. This may be in the form of scar tissue, an arachnoid web, or further descent of the cerebellar tonsils. Imaging with high T 2 resolution protocols is often helpful in detecting flow obstructions.[13] It is, however, known that in some patients the reason for reexpansion of a syrinx cavity, or failure of the cavity to collapse, cannot be ascertained with presently available techniques.[14] Blood in the subarachnoid space and postoperative meningitis following decompression can also give rise to arachnoid adhesions that prevent syrinx collapse. If the persistent syrinx cavity is symptomatic and a structural cause cannot be found, shunting the syrinx cavity may be the only available option.[15]

SUMMARY

The aim of posterior fossa decompression for patients with Chiari malformation, with or without syringomyelia, is to relieve pressure on the brainstem and to restore normal pulsatile CSF flow at the craniocervical junction. There are variations in the anatomical changes that may lead to Chiari malformation resulting in a relatively small posterior fossa and minimal cisterna magna. In correcting this abnormality, it is essential to remove only as much bone as is necessary to visualize the cerebellar tonsils and to restore the CSF compartment securely with regard to water tightness and dural graft properties.

CLINICS CARE POINTS

- Cerebellar tonsillar descent may be the result of several different processes, which must be considered before a diagnosis of Chiari malformation is made.
- Great care should be taken to prevent cerebrospinal fluid leakage from the dural closure site.
- The size of the posterior fossa craniectomy should allow for direct visualization of the cerebellar tonsils, but does not need to expose the cerebellar hemispheres.
- A C 2 laminectomy is generally not required for adequate posterior fossa decompression and may lead to instability.

REFERENCES

1. Greenberg JK, Ladner TR, Olsen MA, et al. Complications and resource use associated with surgery for chiari malformation type 1 in adults: a population perspective. Neurosurgery 2015;77(2):261–8.

2. Atkinson JLD, Weinshenker BG, Miller GM, et al. Acquired Chiari I malformation secondary to spontaneous cerebrospinal fluid leakage and chronic intracranial hypotension syndrome in seven cases. J Neurosurg 1998;(88):237–42.

3. Samii C, Möbius E, Weber W, et al. PseudoChiari type I malformation secondary to cerebrospinal fluid leakage. J Neurol 1999;246:162–4.

4. Banik R, Lin D, Miller NR. Prevalence of Chiari I malformation and cerebellar ectopia in patients with pseudotumor cerebri. J Neurol Sci 2006;247(1):71–5.

5. Holly LT, Batzdorf U. Slitlike syrinx cavities: a persistent central canal. J Neurosurg Spine 2002;97:161–5.

6. Batzdorf U, McArthur DL, Bentson JR. Surgical treatment of Chiari malformation with and without syringomyelia: experience with 177 adult patients. J Neurosurg 2013;118:232–42.

7. Arnautovic A, Splavski B, Boop FA, et al. Pediatric and adult Chiari malformation Type I surgical series 1965-2013: a review of demographics, operative treatment, and outcomes. J Neurosurg Pediatr 2015;15:161–77.

8. Paré LS, Batzdorf U. Syringomyelia persistence after chiari decompression as a result of pseudomeningocele formation: implications for syrinx pathogenesis: report of three cases. Neurosurgery 1988;43(4):945–8.

9. Holly LT, Batzdorf U. Management of cerebellar ptosis following craniovertebral decompression for Chiari I malformation. J Neurosurg 2001;94:21–6.

10. Udani V, Holly LT, Chow D, et al. Posterior fossa reconstruction using titanium plate for the treatment of cerebellar ptosis after decompression for chiari malformation. World Neurosurg 2014;81(5/6):836–41.

11. Grabb PA, Mapstone TB, Oakes WJ. Ventral brain stem compression in pediatric and young adult patients with chiari I malformations. Neurosurgery 1999;44(3):520–8.

12. Milhorat TH, Bolognese PA, Nishikawa M, et al. Syndrome of occipitoatlantal hypermobility, cranial settling and Chiri malformation Type I in patients with hereditary disorders of connective tissue. J Neurosurg Spine 2007;7:601–9.

13. Heiss JD, Suffredini MS, Smith R, et al. Pathophysiology of persistent syringomyelia after decompressive craniocervical surgery. J Neurosurg Spine 2010;13:729–42.

14. Tubbs RS, Webb DB, Oakes WJ. Persistent syringomyelia following pediatric Chiari I decompression: radiological and surgical findings. J Neurosurg Pediatr 2004;100:460–4.

15. Soleman J, Roth J, Bartoli A, et al. Syringo-subarachnoid shunt for the treatment of persistent syringomyelia following decompression for chiari type I malformation: surgical results. World Neurosurg 2017;108:836–43.

Management of Ventral Brainstem Compression in Chiari Malformation Type I

Brian J. Dlouhy, MD*, Arnold H. Menezes, MD

KEYWORDS

- Chiari malformation type I (CM-I) • Ventral brainstem compression • Craniovertebral junction (CVJ)
- Osseoligamentous abnormalities • Crown halo traction • O-arm • Posterior distraction reduction
- Ventral decompression

KEY POINTS

- Ventral brainstem compression (VBC) associated with Chiari malformation type I occurs with craniovertebral junction (CVJ) osseoligamentous abnormalities.
- VBC associated with osseoligamentous abnormalities are either from direct encroachment of ventral structures or due to CVJ instability that leads to posterior displacement of ventral structures or a combination of both.
- Reducible VBC documented by flexion/extension or traction can be stabilized by posterior instrumentation and fusion.
- Crown halo traction under general anesthesia supplemented by neuromuscular blockade (under O-arm computed tomography control) in addition to intraoperative posterior distraction can provide reduction and avoid a ventral decompression in many cases. The realignment can be stabilized by posterior instrumentation and fusion.
- If completely irreducible or posterior reduction is not effective in reducing VBC, a ventral approach (transoral-transpalatal approach, transnasal endoscopic, and transcervical routes) can be effective.

INTRODUCTION

Ventral brainstem compression (VBC) associated with Chiari malformation type I (CM-I) is invariably due to osseoligamentous abnormalities of the craniovertebral junction (CVJ) that disrupt the normal architecture of the CVJ (**Box 1**).[1,2] The CVJ is composed of the occipital bone that surrounds the foramen magnum and the atlas and axis vertebra and their associated ligaments and musculature.[3] The bony anatomy, joint configuration, shape, and orientation at the CVJ are unique in comparison to the rest of the cervical spine.[4] The sophisticated arrangement of structures is critical to allow complex movements of the head and neck and to provide protection to the brainstem and cervical spinal cord. However, this complexity also creates the potential for congenital, developmental, and acquired osseoligamentous pathology.[5] This pathology can be associated with CM-I and result in VBC and instability in patients of all ages from pediatrics to adults.[1,2] Understanding the different CVJ pathology and their pathophysiology in cases of VBC in CM-I leads to a proper treatment strategy and best clinical outcomes.

OSSEOLIGAMENTOUS PATHOLOGY ASSOCIATED WITH VBC AND CM-I

Occipital Condylar Hypoplasia

The occipital condyles are convex and sit on the cup-shaped and concave superior articular

University of Iowa Hospitals & Clinics, University of Iowa Stead Family Children's Hospital, 200 Hawkins Drive, Iowa City, IA 52242, USA
* Corresponding author.
E-mail address: brian-dlouhy@uiowa.edu

Neurosurg Clin N Am 34 (2023) 119–129
https://doi.org/10.1016/j.nec.2022.08.002
1042-3680/23/© 2022 Elsevier Inc. All rights reserved.

Box 1
Osseoligamentous CVJ abnormalities associated with CM-I that cause ventral brainstem compression (VBC)

- Condylar hypoplasia
  - Can result in O-C1 instability and pannus formation
  - Can result in developmental basilar invagination (BI)
- Atlas assimilation
  - Can result in developmental BI
  - Can lead to C1-2 instability with increased atlantodental interval
  - Can lead to C1-2 instability with true BI
- C2-3 segmentation failure
  - Can lead to C1-2 instability with increased atlantodental interval
  - Can lead to C1-2 instability with true BI
- Proatlas segmentation abnormalities
- Bifid anterior and posterior atlas arch with instability
- Os odontoideum with instability
- Syndromic
  - Spondyloepiphyseal dysplasia (SED)
  - Spondylometaphyseal dysplasia (SMD)
  - Mucopolysaccharidosis VI
  - VACTERL syndrome
  - Klippel-Feil syndrome
  - Chondrodysplasia punctata
  - Osteogenesis imperfecta
  - Goldenhar's syndrome
  - Apert's syndrome
  - Robinson's syndrome

surfaces of the atlas to create the O-C1 joint, which is biomechanically important for O-C1 stability.[4] This characteristic structure (ball and cup) of the O-C1 joints limits translation and axial rotation and permits flexion-extension. Occipital condylar hypoplasia[6] is a developmental abnormality in which the occipital condyles are shorter and flatter than normal and, in some cases, results in an abnormal O-C1 joint axis angle.[7] Condylar hypoplasia is often associated with C1 superior articular surfaces that have lost the typical concave shape. Thus, the flattening and shortening of the occipital condyles result in an articulation with C1 that allows for pathologic anterior and posterior translation of the condyles on C1 with

flexion-extension. This is often seen in Down syndrome,[8] and due to the ligamentous laxity in Down syndrome, significant movement can be observed at the O-C1 joint in flexion-extension. Similar findings can also be observed in patients with CM-I.[2,9] In CM-I, condylar hypoplasia can be associated with a shorter and more horizontal clivus, clival hypoplasia, which results in platybasia, and thus, the odontoid is positioned more superiorly than normal. Together, this can lead to an acute clival-axis angle and an odontoid process that is less than 5 mm above the Chamberlain's line, resulting in developmental basilar invagination (BI).[2] Because of this bony configuration, the condylar hypoplasia and resulting BI can lead to VBC in CM-I. If enough laxity is present at O-C1 due to the flattened condyles, a pannus may also form around the clivus and dens, further worsening VBC.[9] This compression is often worse in flexion than in extension. Not all CM-I patients with condylar hypoplasia and BI will have VBC or instability and thus do not require treatment of this ventral abnormality. A complete neurologic examination and proper imaging is required. See **Fig. 1** for illustrative case.

Atlas Assimilation

Atlas assimilation (AA) or occipitalization of the atlas is the congenital fusion of the atlas with the base of the occiput due to segmentation failure.[10] AA can be associated with CM-I and a combination of other osseoligamentous CVJ abnormalities and can lead to instability, neural compression, and ischemia. Because AA prevents flexion-extension at the O-C1 joint, stress is placed on the adjacent C1-2 joint, especially during flexion-extension. Repeated flexion-extension movements over time can weaken the transverse ligament which leads to an increase in the atlantodental interval, instability, and an odontoid that causes VBC.[2] Eventually, this can lead to progressively increasing anterolisthesis of the C1 facets over the C2 facets and vertical translation of C2 through the foramen magnum and true BI.[9] AA can be associated with other CVJ abnormalities such as C2-3 segmentation failure.[9] Without movement at O-C1 and C2-3, the combination of these abnormalities creates even more stress on the C1-2 joint and greater risk of C1-2 instability, increase in the atlantodental interval, vertical C2 subluxation, true BI, and VBC. See **Fig. 2** for illustrative case.

C2-3 Segmentation Failure

C2-3 segmentation failure as discussed above is the congenital fusion of C2 and C3.[9] It can be

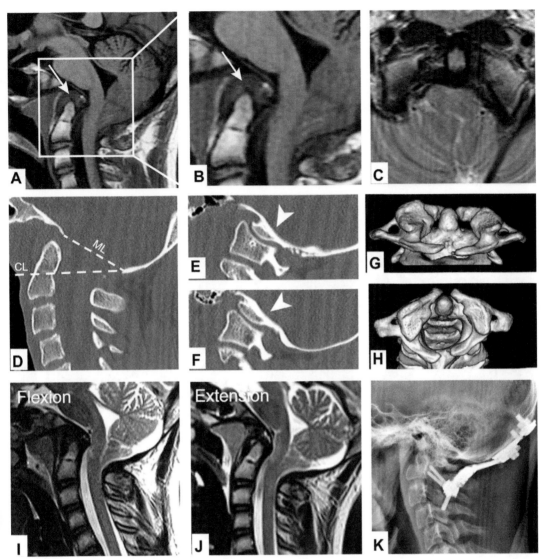

Fig. 1. Condylar hypoplasia with CM-I. A 16-year-old boy with progressive weakness and new-onset weakness of the left leg and broad-based gait with imbalance. On examination, he was found to be hyperreflexic in all 4 extremities with a Hoffman's sign on the left. (*A-C*) MRI of the CVJ revealed ventral pontomedullary junction indentation with deformation and significant brainstem compression with CM-I and tonsillar descent of 17 mm below foramen magnum (down to between C1 and C2). The fourth ventricle is slightly larger than normal with an increase in the fourth ventricle roof angle (FVRA) suggestive of outflow obstruction. The arrowhead is pointing to pannus formation around C1 and the tips of the dens suggestive of CVJ instability. (*D–H*) CT imaging revealed condylar hypoplasia (arrowheads in E and F) with bifid anterior and posterior arch of C1, a shortened clivus (clival hypoplasia), a more horizontal clivus (platybasia), and flatter C1 superior articular surfaces. All these resulted in the odontoid lying more superior than normal consistent with developmental BI. Because of these abnormalities, the clival canal angle was acute (82°), and the clivus and odontoid indented into the pontomedullary junction. (*I, J*) Flexion-extension MRI revealed slightly more ventral compression in flexion than in extension. (*K*) This patient underwent a transoral decompression and posterior extradural decompression with occipitocervical fusion. The patient had significant improvement in gait and strength in the left lower extremity. CL, Chamberlain's line; ML, McRae's line.

associated with Klippel-Feil syndrome and additional segmentation failures throughout the rest of the spine. In isolation without other segmentation failures and without a diagnosis of KFS, it

can be referred to as the Klippel-Feil abnormality.[2] By itself, it places stress on the adjacent C1-2 joint, and like AA, it can result in an increase in the atlantodental interval, vertical C2 subluxation,

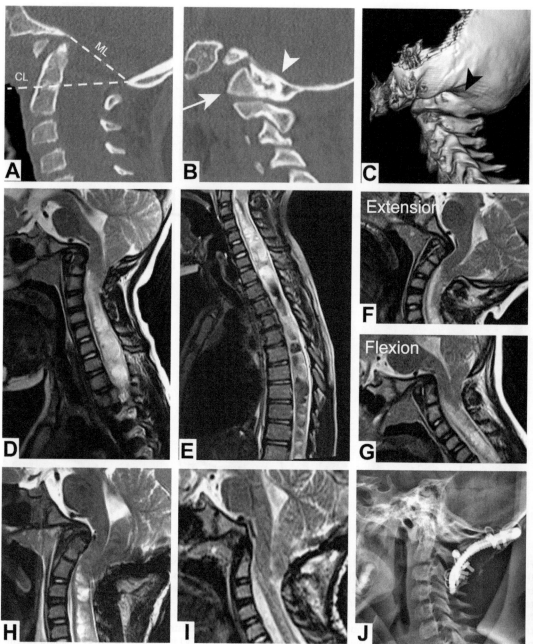

Fig. 2. Atlas assimilation with CM-I. A 5-year-old girl with progressive right arm weakness, bilateral leg weakness, gait difficulty, and imbalance with decreased reflexes in the upper extremities and increased reflexes in the lower extremities. (*A–C*) CT of the CVJ identifying atlas assimilation (AA) in which the atlas (arrow) is congenitally fused to the occiput (arrowhead). This results in the odontoid lying higher than normal and a shorter and more horizontal clivus (clival hypoplasia, platybasia). The C1 anterior arch and dens (atlantodental interval) is separated somewhat more than normal. (*D, E*) MRI of the cervicothoracic spine revealed ventral medulla indentation with deformation and brainstem compression with CM-I and tonsillar descent of 15 mm below foramen magnum (down to top of C2). The fourth ventricle is larger than normal with an increased FVRA. There is a large holocord syrinx. (*F, G*) There is more ventral indentation into the medulla on flexion than on extension with some vertical translocation of C2 as C1 slips anterior to C2. (*H*) Neutral MRI of CVJ preoperatively and (*I*) after transoral decompression and posterior fossa extradural decompression and (*J*) occipitocervical fusion. Decompression and posterior OC fusion with improvement in gait and strength in the left lower extremity. CL, Chamberlain's line; ML, McRae's line.

true BI, and VBC. Because C2-3 segmentation failure does not alter the O-C1 anatomy and joint configuration, it does not cause developmental BI. See **Fig. 3** for illustrative case.

Developmental BI versus True BI

BI most commonly occurs from condylar hypoplasia and AA but may also occur due to many other osseoligamentous abnormalities (see **Box 1**). BI has historically been defined as the odontoid process lying less than 5 mm above the Chamberlain's line.[11] However, the odontoid process can reside above that line in 2 clearly distinct ways with a different pathophysiology.[12] Computed tomography (CT) and MRI imaging have revealed that in many cases, the odontoid may not invaginate through the foramen magnum but still be less than 5 mm above the Chamberlain's line such as that observed in condylar hypoplasia or AA. In these cases, the BI is a developmental abnormality and is not due to C1-2 instability and C2 vertical subluxation through the foramen magnum as is the case with true BI. See **Figs. 1–3** for excellent examples of developmental BI. True BI occurs when stress is placed on the C1-2 joint due to CVJ abnormalities which results in C2 subluxation and an odontoid that invaginates through the foramen magnum..[13] The distinction is important as the pathophysiology between the 2 is different, and thus, treatment strategy differs.

Retroflexed Odontoid

In some patients with CM-I, the dens may be retroflexed.[14] By itself, a retroflexed odontoid will not cause instability because it is not disrupting the normal joint configurations or ligaments of the CVJ. Thus, it is not going to lead to an increase in the atlantodental interval and either type of BI. In the setting of AA or condylar hypoplasia and BI or other osseoligamentous abnormalities, a retroflexed odontoid may increase the risk and degree of VBC.[15,16] See **Fig. 3** for an illustrative case.

Other Osseoligamentous Abnormalities

Many other CVJ osseoligamentous abnormalities and genetic syndromes are associated with CM-I but much less common than those described above (see **Box 1**).[6] See **Fig. 4** for illustrative cases.

SURGICAL TREATMENT STRATEGIES

The treatment of CVJ pathology has undergone remarkable evolution and advancements over the last 100 years.[1] The factors taken into consideration are (1) the reducibility of the lesion with restoration of normal anatomic alignment and relief of neural compression; (2) the direction of encroachment on the neural structures; (3) instability; and (4) presence of Chiari malformation and syringohydromyelia.[1,2,6,17–23] Depending on the location of pathology, surgical approaches to the CVJ are divided into those that use the ventral, lateral, and posterior approaches. The transoral approaches for decompression of irreducible ventral pathology at the CVJ were a mainstay of treatment from the 1980s until the early 2000s.[1] In the last 25 years, the emergence of endoscopic endonasal approaches (EEAs) has provided more options for decompression of irreducible ventral CVJ pathology with much less

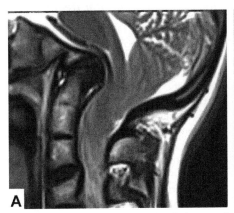
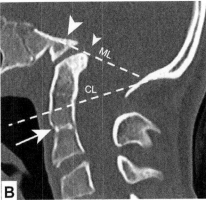

Fig. 3. Atlas assimilation, C2-3 segmentation failure, and retroflexed odontoid with CM-I. A 12-year-old girl with daily occipital headaches that radiate forward with balance difficulty, general weakness, bilateral upper and lower extremity hyperreflexia with absent gag response. (*A*) MRI of the CVJ revealing significant pontomedullary brainstem indentation with CM-I and tonsillar descent of 24 mm below foramen magnum (down to C2). Fourth ventricle is enlarged with an increase in the fourth ventricle roof angle (FVRA). (*B*) CT CVJ reveals the AA and C1 anterior arch fused to the clivus (large arrowhead). There is C2-3 segmentation failure (arrow) and a retroflexed odontoid (smaller arrowhead). Developmental BI causes severe ventral brainstem compression. CL, Chamberlain's line; ML, McRae's line.

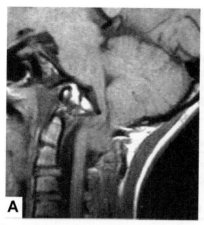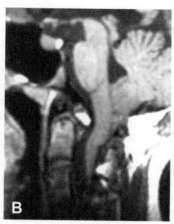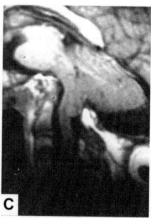

Fig. 4. Other CVJ osseoligamentous abnormalities associated with CM-I. (*A*) Proatlas segmentation abnormality, (*B*) dystopic os odontoideum, and (*C*) osteogenesis imperfecta all causing ventral brainstem compression in 3 patients with CM-I and different degrees of tonsilla herniation.

morbidity.[24] Most importantly, various posterior reduction strategies have evolved using intraoperative traction and intraoperative distraction-reduction techniques.[21,25–28] The ability to properly reduce ventral CVJ lesions and avoid a ventral approach has increased over the last 50 years due to improvements in occipitocervical instrumentation, preoperative and intraoperative imaging, and a better understanding of CVJ pathology and pathophysiology. Over the last 50 years at the University of Iowa Hospitals and Clinics, more than 7000 children and adults have been treated for wide-ranging CVJ pathology.

Clinical Presentation

Patients with CM-I and VBC may present with the classic signs and symptoms of Valsalva-induced occipital headache.[2] Because of the associated osseoligamentous CVJ abnormality causing VBC, patients will often present with signs and symptoms of brainstem dysfunction and myelopathy.[29] Brainstem dysfunction may include facial numbness, ataxia, sleep apnea, and nystagmus. Myelopathic symptoms of weakness, sensation changes, and hyperreflexia on neurologic examination may be observed. Syringomyelia may also be present complicating the clinical presentation as it may overshadow the myelopathy.[9] If the CVJ abnormality has created instability, the patient may also present with occipitocervical headache and neck pain that is relieved with lying down, neck stabilizing (placing the head against a wall or back of a chair), or cervical orthosis.

Preoperative Imaging

MRI of the brain and spine should be performed in all patients who present with CM-I to evaluate the

tonsillar herniation, rule out supratentorial masses as the actual cause of the tonsillar descent, evaluate for hydrocephalus, and assess for syringomyelia.[1,2] If VBC is observed or the typical CVJ configuration appears abnormal in MRI, a CT of the CVJ is critical for full assessment of the osseous anatomy which may not be easily identifiable on MRI.[1] In addition, a flexion-extension MRI of the cervical spine will evaluate for instability and whether reduction is obtained in extension, thus signifying that the abnormality is reducible easily with neck maneuvers and thus will be reducible with crown halo traction.[1] Obtaining upright cervical radiographs is also important to evaluate CVJ and cervical alignment.

Indications for Surgical Treatment

A proper clinical history and neurologic examination is of utmost importance in determining whether a patient is symptomatic from the CM-I or the ventral brainstem CVJ abnormality and/or instability.[2] If completely asymptomatic and no gross instability, the patient can be managed conservatively without surgical treatment. If syrinx present and asymptomatic, there should be a discussion with the patient and their family of the risks and benefits of surgical intervention versus conservative management. However, if symptomatic, one needs to determine if the ventral CVJ abnormality is the cause or part of the cause. This determination helps support the need for treatment of the CVJ abnormality.

Treatment Algorithm

The treatment of CVJ pathology has improved based on evolutions in transoral approaches and EEAs to the CVJ, better strategies to reduce and decompress neural structures by using various forms of traction and distraction-reduction techniques, and better preoperative and intraoperative imaging.[1] Incorporating the advances mentioned above, we have updated the treatment algorithm[1] here for osseoligamentous CVJ pathology that results in VBC and/or CVJ instability (occipitoatlantal instability, atlantoaxial instability, or occipitoatlantoaxial instability) with CM-I (**Fig. 5**). Although posterior reduction or ventral decompression may treat the osseoligamentous pathology, a posterior decompression is often still warranted in each case to treat the tonsillar herniation and to ensure complete brainstem decompression.[1,2] The algorithm is a general guide for CVJ pathology and should be used as such when determining the appropriate treatment strategy for each patient. The treatment strategy for each pathology does vary somewhat, and the details required for each go beyond the scope of this review.

The relief of VBC due to CVJ abnormalities in CM-I can be achieved by (1) flexion-extension MRI and evaluating whether extension assists in reduction; (2) crown halo traction in the operating room under general anesthesia with neuromuscular

blockade and documentation with O-arm; (3) intraoperative distraction with posterior instrumentation for reduction; (4) lateral joint drilling of C1 and distraction of facets using spacers in BI; and (5) lateral joint drilling, spacer placement, and compression to pivot off the spacer to pull the odontoid down in BI. This leads to improved position of the ventral bony compression which requires posterior instrumentation for stabilization and autograft and/or allograft for fusion.

Crown Halo Traction Under Anesthesia with Intraoperative CT

The ability to reduce ventral CVJ lesions and avoid a ventral approach has increased since the late 1970s due to improvements in occipitocervical instrumentation, preoperative and intraoperative imaging, and a better understanding of CVJ pathology.[1] This has resulted in a decrease in the number of cases requiring a ventral (transoral, transnasal, or transcervical) approach over the last 50 years. Bedside preoperative skeletal traction has been the most common method for reduction, but reduction may take days while the

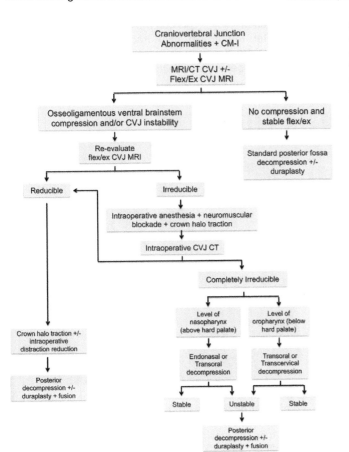

Fig. 5. Updated treatment algorithm for CVJ osseoligamentous abnormalities associated with CM-I. This is an updated treatment algorithm. The ability to use crown halo tract under general anesthesia and neuromuscular blockade with O-arm visualization and intraoperative distraction reduction has made this approach much more common than the previously used ventral decompression. Of note, a posterior fossa decompression is still used in all cases. This entails a suboccipital craniectomy, foramen magnum widening, C1 laminectomy, excision of the atlantooccipital membrane, and use of intraoperative ultrasound to verify adequate decompression. If needed, an intradural decompression and duraplasty may be required.

patient is admitted and bedbound. In children, skeletal traction often requires intubation and sedation. Being immobile and confined to the bed, in addition to the use of narcotics, sedation, and intubation, increase morbidity. Because of this morbidity, improved techniques for reduction have been developed.

We have established an intraoperative rather than preoperative approach to reduce CVJ pathology (**Fig. 6**).[21] The patient is brought to the operating room where fiberoptic intubation is performed and general anesthesia is induced. Complete neuromuscular blockade is achieved using rocuronium, and somatosensory evoked potential monitoring is used. The crown halo is applied with the patient supine, and the head is placed on a horseshoe headrest with traction (see **Fig. 6**A). Using the O-arm (Medtronic, Inc, Minneapolis, MN), an intraoperative 3D CT of the CVJ is obtained in traction, and the amount of reduction and decompression of the ventral brainstem, along with the new alignment, are all evaluated. If there is adequate reduction and decompression with the neck in proper alignment, a ventral decompression is not needed. The patient is placed prone, and another intraoperative 3D CT is obtained to verify adequate reduction, distraction of the odontoid process from the basiocciput, reduction of deformity, reduction of an increased atlantodental interval if present, reduction of O-C1 subluxation/dislocation, and an appropriate

ventral decompression. If this is satisfactory, a posterior fusion is performed to maintain the reduced and realigned position. The amount of traction can vary based on the age and weight of the patient, degree of reduction needed, and type of CVJ pathology. This approach and technique for reduction has now been used for developmental and true BI, acute and chronic rotatory subluxation in children and adults, chronic dystopic os odontoideum, and many other pathologies.

In addition to the reduction provided above, a posterior fossa suboccipital craniectomy, C1 laminectomy, and excision of the atlantooccipital membrane may still be critical to treating the tonsillar herniation.[1] The use of intraoperative ultrasound will then assist in evaluating the degree of decompression. If the tonsils remain herniated with decreased cerebrospinal fluid (CSF) flow, intradural scarring may be present,[30] and an intradural decompression and duraplasty should be performed.[31]

Posterior Distraction and Reduction

Distraction using the occipitocervical instrumentation intraoperatively for reduction has also been used.[21,25–28] This can provide further reduction after the crown halo traction described above. Distraction may be conducted using instrumentation between the occipital bone plate/screws and

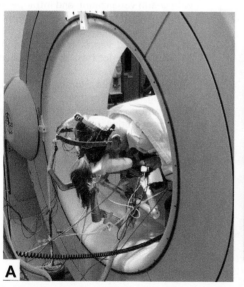
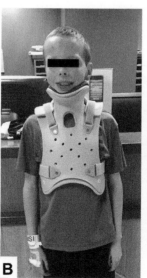
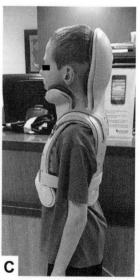

Fig. 6. Crown halo traction under general anesthesia with neuromuscular blockade and O-arm confirmation. (*A*) Crown halo tract under general anesthesia and neuromuscular blockade with O-arm visualization. If there is any reducibility, a posterior approach is used with intraoperative distraction assisting in further reduction. This approach has been much more used in the last 10 years than the previously used ventral decompression. (*B, C*) Postoperative molded Minerva is used for almost all pediatric patients, whereas a cervical orthosis is used for adults.

C1–2 vertebral instrumentation or with distraction between C-1 and C-2 when C-1 is congenitally fused with the occiput (AA) to reduce BI and bring the dens in proper position next to the anterior arch of C1 and clivus.[1,26] This is most often utilized in cases of true BI and dens invagination through foramen magnum or increased atlantodental interval and posterior displacement of the dens relative to the C1 arch. Thus, the movement of the distraction is both inferior and anterior. Others have used spacers and bone graft to distract between the joints of C-1 and C-2 to treat BI.[28] Taking advantage of the biomechanics of the CVJ, more recently others have used spacers between the joints of the CVJ to act as a pivot while compressing posteriorly between the occiput and C2 and thus reducing the dens invagination by essentially pulling the odontoid down into a more normal position in cases of BI.[27] There is no best posterior reduction method; however, the combination of the aforementioned techniques in addition to intraoperative crown halo traction under general anesthesia and neuromuscular blockade has become a much more common approach we have taken as well as others to treat ventral pathology over the last 15 years. These approaches necessitate proper reduction prior to occipitocervical fixation. Instrumentation and fixation with improper reduction and therefore persistence of ventral compression may necessitate a subsequent ventral decompressive approach. As with the above, a standard CM-I decompression should also be performed with or without intradural decompression and duraplasty depending on ultrasound findings.

Ventral Decompression

Ventral decompression via the transoral, endoscopic transnasal, or transcervical approaches has been a mainstay of treatment for VBC in the setting of CVJ osseoligamentous abnormalities.[1] The utilization of these techniques in the last 15 years has decreased significantly due to the advances in posterior reduction methods. However, developmental CVJ abnormalities that cause VBC in CM-I may be completely irreducible, thus necessitating a ventral decompression, especially in cases of CM-I with syringomyelia. Studies have shown that a ventral decompression will increase posterior fossa volume and the foramen magnum diameter.[29] Thus, it will assist in treating the tonsillar herniation and syrinx if present and increase the CSF outflow through the foramen of Magendie and foramen magnum.[29] However, it may not entirely be effective at relieving posterior compression from tonsillar herniation and CSF flow block. Most ventral decompressions should

also be stabilized posteriorly with occipitocervical fusion. While conducting the fusion, like above, we recommend also performing a standard CM-I decompression.

Postoperative Management

All patients are maintained in a cervical orthosis or molded Minerva brace postoperatively (see **Fig. 6**B, C). Follow-up imaging with MRI and CT is conducted at 6 to 12 months postoperatively to confirm adequate decompression, resolution of syrinx, and proper fusion.

CLINICS CARE POINTS

- Ventral brainstem compression associated with CM-I occurs due to osseoligamentous craniovertebral junction (CVJ) bony abnormalities.
- CVJ osseoligamentous abnormalities differ in their pathophysiology and may result in ventral brainstem compression and instability.
- Crown halo traction under general anesthesia supplemented by neuromuscular blockade (under O-arm CT control) can provide reduction. Intraoperative distraction using occipitocervical instrumentation will further reduce the abnormality.
- Ventral brainstem compression may be required in completely irreducible abnormalities. These approaches include the endoscopic transnasal, transoral, and transcervical routes.

ACKNOWLEDGMENTS

Funding providng by NIH NINDS K08 NS112573 01 A1, the Moss family, and the Carver Trust at the University of Iowa.

DISCLOSURE

The authors have nothing to disclose.

REFERENCES

1. Dlouhy BJ, Dahdaleh NS, Menezes AH. Evolution of transoral approaches, endoscopic endonasal approaches, and reduction strategies for treatment of craniovertebral junction pathology: a treatment algorithm update. Neurosurg Focus 2015;38(4):E8.

2. Fenoy AJ, Menezes AH, Fenoy KA. Craniocervical junction fusions in patients with hindbrain herniation and syringohydromyelia. J Neurosurg Spine 2008; 9(1):1–9.

3. Menezes AH, Traynelis VC. Anatomy and biomechanics of normal craniovertebral junction (a) and biomechanics of stabilization (b). Childs Nerv Syst 2008;24(10):1091–100.

4. Lopez AJ, Scheer JK, Leibl KE, et al. Anatomy and biomechanics of the craniovertebral junction. Neurosurg Focus 2015;38(4):E2.

5. Menezes AH, Vogel TW. Specific entities affecting the craniocervical region: syndromes affecting the craniocervical junction. Childs Nerv Syst 2008; 24(10):1155–63.

6. Menezes AH. Craniovertebral junction database analysis: incidence, classification, presentation, and treatment algorithms. Childs Nerv Syst 2008; 24(10):1101–8.

7. Oba H, Oda I, Takahashi J, et al. Occipitoatlantal Anteroposterior Subluxation Associated with Condylar Hypoplasia and Congenital Atlantoaxial Fusion: Clinical Correspondence. Spine Surg Relat Res 2022;6(2):185–8.

8. Hankinson TC, Anderson RC. Craniovertebral junction abnormalities in Down syndrome. Neurosurgery 2010;66(3 Suppl):32–8.

9. Menezes AH. Primary craniovertebral anomalies and the hindbrain herniation syndrome (Chiari I): data base analysis. Pediatr Neurosurg 1995;23(5): 260–9.

10. Menezes AH, Dlouhy BJ. Atlas assimilation: spectrum of associated radiographic abnormalities, clinical presentation, and management in children below 10 years. Childs Nerv Syst 2020;36(5): 975–85.

11. Chamberlain WE. Basilar Impression (Platybasia): A Bizarre Developmental Anomaly of the Occipital Bone and Upper Cervical Spine with Striking and Misleading Neurologic Manifestations. Yale J Biol Med 1939;11(5):487–96.

12. Shah A, Serchi E. Management of basilar invagination: A historical perspective. J Craniovertebral Junction Spine 2016;7:96–100.

13. Goel A. Basilar invagination, Chiari malformation, syringomyelia: a review. Neurol India 2009;57(3): 235–46.

14. Ishak B, Dhaliwal G, Rengifo R, et al. The Retroverted Dens: A Review of its Anatomy, Terminology, and Clinical Significance. World Neurosurg 2020; 137:304–9.

15. Grabb PA, Mapstone TB, Oakes WJ. Ventral brain stem compression in pediatric and young adult patients with Chiari I malformations. Neurosurgery 1999;44(3):520–7. ; discussion 527-528.

16. Salunke P, Sura S, Futane S, et al. Ventral compression in adult patients with Chiari 1 malformation sans basilar invagination: cause and management. Acta Neurochir (Wien) 2012; 154(1):147–52.

17. Menezes AH. Honored guest presentation: conception to implication: craniocervical junction database and treatment algorithm. Clin Neurosurg 2005;52: 154–62.

18. Milhorat TH, Chou MW, Trinidad EM, et al. Chiari I malformation redefined: clinical and radiographic findings for 364 symptomatic patients. Neurosurgery 1999;44(5):1005–17.

19. Menezes AH. Nosographic identification and management of pediatric craniovertebral junction anomalies: evolution of concepts and modalities of treatment. Adv Tech Stand Neurosurg 2014;40: 3–18.

20. Hankinson TC, Grunstein E, Gardner P, et al. Transnasal odontoid resection followed by posterior decompression and occipitocervical fusion in children with Chiari malformation Type I and ventral brainstem compression. J Neurosurg Pediatr 2010; 5(6):549–53.

21. Dahdaleh NS, Dlouhy BJ, Menezes AH. Application of neuromuscular blockade and intraoperative 3D imaging in the reduction of basilar invagination. J Neurosurg Pediatr 2012;9(2):119–24.

22. CreveCoeur TS, Yahanda AT, Maher CO, et al. Occipital-Cervical Fusion and Ventral Decompression in the Surgical Management of Chiari-1 Malformation and Syringomyelia: Analysis of Data From the Park-Reeves Syringomyelia Research Consortium. Neurosurgery 2021;88(2):332–41.

23. Alalade AF, Ogando-Rivas E, Forbes J, et al. A Dual Approach for the Management of Complex Craniovertebral Junction Abnormalities: Endoscopic Endonasal Odontoidectomy and Posterior Decompression with Fusion. World Neurosurg X 2019;2:100010.

24. Kassam AB, Snyderman C, Gardner P, et al. The expanded endonasal approach: a fully endoscopic transnasal approach and resection of the odontoid process: technical case report. Neurosurgery 2005;57(1 Suppl):E213. ; discussion E213.

25. Dahdaleh NS, Dlouhy BJ, Menezes AH. One-step fixation of atlantoaxial rotatory subluxation: technical note and report of three cases. World Neurosurg 2013;80(6):e391–5.

26. Hsu W, Zaidi HA, Suk I, et al. A new technique for intraoperative reduction of occipitocervical instability. Neurosurgery 2010;66(6 Suppl Operative):319–23. ; discussion 323-314.

27. Chandra PS, Prabhu M, Goyal N, et al. Distraction, Compression, Extension, and Reduction Combined With Joint Remodeling and Extra-articular Distraction: Description of 2 New Modifications for Its Application in Basilar Invagination and Atlantoaxial Dislocation: Prospective Study in 79

Cases. Neurosurgery 2015;77(1):67–80. ; discussion 80.

28. Goel A. Treatment of basilar invagination by atlantoaxial joint distraction and direct lateral mass fixation. J Neurosurg Spine 2004;1(3):281–6.

29. Menezes AH. Craniovertebral junction abnormalities with hindbrain herniation and syringomyelia: regression of syringomyelia after removal of ventral craniovertebral junction compression. J Neurosurg 2012; 116(2):301–9.

30. Dlouhy BJ, Dawson JD, Menezes AH. Intradural pathology and pathophysiology associated with Chiari I malformation in children and adults with and without syringomyelia. J Neurosurg Pediatr 2017; 20(6):526–41.

31. Dlouhy BJ, Menezes AH. Autologous cervical fascia duraplasty in 123 children and adults with Chiari malformation type I: surgical technique and complications. J Neurosurg Pediatr 2018;22(3):297–305.

Craniovertebral Junction Instability in the Setting of Chiari Malformation

Yosef M. Dastagirzada, MD[a],*, David B. Kurland, MD, PhD[a],
Todd C. Hankinson, MD[b], Richard CE. Anderson, MD[a]

KEYWORDS

- Chiari I malformation • Complex Chiari • Basilar invagination • Craniovertebral • Craniocervical
- Instability • Occipitocervical fusion

KEY POINTS

- Despite its rarity, clinicians should be cognizant of the possibility of craniovertebral junction (CVJ) instability in the setting of Chiari I malformation (CMI), as the surgical management in this situation is significantly different.
- This manuscript discusses the basic anatomy/biomechanics of the CVJ and various factors (radiographic, etiologic, and clinical) demonstrated to be associated with instability in the setting of CMI.
- In addition, the surgical techniques of CVJ stabilization, perioperative care, and outcomes are reviewed. Preoperative considerations for traction, feasibility of hardware placement, and possible ventral decompression are emphasized.
- If CVJ instability is unrecognized and not addressed, clinical outcomes are likely to be suboptimal.

INTRODUCTION

Described in the seminal paper by Hans Chiari in 1891, the Chiari I malformation (CMI) is a radiographic diagnosis commonly encountered by neurosurgeons and is often treated surgically with generally positive clinic outcomes.[1–3] Studies have documented that 1% to 4% of patients undergoing MRI of the brain or cervical spine will be diagnosed with CMI, characterized by greater than 5 mm tonsillar herniation below the foramen magnum. More recently CMI has been described as a spectrum of disease, which includes Chiari 0, Chiari 1.5, and the complex Chiari.[4–7] Primarily through multicenter clinical outcomes research, our understanding of the pathology continues to evolve, as does the drive for delineating optimal clinical management strategies and surgical treatment.

Most patients with symptomatic CMI, including those with symptoms associated with basilar invagination and syringomyelia, will improve following standard posterior fossa decompression, with or without expansile duraplasty. Although up to 80% of patients will show symptomatic improvement after posterior fossa decompression (PFD) alone,[3] clinical experience has led to the identification of more complex phenotypes of CMI that may necessitate a different surgical approach, typically requiring additional ventral decompression and/or occipitocervical stabilization. These patients typically fall into 3 main categories.

1. Patients who present with craniovertebral junction (CVJ) instability on presentation with CMI-associated symptoms (*macroinstability*).[8–12]
2. Patients who fail to improve significantly after posterior decompression alone and then develop CVJ instability (*macroinstability*).[13]
3. Patients who transiently improve after decompression but subsequently develop brainstem

[a] Department of Neurological Surgery, Hassenfeld Children's Hospital, NYU Langone Health, NY 462 1st Avenue, Suite 7S4, New York, NY 10016, USA; [b] Department of Neurological Surgery, University of Colorado School of Medicine, 13123C E16th Avenue, Box 330, Aurora, CO 80045, USA
* Corresponding author.
E-mail address: Yosef.dastagirzada@nyulangone.org

Neurosurg Clin N Am 34 (2023) 131–142
https://doi.org/10.1016/j.nec.2022.09.006
1042-3680/23/© 2022 Elsevier Inc. All rights reserved.

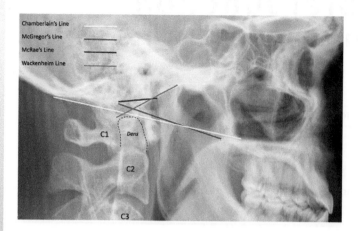

Fig. 1. Lateral radiograph with lines used to assess for basilar invagination.

compression symptoms without overt findings of CVJ instability *(potential microinstability)*.[14]

The concept of the "complex Chiari" was introduced by Brockmeyer in 2011. This concept differentiated patients by radiographic and clinical criteria as more likely to require surgical interventions beyond a standard PFD because of the higher likelihood of ventral compression and/or craniovertebral junction instability.[15] These criteria include brainstem herniation through the foramen magnum (Chiari 1.5 malformation), kinking of the medulla, retroflexed odontoid, abnormalities of the clival-cervical angle, occipitalization of C1, basilar invagination, presence of a syrinx, scoliosis, and signs and symptoms of brainstem compression.[16]

Despite the very low incidence of CVJ instability in the CMI population at large, clinicians must be aware of the important radiographic and clinical factors that are associated with various versions of Chiari malformations so the best clinical management decisions can be made. In this report, the authors (1) briefly describe the important anatomic, embryologic, and biomechanical properties of the craniovertebral junction, (2) review the radiographic and clinical parameters most commonly used to assess for CVJ instability, (3) identify different phenotypes of patients with CMI in which craniocervical stabilization is more likely to be necessary, and (4) discuss common surgical techniques for posterior decompression and stabilization with rigid internal fixation and fusion.

EMBRYOLOGY, ANATOMY, AND BIOMECHANICS OF THE CRANIOVERTEBRAL JUNCTION

The CVJ is an osteoligamentous complex that houses and protects vital neurovascular structures at the transition point between the brainstem and the spinal cord. It is composed of 2 pairs of joints, the occipitoatlantal and atlantoaxial joints—the former known to be the most stable and the latter the most mobile of all joints in the body.[17] The CVJ is of mesodermal origin (appearing in the third week of gestation), which eventually divides into somites—a transient structure with precursor cells for development of the vertebral column.[18,19]

The cuplike joint of the occipital condyles provides bony articulation with the cervical spine that is designed to permit flexion and extension of the neck while limiting excessive axial rotation.[20] The atlantoaxial joint, on the other hand, is primarily responsible for axial rotation of the neck, with limited flexion or extension. Biomechanical studies have demonstrated that these joints work in synchrony to guide these overall movements. For example, Panjabi and colleagues attributed about 23° to 25° of flexion/extension of the skull to the occipitoatlantal junction and about

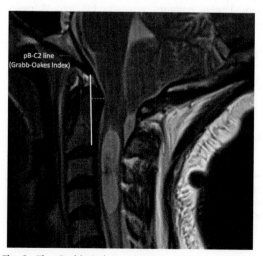

Fig. 2. The Grabb-Oakes Index (pB-C2 line).

10° to 22° to the atlantoaxial joint.[21] Their study discovered that the movement of axial rotation was found to be predominantly dictated by the atlantoaxial joint (38.9°) and less so the occipitoatlantal joint (7°).

Multiple studies have tried to ascertain the primary determinants of stability at the CVJ. At O-C1, capsular ligaments enclose the articulations. The atlantooccipital membranes connecting the foramen magnum to the anterior/posterior arches of the atlas have not been thought to contribute to the stability of the CVJ. At the C1-C2 joint, the integrity of the odontoid and the transverse ligament have long been considered primarily responsible for maintaining stability. More recent finite element models (FEM) have suggested, however, that other ligaments contribute to stabilization of the joints in the craniocervical junction.[22,23] For example, the occipitoatlantal capsular ligaments were shown to contribute significantly to the stabilization of the O-C1 joint, whereas the atlantoaxial capsular ligaments and transverse ligament were deemed primary stabilizers of the C1-2 joint.[24,25] Before the use of FEM, pediatric cervical spine biomechanics were largely assessed with adult and very limited pediatric cadaveric testing.[26] Understanding the biomechanical properties and motion of the CVJ allow for an accurate and productive conversation when counseling patients about postoperative expectations.

SCOPE OF THE PROBLEM

The incidence of asymptomatic CMI has been estimated to be 1% to 2% of the general population and among the pediatric literature, around 3.6% of brain imaging obtained.[4,5] Of those with the characteristic tonsillar descent, 32% were symptomatic and an even smaller proportion had an associated syringomyelia (0.83%) or bony anomalies (platybasia and basilar invagination, 1.8% and 4.7%) thought to potentially contribute to craniovertebral instability.[4] Descriptions of Chiari 1.5 malformations and complex Chiari malformations have also provided insights to Chiari phenotypes that have a higher risk for associated CVJ instability and may necessitate stabilization in addition to decompression. For instance, Tubbs and colleagues reported that among patients with Chiari 1.5 undergoing posterior fossa decompression, 13.6% required further decompression and unilateral tonsillar coagulation in light of persistent syringomyelia and progressive scoliosis.[27] Furthermore, Bollo and colleagues described in 2012 that basilar invagination, Chiari 1.5, and a clivoaxial angle (CXA) less than 125° are high-risk

indicators of patients necessitating future occipitocervical fusion.[28] Based on this work, the combination of brainstem herniation through the foramen magnum (CM1.5), retroflexed odontoid, medullary kink, abnormal clival-cervical angle, occipitalization of the atlas, basilar invagination (BI), syringomyelia, and scoliosis has been labeled as "complex Chiari malformation." Further work by Brockmeyer's group has demonstrated that patients with complex Chiari malformation with a CXA less than 125° are 11.3 times more likely to fail a standard posterior decompression and require posterior stabilization.[29] The complex Chiari population has been extensively analyzed, and specific radiographic parameters to identify this cohort have been created, along with management algorithms for consideration of occipitocervical fusion (OCF) and endoscopic transnasal odontoidectomy.[16,29]

RADIOGRAPHIC, ETIOLOGIC, AND CLINICAL FACTORS ASSOCIATED WITH CHIARI/ CRANIOVERTEBRAL JUNCTION INSTABILITY

Defining CVJ instability among patients with CMI is often challenging. Although some clinical management algorithms have been created to help guide surgeons, specific indications for CVJ stabilization are lacking and significant clinical equipoise remains. The distinction between vertical and translational instability is important to make on initial assessment. The former is more common among the Chiari population and is typically diagnosed on traditional craniocervical imaging (eg, basilar invagination, CXA <125°, and so forth). On the other hand, translational instability is a finding seen on dynamic imaging that is more typical of traumatic or different congenital disorders (eg, Down syndrome). Here the authors describe the clinical and radiographic findings associated with CVJ instability in the setting of CMI.

Prevalence of Craniovertebral Junction Instability with Chiari I Malformation

Overall, among surgical patients with CMI and syrinx, the prevalence of coexisting CVJ instability is extremely low. In a multicenter study of 637 patients who underwent posterior fossa decompression for CMI and syrinx, only 1.9% went on to have OCF for instability.[30]

Radiographic Findings Among Patients with Chiari I Malformation with Craniovertebral Junction Instability

Unfortunately, there are no radiographic findings that are present in all patients with CMI with CVJ instability. However, several measurements have been reported to help define patients with CMI with a higher likelihood of instability requiring stabilization. The presence of various techniques has the potential to lead to inconsistency in the assessment of instability, and no standard measurement has been established. The reported incidence of bony anomalies associated with the CMI has been estimated to affect about 7% to 11% of patients[31]; this is likely an overestimate due to practice patterns from single centers including Brockmeyer, Menezes, Goel, and others.[16,31,32] Certain osseous abnormalities are associated with a higher incidence of CVJ instability and are critical to identify in the preoperative workup, as they may be indicators of potential instability (**Table 1**).

Basilar invagination

Although dynamic imaging with computed tomography (CT) and MRI has become increasingly important, CVJ instability due to basilar invagination was initially diagnosed with plain radiographs and static imaging. Basilar invagination is among the most common findings in patients with CMI with CVJ instability.[10,12,34,35,38–45] It is defined as a developmental anomaly in which the odontoid prolapses into the foramen magnum and is distinguished from basilar impression, an acquired form as a result of skull base bony softening (ie, Paget disease, osteogenesis imperfecta, and so forth).[34] Basilar invagination has the potential to be associated with cerebrospinal fluid (CSF) obstruction, ventral brainstem compression, vertebrobasilar insufficiency, reduction of the posterior fossa cranial volume, and compromised spinal cord/medulla. Historically, the imaging parameters (Chamberlain, McGregor, McRae, and Wackenheims lines) used to evaluate for this abnormality were measured on lateral skull radiographs but they have been also validated on CT imaging (**Fig. 1**).[45,46] **Table 2** further explains these lines and the numerical parameters that indicate basilar invagination. In a series of patients with CMI, all patients with basilar invagination required eventual occipitocervical fusion; these patients were 10x more likely to require surgical fusion than their counterparts.[28]

Ventral brainstem compression

Grabb and colleagues reported the pB-C2 line (Grabb-Oakes Index) in 1999,[33] which defined a parameter to assess for ventral brainstem compression in patients with CMI (**Fig. 2**). Specifically, the line identified patients who had symptomatic ventral compression without the

Table 1
Osseous abnormalities associated with Chiari I malformation and craniovertebral junction instability

Abnormality	Definition
Retroflexed odontoid process	Odontoid process is angled toward the brainstem, can use pBC2 distance (>9 mm)[33]
Basilar invagination	Prolapse of odontoid into the foramen magnum[34]
Occipital condyle hypoplasia	Flattening of the condyles with elevation of the atlas-axis
Platybasia	Flattening of the skull base (Welcher basal angle >140°)[35]
Proatlas segmentation failures	Embryologic failure of segmentation (somite > vertebra); can affect foramen magnum, occipital condyles, cruciate/alar ligaments, lateral atlantal masses, posterior arch of atlas[36]
Basioccipital/clivus hypoplasia	Shortened clivus, associated with CHARGE syndrome[37]
Atlas assimilation	Partial or complete congenital fusion of the atlas with occiput

presence of basilar invagination. The line is defined as the perpendicular distance from the posterior dens or soft tissue to a line connecting the basion (most caudal point of the clivus) to the inferoposterior aspect of the C2 vertebral body. Although based on only a few cases, the investigators reported that patients who had a distance greater than 9 mm were at increased risk to fail a standard posterior decompression and require ventral decompression.

Since then, others have investigated additional associations and have outlined mixed results regarding its application for risk stratification. Bollo found 74% of patients with CMI who required CVJ fusion met the original pB-C2 parameter (>9 mm) but this was associated with CVJ instability only on univariate analysis and not multivariate.[28] More recently, using the Park-Reeves

Table 2
Radiographic lines used to assess for basilar invagination

Line	Landmarks	Basilar Invagination is Considered if...
Chamberlains	Hard palate to opisthion	Odontoid tip >5 mm above line
McGregor	Hard palate to most caudal part of occipital bone	Odontoid tip >7 mm above line
McRae's	Basion to opisthion (AP diameter of foramen magnum)	Odontoid tip is above line
Wackenheims (clivus canal line)	Along the clivus, extending into cervical canal	Odontoid tip transects line

Syringomyelia Research Consortium database, Hankinson and colleagues reported an intraclass correlation coefficient of 0.72 to 0.76, indicating a strong agreement of measuring the pB-C2 parameter among multiple observers and various imaging modalities (T1-weighted MRI and CT).[47] Furthermore, pB-C2 has been reported as a strong indicator of Chiari-related scoliosis progression.[48]

A more recently described radiographic parameter to evaluate the need for potential occipitocervical fusion or ventral brainstem decompression among patients with CMI is the occipital condyle-C2 sagittal vertical alignment (C-C2SVA).[49] The investigators describe using more of a deformity and global alignment lens when assessing the role of the occipitocervical joint position (C0-C1) to the load bearing structures (C2-3 disc space). The C-C2SVA is delineated by the following steps (**Fig. 3**): (1) draw a line parallel to the C2 inferior endplate (on midline MR sequence, *blue line*), (2) identify and mark the midpoint of the C0-1 joint on a parasagittal MRI (*green star*), (3) using the joint reference point, draw a perpendicular line (*red arrow*) to the C2 horizontal line (*blue line*), (4) measure the distance from the posterior aspect of the C2-3 disc space to the plumb line (mm, *orange dashed line*). After measuring the C-C2SVA in 60 patients with CM1, the parameter was discovered to be potentially helpful as a screening tool given the 100% sensitivity and 74% specificity in recognizing patients needing ventral decompression-occipitocervical fusion (C-C2SVA ≥ 5 mm).[49] The advantage of this measurement over the pB-C2 is that it accounts for craniocervical load-bearing roles as well as overall craniocervical alignment. Furthermore, the study identified a strong Pearson correlation coefficient as well as substantial agreement on interrater reliability testing. Given the rarity of the pathology and the single-institution nature of this investigation, a Park-Reeves study was done as a follow-up in 206 patients among multiple centers and external cohorts. The results from this study, including

more than 36 participating centers and a registry of more than 1200, validated the use of the parameter with 100% sensitivity, 86% specificity, and a 12.6% misclassification rate.[50] Lastly, because this was found to be a potential screening tool for identifying higher risk patients with CMI needing stabilization, the investigators recommend using the CXA less than 125° as a confirmatory measurement.

Craniocervical angulation

The CXA—normally varying from 144° in flexion to 170° in extension—has been recognized as an important parameter for assessing the degree of craniocervical angulation and the subsequent risk of brainstem deformity and/or craniovertebral instability among patients with CMI.[51] The angle is formed by a line drawn along the clivus into the cervical canal and a line drawn along the posterior side of the axis (**Fig. 4**).[52] As mentioned earlier, a kyphotic CXA (<125°) has been associated with the increased risk of CVJ instability but there has been no universally accepted cutoff for this measurement. In 1983, Nagashima and Kubota advocated for surgical correction of CXA in cases less than 130°, as these patients were more prone to ventral brainstem compression.[53] Van Gilder reported that angles less than 150 were associated with neurologic compromise.[54] The multicenter, Park-Reeves Syringomyelia Research consortium has also identified the CXA to be significantly lower among patients with CMI requiring occipitocervical fusion ± ventral decompression in comparison to those with PFD only.[30] On the contrary, surgical outcome data have shown that a preoperative CXA greater than 135° can be an independent predictor for favorable outcomes after posterior fossa decompression alone among patients with CMI.[55] Deformative stress at multiple neuroanatomic levels (corticospinal tracts, dorsal columns, nucleus solitarius, and dorsal motor nucleus) in conjunction with axonal stretch injury have been thought to be major

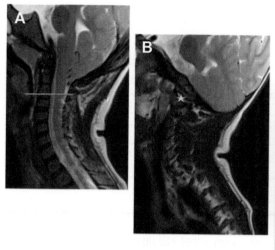
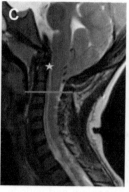
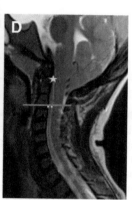

Fig. 3. Steps to measuring the C-C2SVA.

contributors to morbidity in patients with a kyphotic CXA.[56] The contemporary development of the SCOSIA (Spinal Cord Stress Injury Analysis) technology—using finite element analysis—quantifies the neuraxial stress at various levels in cases of abnormal CXA and has found positive associations with disability and Karnofsky scores after its surgical correction.[57]

Etiologic associations

Genetic syndromes may also present with CMI and/or CVJ instability, as numerous heritable disorders are known to predispose patients to musculoligamentous instability (**Box 1**). Hereditary disorders of connective tissue (HDCT) including Ehlers-Danlos and Marfan syndrome have joint hypermobility as a defining feature and have been associated with hyperlaxity of the

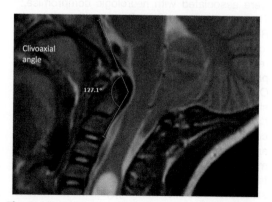

Fig. 4. Measurement of the clivoaxial angle.

occipitoatlantal and atlantoaxial joints; interestingly, both are mesodermal disorders.[58] Milhorat and colleagues noted a 12.7% coincidence with CMI with HDCT, of which Ehlers-Danlos was the most common disorder.[38]

Clinical Findings

Given the low prevalence of coexisting CVJ instability and CMI, it is difficult to define a universal clinical picture among these patients. Furthermore, the symptoms commonly seen are often not distinct from patients with CMI alone (with or without associated syringomyelia). Although much of the data reported in the literature are skewed by single-center, unique practice patterns, increasing publications from multicenter registries including the Park Reeves Syringomyelia Research Consortium are helping to generalize reported findings.

Headache and neck pain are the most common symptoms among children with CVJ abnormalities, accounting for up to 85% of children with CVJ instability.[60] Basilar migraine has also been described due to compression of the medulla from basilar invagination. Furthermore, among 2000 children with CVJ abnormalities, myelopathy was the most common neurologic deficit, and hearing loss was the most common cranial nerve deficit.[60] Other symptoms and signs include nystagmus, hyperreflexia, dysphagia, ataxia, dysmetria, sensory dysfunction (posterior columns), and bowel/bladder dysfunction.[39] Among the Fenoy series, a decreased gag reflex was

---

Box 1
Genetic syndromes associated with craniovertebral junction instability[8,59]

Ehlers-Danlos syndrome

    Marfan syndrome

    Down syndrome

    VACTERL

    Klippel-Feil syndrome

    Achondroplasia

    Down syndrome

    Osteogenesis imperfecta

    Skeletal dysplasia

    Goldenhar syndrome

    Crouzon syndrome

    Conradi syndrome

    Morquio syndrome

    Hurler syndrome

    Noonan syndrome

    Kniest syndrome

---

appreciated in up to 39% of patients.[8] Gait instability, dysphagia, and weak neck rotation were found to be statistically greater in patients with CMI requiring occipitocervical fusions among a multicenter study of the Park-Reeves Syringomyelia Research Consortium.[30] In regard to the acuity of symptom presentation, Goel and colleagues found that symptoms in patients with basilar invagination and CMI were typically long-standing and progressive as opposed to acute courses in those with basilar invagination without CMI.[32(p190)]

SURGICAL TECHNIQUE

Surgical goals for patients with CMI and coexisting CVJ instability are to relieve compression and stabilize the craniovertebral junction. Although there is no universally accepted treatment for this study population, likely as a result of the various CVJ abnormalities and low prevalence, investigators have created helpful algorithms for the various pathologies and presentations (**Fig. 5**).

Preoperative Planning

Patients with symptomatic CMI and CVJ instability (defined by one or multiple of the aforementioned radiographic parameters) who are being evaluated for surgical intervention should get a brain and total spine MRI as well as dynamic cervical spine radiographs. If a patient is to undergo rigid instrumentation and fusion, CT is recommended with fine-cuts and reconstructions for feasibility and technical details (screw length, width, location, and so forth) of screw placement and evaluation of the vertebral artery course. CT is especially important in patients with genetic syndromes as it can identify dysplastic cervical bony anatomy.

For patients with basilar invagination and symptomatic ventral brainstem compression, a trial of halo traction should be considered. Using a modified Delphi Method, best practice guidelines have been created for the use of halo gravity traction in both pediatric spinal deformity and pediatric cervical trauma/deformity.[61,62] Although the process can be quite difficult and uncomfortable for pediatric patients, it is important to establish reducibility and potentially avoid the need for an additional anterior approach for ventral decompression. The number of halo pins and torque are based on the patients age, with serial radiographs obtained to evaluate for migration of the odontoid process out of the foramen magnum. Further details and technical indications can be found in a prior Delphi study.[61]

Preparation and Positioning

Communication with the anesthesia team is germane to obtaining safe outcomes in these cases. Awake fiber-optic intubation is generally recommended for cases of CMI and CVJ instability undergoing surgical correction in hopes of minimizing risk of acute injury to the spinal cord/cervicomedullary junction. Neuromonitoring with brainstem auditory evoked potentials and motor-evoked potentials are routinely used, and preposition baseline recordings are obtained to evaluate for changes during positioning. After placing the patient prone on gel pads, the head is fixated into a Mayfield skull clamp or with continuation of cervical traction. A lateral fluoroscopic image is subsequently obtained to assess for alignment before incision. Posterior iliac crest bone (children older than 3 years) or rib graft for autograft bone can be considered and draped accordingly.

Surgical Approach

Regarding the aforementioned surgical algorithms that have previously been created, many advocate for posterior midline approaches for most of the patients with symptomatic CMI and CVJ instability. Klekamp demonstrated positive long-term outcomes after posterior decompression and fusion for a very specific group of patients with CM1 and basilar invagination.[46] More specifically, PFD alone was used for cases without CVJ instability or ventral brainstem compression, regardless

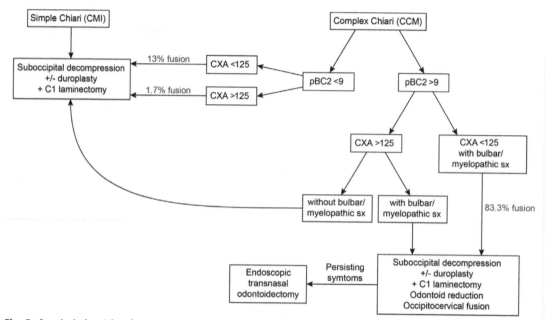

Fig. 5. Surgical algorithm for patients with complex Chiari[16]

of the presence of basilar invagination. Fusion would be added to a standard PFD in any other cases, and transoral decompression was used for patients presenting with cranial nerve deficits. Menezes has developed management algorithms for when to use anterior, posterior, or combined approaches for this specific patient population; anterior transoral approaches are reserved for irreducible cases and always followed by posterior stabilization with a morbidity of approximately 2.6%.[47,63] That being said, the transoral approach has the disadvantages of dysphagia and need for postoperative intubation/nasogastric tube; this has led to the popularization of transnasal approaches for odontoidectomy when needed. Others have advocated avoiding anterior approaches by using preoperative traction or intraoperative cervical distraction and extension to facilitate occipitocervical fusion after posterior fossa decompression.

The posterior midline approach allows for a direct approach to decompressing the foramen magnum and stabilizing the CVJ, specifically the occiput to atlas (O-C2). A skin incision is initially made from the inion to the spinous process of C2. Using midline avascular dissection, a subperiosteal dissection is used to expose the occiput, foramen magnum, the C1 posterior arch, and the C2 spinous process/lamina (without exposing the C2-3 joint to prevent unintended fusion). A standard posterior fossa decompression (suboccipital craniectomy and C1 laminectomy) is now performed with strong consideration of integrating an expansile duraplasty to minimize recurrence.

Ultrasound can be used as an important tool, as it can guide assessment of adequate decompression by locating the caudal end of the tonsils and establishing pulsatile flow of CSF through the foramen magnum. Bond and colleagues have noted that the use of intraoperative imaging (ultrasound or intraoperative MRI) may be limited by flow at the foramen magnum that can change significantly based on patient positioning.[64]

After an adequate decompression has been established (first surgical goal), craniovertebral fixation is addressed (second surgical goal). Using the preoperative imaging, notably the fine-cut CT of the cervical spine, the instrumentation construct must be determined. The most common fixation points are C1 lateral mass screws and C2 pars or pedicle screws. The sagittal and axial CT cuts are helpful in assessing the feasibility of C2 pars and pedicle screws, respectively. Fluoroscopy or intraoperative navigation can be used to place atlantoaxial screws, and a midline occipital plate is subsequently placed using midline screws in the occipital keel, approximately 1 cm above the craniectomy site. Rods are then sized, cut, and bent to size with placement of set screws. If a structural autograft is being used (rib or iliac crest), one can size it between the occipital plate and the superior edge of the C2 spinous process. Titanium cables are typically used to secure the graft. Cortical bony drilling is then performed to increase bony fusion surface area. Meticulous hemostasis is achieved, and the muscle, fascia, and subcutaneous tissues are closed in layers. Drains are not typically left in and are used at the discretion of the surgeon.

Surgical complications to be aware of include vertebral artery injury (more prevalent with C1-C2 transarticular screws in comparison to C2 pedicle screws),[65] screw violation of the spinal canal, dural tears, wound infection, CSF leak, graft site hematoma, and pseudoarthrosis.

Surgical Outcome Data

Historically, the surgical literature regarding occipitocervical fixation revolved around traumatic and congenital causes and described results following wiring-based stabilization. During the early 1990s, the Brooks-type fusion was commonly used[66]; this included bilateral sublaminar wires with an interlaminar bicortical bone and carried an approximately 80% success rate. However, contemporary pediatric spine data have shown that rigid fixation with structural autografts provides the best fixation rates.[67–69] Wiring/graft techniques were favored for younger patients given their bony anatomy, but investigators have described successful screw-rod constructs in patients as young as 15 to 18 months.[68,70,71] Hwang and colleagues reported a fusion rate of 99% after 3 months among a systematic review of 287 patients.[72] Furthermore, autograft as the bone substrate and occiput inclusion have been associated with higher fusion rates.[73] Patient-reported outcomes and health-related quality of life data have also established acceptable parameters in the pediatric population after occipitocervical fusion as well as preserved neurologic function.[74]

Postoperative Care

Patients are typically brought to the intensive care unit postoperatively for close neuromonitoring. Antibiotics are continued for 24 hours postoperatively, and pain control regimens include scheduled acetaminophen, ketorolac, and diazepam with opioids (morphine, Dilaudid, and so forth) for breakthrough pain. Patient-controlled analgesia pumps are not typically used but can be used for patients with refractory pain. Early mobilization (postoperative day 1) is encouraged with the physical therapy team. Effective transition to oral pain medication occurs at 24 to 48 hours in preparation for discharge. Hard cervical collars are used when upright and ambulating for approximately 6 to 8 weeks, and standing anteroposterior/lateral radiographs with flexion/extension views are obtained at 3-, 6-, and 12-month intervals to assess for hardware competency, fusion evaluation, and adjacent segment disease.

DISCUSSION

The CMI, characterized as tonsillar descent below the foramen magnum, is commonly discovered incidentally in asymptomatic patients. When patients with CMI present with, or develop symptoms, standard posterior fossa decompression with or without expansile duraplasty is a safe, effective surgical option that confers a high rate of clinical improvement. Infrequently, patients with symptomatic CMI present with concurrent craniovertebral junction instability.

Recent efforts have described radiographic and clinical criteria that define a spectrum of CMI phenotypes that may predispose to CVJ instability requiring stabilization along with PFD. Radiographically, the pBC2 and CXA parameters seem to be the most robust indicators of high-risk CMI, and abnormal values should engender caution to proceed with PFD alone. Several genetic syndromes predispose to musculoligamentous laxity and CMI, and when evaluating these patients, clinicians should have a high index of suspicion for coincident CVJ instability. In addition, more pronounced bulbar and myelopathic symptoms on presentation or follow-up should raise concern for the presence of micro- and/or macroinstability.

A surgical algorithm for patients with complex CMI has been developed to aid in decision-making, which incorporates the aforementioned criteria. Preoperative considerations for traction, feasibility of hardware placement, and need for ventral decompression are paramount. Multicenter studies are currently ongoing to determine the factors associated with successful outcomes in pediatric patients undergoing OCF, although modern constructs commonly include occipital plating with segmental instrumentation and autograft. Immobilization in a hard cervical collar is typically recommended postoperatively, and patient-reported outcomes are generally good.

CLINICS CARE POINTS

- Understanding the biomechanical properties and normal motion at the CVJ allow a greater understanding of abnormal pathologies and instability.
- Descriptions of atypical Chiari malformations (Chiari 1.5, complex Chiari, and so forth) have provided insights to Chiari phenotypes that have a higher risk for associated CVJ instability and may necessitate stabilization in addition to decompression.

- Osseous craniocervical abnormalities (retroflexed odontoid process, basilar invagination, platybasia, and so forth) often raise suspicion for CVJ instability among patients with CM1.

- Radiographic measurements including the Grabb-Oakes Index (pB-C2 line), CXA, and the occipital condyle-C2 sagittal vertical alignment (C-C2SVA), can help physicians to make decisions whether to include craniocervical arthrodesis in surgical management.

- Surgical goals for patients with CMI and coexisting CVJ instability are to relieve compression and stabilize the craniovertebral junction.

DISCLOSURE

The authors have nothing to disclose.

REFERENCES

1. Chiari H. Ueber veränderungen des kleinhirns infolge von hydrocephalie des grosshirns1. Dmwdtsch Med Wochenschr 1891;17(42):1172–5.

2. Carmel PW, Markesbery WR. Early descriptions of the Arnold-Chiari malformation: the contribution of John Cleland. J Neurosurg 1972;37(5):543–7.

3. Tubbs RS, Beckman J, Naftel RP, et al. Institutional experience with 500 cases of surgically treated pediatric Chiari malformation Type I. J Neurosurg Pediatr 2011;7(3):248–56.

4. Meadows J, Kraut M, Guarnieri M, et al. Asymptomatic Chiari Type I malformations identified on magnetic resonance imaging. J Neurosurg 2000;92(6):920–6.

5. Strahle J, MuraSzKo KM, Kapurch J, et al. Chiari malformation Type I and syrinx in children undergoing magnetic resonance imaging. J Neurosurg Pediatr 2011;8(2):205–13.

6. Albright AL, Pollack IF, Andelson PD. Principles and Practice of Pediatric Neurosurgery. Thieme 2015; 217–33.

7. Tubbs RS, Elton S, Grabb P, et al. Analysis of the posterior fossa in children with the Chiari 0 malformation. Neurosurgery 2001;48(5):1050–5.

8. Fenoy AJ, Menezes AH, Fenoy KA. Craniocervical junction fusions in patients with hindbrain herniation and syringohydromyelia. J Neurosurg Spine 2008; 9(1):1–9.

9. Nishikawa M, Ohata K, Baba M, et al. Chiari I malformation associated with ventral compression and instability: one-stage posterior decompression and fusion with a new instrumentation technique. Neurosurgery 2004;54(6):1430–5.

10. Kim LJ, Rekate HL, Klopfenstein JD, et al. Treatment of basilar invagination associated with Chiari I

malformations in the pediatric population: cervical reduction and posterior occipitocervical fusion. J Neurosurg Pediatr 2004;101(2):189–95.

11. Bonney PA, Maurer AJ, Cheema AA, et al. Clinical significance of changes in pB–C2 distance in patients with Chiari type I malformations following posterior fossa decompression: A single-institution experience. J Neurosurg Pediatr 2016;17(3):336–42.

12. Ridder T, Anderson RC, Hankinson TC. Ventral decompression in Chiari malformation, basilar invagination, and related disorders. Neurosurg Clin 2015;26(4):571–8.

13. Klekamp J. Neurological deterioration after foramen magnum decompression for Chiari malformation type I: old or new pathology? J Neurosurg Pediatr 2012;10(6):538–47.

14. Sunshine KS, Elder TA, Tomei KL. Noninvasive evaluation of craniovertebral junction instability in 2 patients following Chiari decompression with rigid C-collar immobilization: illustrative cases. J Neurosurg Case Lessons 2021;1(6).

15. Brockmeyer DL. The complex Chiari: issues and management strategies. Neurol Sci 2011;32(3): 345–7.

16. Brockmeyer DL, Spader HS. Complex Chiari malformations in children: diagnosis and management. Neurosurg Clin 2015;26(4):555–60.

17. Goel A. Craniovertebral junction instability: a review of facts about facets. Asian Spine J 2015;9(4):636.

18. Offiah CE, Day E. The craniocervical junction: embryology, anatomy, biomechanics and imaging in blunt trauma. Insights Imaging 2017;8(1):29–47.

19. Gilbert SF. Developmental biology. Sunderland, MA: Sinauer Associates, Inc; 2000. p. 301–5.

20. Noble ER, Smoker WR. The forgotten condyle: the appearance, morphology, and classification of occipital condyle fractures. Am J Neuroradiol 1996; 17(3):507–13.

21. Panjabi M, Dvorak J, Duranceau J, et al. Three-dimensional movements of the upper cervical spine. Spine 1976;613:726–30.

22. Finley SM, Astin JH, Joyce E, et al. FEBio finite element model of a pediatric cervical spine. J Neurosurg Pediatr 2021;1(aop):1–7.

23. Phuntsok R, Mazur MD, Ellis BJ, et al. Development and initial evaluation of a finite element model of the pediatric craniocervical junction. J Neurosurg Pediatr 2016;17(4):497–503.

24. Phuntsok R, Provost CW, Dailey AT, et al. The atlantoaxial capsular ligaments and transverse ligament are the primary stabilizers of the atlantoaxial joint in the craniocervical junction: a finite element analysis. J Neurosurg Spine 2019;31(4):501–7.

25. Phuntsok R, Ellis BJ, Herron MR, et al. The occipitoatlantal capsular ligaments are the primary stabilizers of the occipitoatlantal joint in the

craniocervical junction: a finite element analysis. J Neurosurg Spine 2019;30(5):593–601.

26. Luck JF, Nightingale RW, Song Y, et al. Tensile failure properties of the perinatal, neonatal, and pediatric cadaveric cervical spine. Spine 2013;38(1):E1–12.

27. Tubbs RS, Iskandar BJ, Bartolucci AA, et al. A critical analysis of the Chiari 1.5 malformation. J Neurosurg Pediatr 2004;101(2):179–83.

28. Bollo RJ, Riva-Cambrin J, Brockmeyer MM, et al. Complex Chiari malformations in children: an analysis of preoperative risk factors for occipitocervical fusion. J Neurosurg Pediatr 2012;10(2):134–41.

29. Ho WS, Brockmeyer DL. Complex Chiari malformation: using craniovertebral junction metrics to guide treatment. Childs Nerv Syst 2019;35(10):1847–51.

30. CreveCoeur TS, Yahanda AT, Maher CO, et al. Occipital-cervical fusion and ventral decompression in the surgical management of Chiari-1 malformation and syringomyelia: analysis of data from the Park-Reeves Syringomyelia Research Consortium. Neurosurgery 2021;88(2):332–41.

31. Menezes AH. Associated Bony Malformations and Instability in the Chiari I Malformation. In: The Chiari malformations. New York, NY: Springer; 2013. p. 181–9.

32. Goel A, Bhatjiwale M, Desai K. Basilar invagination: a study based on 190 surgically treated patients. J Neurosurg 1998;88(6):962–8.

33. Grabb PA, Mapstone TB, Oakes WJ. Ventral brain stem compression in pediatric and young adult patients with Chiari I malformations. Neurosurgery 1999;44(3):520–7.

34. Smith JS, Shaffrey CI, Abel MF, et al. Basilar invagination. Neurosurgery 2010;66(suppl_3):A39–47.

35. Pinter NK, McVige J, Mechtler L. Basilar invagination, basilar impression, and platybasia: clinical and imaging aspects. Curr Pain Headache Rep 2016;20(8):1–8.

36. Muhleman M, Charran O, Matusz P, et al. The proatlas: a comprehensive review with clinical implications. Childs Nerv Syst 2012;28(3):349–56.

37. Fujita K, Aida N, Asakura Y, et al. Abnormal basiocciput development in CHARGE syndrome. Am J Neuroradiol 2009;30(3):629–34.

38. Milhorat TH, Bolognese PA, Nishikawa M, et al. Syndrome of occipitoatlantoaxial hypermobility, cranial settling, and chiari malformation type I in patients with hereditary disorders of connective tissue. J Neurosurg Spine 2007;7(6):601–9.

39. Liao C, Visocchi M, Zhang W, et al. The relationship between basilar invagination and Chiari malformation type I: a narrative review. New Trends Craniovertebral Junction Surg 2019;125:111–8. Published online.

40. Kyoshima K, Kakizawa Y, Tokushige K, et al. Odontoid compression of the brainstem without basilar impression—"odontoid invagination. J Clin Neurosci 2005;12(5):565–9.

41. Wang S, Huang Z, Xu R, et al. Chiari Malformations Type I without Basilar Invagination in Adults: Morphometric and Volumetric Analysis. World Neurosurg 2020;143:e640–7.

42. Goel A, Jain S, Shah A. Radiological evaluation of 510 cases of basilar invagination with evidence of atlantoaxial instability (Group A basilar invagination). World Neurosurg 2018;110:533–43.

43. Song GC, Cho KS, Yoo DS, et al. Surgical treatment of craniovertebral junction instability: clinical outcomes and effectiveness in personal experience. J Korean Neurosurg Soc 2010;48(1):37.

44. Pindrik J, Johnston JM. Clinical presentation of Chiari I malformation and syringomyelia in children. Neurosurg Clin 2015;26(4):509–14.

45. Milhorat TH, Chou MW, Trinidad EM, et al. Chiari I malformation redefined: clinical and radiographic findings for 364 symptomatic patients. Neurosurgery 1999;44(5):1005–17.

46. Klekamp J. Chiari I malformation with and without basilar invagination: a comparative study. Neurosurg Focus 2015;38(4):E12.

47. Hankinson TC, Tuite GF, Moscoso DI, et al. Analysis and interrater reliability of pB-C2 using MRI and CT: data from the Park-Reeves Syringomyelia Research Consortium on behalf of the Pediatric Craniocervical Society. J Neurosurg Pediatr 2017;20(2):170–5.

48. Ravindra VM, Onwuzulike K, Heller RS, et al. Chiari-related scoliosis: a single-center experience with long-term radiographic follow-up and relationship to deformity correction. J Neurosurg Pediatr 2017;21(2):185–9.

49. Ravindra VM, Iyer RR, Awad AW, et al. Defining the role of the condylar–C2 sagittal vertical alignment in Chiari malformation type I. J Neurosurg Pediatr 2020;26(4):439–44.

50. Ravindra VM, Iyer RR, Yahanda AT, et al. A multicenter validation of the condylar–C2 sagittal vertical alignment in Chiari malformation type I: a study using the Park-Reeves Syringomyelia Research Consortium. J Neurosurg Pediatr 2021;1(aop):1–7.

51. Sayah A, Farley AD, Munoz EC, et al. Normal range of clivoaxial angle in adults using flexion and extension cervical magnetic resonance imaging scans. Neuroradiol J 2021;34(4):348–54.

52. Henderson FC, Wilson WA, Mark AS, et al. Utility of the clivo-axial angle in assessing brainstem deformity: pilot study and literature review. Neurosurg Rev 2018;41(1):149–63.

53. Nagashima C, Kubota S. Craniocervical abnormalities. Neurosurg Rev 1983;6(4):187–97.

54. Van Gilder JC, Menezes AH, Dolan KD. The craniovertebral junction and its abnormalities. Futura Publishing Company; 1987. p. 209–23.

55. Sangwanloy P, Vaniyapong T, Norasetthada T, et al. Influence of clivo-axial angle on outcome after foramen magnum decompression in adult symptomatic Chiari type 1 malformation. Clin Neurol Neurosurg 2022;216:107214.

56. Chung RS, Staal JA, McCormack GH, et al. Mild axonal stretch injury in vitro induces a progressive series of neurofilament alterations ultimately leading to delayed axotomy. J Neurotrauma 2005;22(10): 1081–91.

57. Henderson FC, Wilson WA, Mott S, et al. Deformative stress associated with an abnormal clivo-axial angle: a finite element analysis. Surg Neurol Int 2010;1.

58. Zhao DY, Rock MB, Sandhu FA. Craniocervical Stabilization After Failed Chiari Decompression: A Case Series of a Population with High Prevalence of Ehlers-Danlos Syndrome. World Neurosurg 2022; 161:e546–52.

59. Menezes AH. Craniocervical developmental anatomy and its implications. Childs Nerv Syst 2008; 24(10):1109–22.

60. Menezes AH. Craniovertebral junction database analysis: incidence, classification, presentation, and treatment algorithms. Childs Nerv Syst 2008; 24(10):1101–8.

61. Alexiades NG, Shao B, Braga BP, et al. Development of best practices in the utilization and implementation of pediatric cervical spine traction: A modified Delphi study. J Neurosurg Pediatr 2021; 27(6):649–60.

62. Roye BD, Campbell ML, Matsumoto H, et al. Establishing consensus on the best practice guidelines for use of halo gravity traction for pediatric spinal deformity. J Pediatr Orthop 2020;40(1):e42–8.

63. Ladner TR, Dewan MC, Day MA, et al. Evaluating the relationship of the pB–C2 line to clinical outcomes in a 15-year single-center cohort of pediatric Chiari I malformation. J Neurosurg Pediatr 2015;15(2): 178–88.

64. Bond AE, Jane JA, Liu KC, et al. Changes in cerebrospinal fluid flow assessed using intraoperative MRI during posterior fossa decompression for Chiari malformation. J Neurosurg 2015;122(5):1068–75.

65. Yeom JS, Buchowski JM, Kim HJ, et al. Risk of vertebral artery injury: comparison between C1–C2 transarticular and C2 pedicle screws. Spine J 2013;13(7): 775–85.

66. Lowry DW, Pollack IF, Clyde B, et al. Upper cervical spine fusion in the pediatric population. J Neurosurg 1997;87(5):671–6.

67. Martinez-del-Campo E, Turner JD, Rangel-Castilla L, et al. Pediatric occipitocervical fixation: radiographic criteria, surgical technique, and clinical outcomes based on experience of a single surgeon. J Neurosurg Pediatr 2016;18(4):452–62.

68. Anderson RC, Ragel BT, Mocco J, et al. Selection of a rigid internal fixation construct for stabilization at the craniovertebral junction in pediatric patients. J Neurosurg Pediatr 2007;107(1):36–42.

69. Bambakidis NC, Feiz-Erfan I, Horn EM, et al. Biomechanical comparison of occipitoatlantal screw fixation techniques. J Neurosurg Spine 2008;8(2): 143–52.

70. Anderson RC, Kan P, Gluf WM, et al. Long-term maintenance of cervical alignment after occipitocervical and atlantoaxial screw fixation in young children. J Neurosurg Pediatr 2006;105(1):55–61.

71. Gluf WM, Schmidt MH, Apfelbaum RI. Atlantoaxial transarticular screw fixation: a review of surgical indications, fusion rate, complications, and lessons learned in 191 adult patients. J Neurosurg Spine 2005;2(2):155–63.

72. Hwang SW, Gressot LV, Rangel-Castilla L, et al. Outcomes of instrumented fusion in the pediatric cervical spine. J Neurosurg Spine 2012;17(5):397–409.

73. Reintjes SL, Amankwah EK, Rodriguez LF, et al. Allograft versus autograft for pediatric posterior cervical and occipito-cervical fusion: a systematic review of factors affecting fusion rates. J Neurosurg Pediatr 2016;17(2):187–202.

74. Vedantam A, Hansen D, Briceño V, et al. Patient-reported outcomes of occipitocervical and atlantoaxial fusions in children. J Neurosurg Pediatr 2017;19(1): 85–90.

Complex Chiari Malformations
Diagnosis, Evaluation, and Treatment

Vijay M. Ravindra, MD, MSPH[a,b,c], Douglas L. Brockmeyer, MD[b,d],*

KEYWORDS

- Chiari malformations • Basilar invagination • Clivoaxial angle (CXA) • Retroflexed odontoid
- Condylar-C2 sagittal vertical alignment (C-C2SVA) • Complex Chiari malformation (CCM)

KEY POINTS

- Accurate and timely diagnosis of Complex Chiari malformation can aid in the management of this complex disease process.
- Radiographic measurements focused on craniocervical kyphosis can help identify Complex Chiari malformation.
- Evidence-based algorithms can help direct the management of affected patients but clinical judgment is important, with focus on presenting symptoms and reducing neurologic morbidity.

INTRODUCTION

The initial description of the group of conditions currently known as "Chiari malformation" (CM) was developed in 1896 purely based on anatomic findings.[1] Over time, it has become clear that the 2 most commonly encountered variations of that classification are CM Type 1 (CM1) and CM Type 2 (CM2). CM1 is traditionally described as herniation of the cerebellar tonsils and lower part of the medulla into the foramen magnum without displacement of the fourth ventricle. CM2 describes spina bifida–associated caudal migration of the cerebellum with downward displacement of the brainstem and fourth ventricle.

Currently, the most popular definition for CM1 dictates that 5 mm or greater of tonsillar herniation below the foramen magnum must be present. It is estimated that the prevalence of CM1 may be as high as 3.7%[2]; however, only a small percentage of affected children, approximately 10% to 20%, ultimately require surgical decompression. The decision to proceed with surgery is often based on clinical presentation, neurologic symptoms, headache chronicity and severity, and presence of syringomyelia or scoliosis. The surgical treatment of symptomatic CM1 typically includes posterior fossa decompression (PFD), that is, suboccipital decompression and C1 laminectomy, with (PFDD) or without (PFD) duraplasty. Both procedures are thought to be effective in relieving symptoms including headaches or neck pain as well as syringomyelia.[3–5]

There is, however, a subset of children with pathologic findings that have a more severe form of CM1 that may not benefit from simple PFD/PFDD. These patients have more severe symptoms caused by skull base and upper cervical anomalies due to direct brainstem compression and cervicomedullary crowding. This phenomenon has been termed the "Complex Chiari malformation" (CCM).[6] In this article, we discuss the pathologic processes involved in CCM, with focus on the current diagnosis, evaluation, and treatment of this finding.

Defining the Complex Chiari Malformation

Since the designation of the CCM phenotype, there has been active investigation to define a set of criteria to diagnose this condition. Previous

a Department of Neurosurgery, Naval Medical Readiness Training Command, San Diego, CA, USA;
b Department of Neurosurgery, Clinical Neurosciences Center, University of Utah, Salt Lake City, UT, USA;
c Department of Neurosurgery, University of California San Diego, San Diego, CA, USA; d Division of Pediatric Neurosurgery, Intermountain Primary Children's Hospital, Salt Lake City, UT, USA
* Corresponding author.
E-mail address: neuropub@hsc.utah.edu

Neurosurg Clin N Am 34 (2023) 143–150
https://doi.org/10.1016/j.nec.2022.08.009
1042-3680/23/© 2022 Elsevier Inc. All rights reserved.

attempts have aimed to identify criteria to determine morphologic features that represent a higher risk for repeat surgery. In 1999, Grabb and colleagues[7] and Oakes and colleagues[8] described odontoid retroflexion, defined as pBC2 distance (maximum perpendicular distance to the basion-inferoposterior point of the C2 body) greater than 9 mm, as one possible component of a more severe phenotype that was associated with the need for occipitocervical fusion (OCF; **Fig. 1**A). Tubbs and colleagues[8] described patients with caudal descent of the brainstem in addition to the cerebellar tonsils, a finding coined the Chiari 1.5 malformation (CM 1.5). The finding of a CM 1.5 represented a risk factor for persistent syringomyelia after initial posterior fossa decompression and predicted the need for reoperation. Another measurement, the clivoaxial angle (CXA), was initially described by Nagashima and Kubota[9] and later by Smoker.[10] The CXA is now commonly used to understand relationships between the skull base and cervical spine (**Fig. 1**B).

Bollo and colleagues[6] synthesized the above radiographic parameters and used them to identify risk factors related to the need for delayed OCF in CM1 patients. On multivariate analysis of 102 surgical patients, the risk factors were identified as CM 1.5, basilar invagination, and a CXA less than $125°$,[6] thus establishing the use of these parameters in the definition of CCM. In 2021, using the Park-Reeves Syringomyelia Research Consortium (PRSRC) database, CreveCoeur and colleagues[11] showed that the CXA was the factor most predictive of the need for OCF and ventral brainstem decompression (VBD), thus solidifying the concept that craniocervical kyphosis defines a more complex subset of Chiari patients.

A new measurement, the condylar-C2 sagittal vertical alignment (C-C2SVA; **Fig. 1**C-F), was recently introduced to help predict the need for OCF and/or VBD in CCM patients.[12] The results of a retrospective single-center study demonstrated that a C-C2SVA of 5 mm or greater was 100% sensitive and 86% specific in predicting the need for OCF and/or VBD. In comparison, a CXA less than $125°$ was 55% sensitive and 99% specific, and a pBC2 of 9 mm or greater was 20% sensitive and 88% specific. The initial C-C2SVA study was subsequently validated using the PRSRC database.[13]

Thus, at the present time, it seems that in the presence of a CM 1.5 diagnosis, a CXA less than $125°$ and a C-C2SVA greater than 5 mm are the most helpful radiographic parameters in determining the presence or absence of a CCM (**Table 1**). Nevertheless, it should be kept in mind that these parameters are meant to only guide clinical decision-making and educate patients and parents. They are not meant to be dogmatic guidelines for patient care.

CLINICAL DECISION-MAKING
Clinical Presentation

As previously mentioned, although radiographic measurements contribute to clinical decision-making, the decision to undertake surgery must be made based on the overall clinical picture. As with CM1, the most common symptom related to CCM is suboccipital, Valsalva-induced headache but additional neurologic sign and symptoms, often localized to the brainstem and spinal cord, are also common. These may include dysphagia, dysarthria, sleep apnea, eye movement abnormalities, paresthesias, and ataxia, to name a few. Children aged younger than 4 years with CCM typically present with oropharyngeal apraxia, including central sleep apnea, snoring, and dysphagia.[6,14] These symptoms are typically thought to arise because of severe crowding of the cervicomedullary structures around the foramen magnum area.

Incidental diagnoses of CCM can also be made. Many patients with incidental CCM have several of the high-risk radiographic features described above; however, it is critical to tease out symptoms and focus clinical decisions on presentation rather than radiographic findings. A common exception is the finding of a moderate or large syrinx on radiographic imaging.[15] The presence of a moderate to large syrinx with or without scoliosis should trigger surgical consultation and treatment because the natural history of this finding is unfavorable without intervention.[16,17]

Another clinical scenario that may be underappreciated is the delayed onset of severe, lifestyle-limiting headaches, particularly with neck motion, after traditional PFDD in a patient with severe CCM risk factors. It is hypothesized that this scenario occurs because surgical release of the posterior musculo-ligamentous tension band in patients with preexisting craniocervical kyphosis may create biomechanical imbalance and abnormal motion in the occipitocervical structures. This abnormal balance may cause severe headaches and neck pain that is often only relieved by craniocervical fusion. Our clinical experience has shown that symptomatic improvement can be sudden and dramatic after surgery, although the biomechanical underpinnings and underlying pathophysiology of this condition are incompletely understood.

Diagnostic Evaluation

Patients presenting for neurosurgical evaluation have typically already had MRI of the brain, often

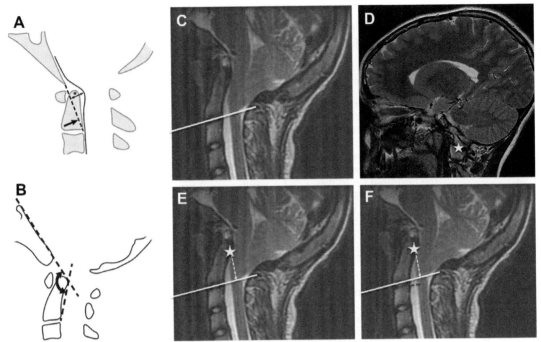

Fig. 1. The most frequently used craniocervical parameters. (*A*) The pBC2 is represented by a line from the inferior aspect of the clivus to the posterior inferior aspect of the C2 vertebral body. The pBC2 distance is defined as the maximum perpendicular distance from the posterior-superior aspect of the odontoid process to the line joining the basion to the posterior-inferior aspect of the C2 vertebral body. (*B*) The CXA is an angle (indicated by the *double-sided arrow*) obtained by creating a line from the inferior two-thirds of the clivus and a second line drawn from the posterior-inferior C2 body to the superior-posterior aspect of the odontoid. (*C-F*) The C-C2SVA is measured on sagittal and parasagittal MRI by drawing a line parallel to the C2 inferior endplate on a midline, sagittal image (*C*) and then identifying the midpoint of the C0-1 joint on a parasagittal image(*star, D*). Using the corresponding C0-1 reference point on the midline MR image, a line is created perpendicular to the C2 horizontal line in the midline (*E*) and then the distance from the posterior aspect of the C2-C3 disc space to the plumb line is measured in millimeters (*dashed red lines, F*). (Panels A, B reproduced with permission from Brockmeyer DL, Spader HS. Complex Chiari malformations in children: diagnosis and management. *Neurosurg Clin N Am.* 2015;26(4):555-560. Panels C–F reproduced with permission from Ravindra et al. Defining the role of the condylar-C2 sagittal vertical alignment in Chiari malformation type I. J Neurosurg Pediatr 26: 439-444, 2020.)

as part of prior workup for headaches. Sometimes, a spinal MRI has been performed as well. MRI scanning should be performed in a neutral position to accurately determine the patient's craniocervical anatomic relationships. The radiographic measures described previously should be made to stratify patients into the simple CM1 or CCM categories.

Congenital anomalies may also be present, including axis assimilation, pro-atlas segmentation abnormalities, and vascular dysgenesis. Depending on their severity, these findings may or may not directly influence surgical decision but they should be noted as part of surgical planning. The use of computed tomography (CT) imaging to delineate further bony anatomy is at the discretion of the treating surgeon/care team. Additional dynamic imaging of the cervical spine may be warranted if there is concern regarding occipitocervical instability or atlantoaxial instability in addition to the pathologic spectrum of CCM. In younger children who present with scoliosis, full 36-inch cassette films are needed to understand global spinal alignment. In patients with bulbar symptomatology, sleep and swallow studies may be indicated to help determine their existence and severity.

An Algorithmic Approach

An evidence-based evaluation for CCM patients should be used. A specific tailored approach should be chosen from among the multiple surgical procedures available for patients with symptomatic CCM. The treatment algorithm presented in **Fig. 2** demonstrates how to combine clinical presentation with radiographic measurements to inform decision-making.

Table 1 Measurements used in describing the morphology of the craniocervical junction in children with CCM	
Measurement	**Description with Potential Downfalls**
pBC2	Line drawn between the basion and posterior-inferior aspect of the C2 body. A line perpendicular to this line drawn through the odontoid tip to the ventral dura ($\geq$9 mm associated with symptoms) • May overestimate soft tissue contribution to craniocervical junction morphology
CXA	Line drawn along the clivus and inferiorly. Line falls tangent to the posterior aspect of the odontoid process (<125° associated with basilar invagination) • May be measured on neutral MRI/CT
C-C2SVA	Parasagittal midpoint of the occipital-C1 joint to the C2-C3 disc space. Continuous variable measured in millimeters • Requires neutral MRI scan • Difficult to measure in cervical scoliosis

Previous treatment algorithms focused on the pBC2 value of 9 mm as a decision point, but in the current model, we emphasize the presence of symptoms. If there are no symptoms present, then close observation with clinical and radiographic follow-up may be appropriate. For symptomatic children, evaluation of the degree of tonsillar herniation, as well as the pBC2, CXA, and C-C2SVA, is appropriate. In low-risk children, where the pBC2 is less than 9 mm, the C-C2SVA is less than 5 mm, and the CXA is greater than 125° with the absence of bulbar or myelopathic symptoms, the patient should undergo PFDD with C1 laminectomy. It is important to realize that even when proceeding with traditional decompression, documentation and tracking of these 3 measurements should be done. According to one study, patients with a CXA greater than 125° have a 1.7% future risk of requiring OCF, whereas those with a CXA less than 125° have a 13% of risk of needing OCF.[6]

Patients with bulbar symptoms and myelopathy should be evaluated carefully. Traditional PFDD may be enough to alleviate their symptoms but that may depend on the type and extent of manipulations done with the cerebellar tonsils (ie, tonsillar reduction with cautery vs tonsillopexy) and the size of the duraplasty during surgery. Only in patients with severe, intractable bulbomyelopathy due to bony compression and in whom intradural manipulations alone are unlikely to improve symptoms should upfront odontoid reduction and OCF be considered.[6,18] Bollo and colleagues[6] reported that patients with a pBC2 greater than 9 and CXA less than 125° with bulbar and myelopathy symptoms were most likely to benefit from an upfront fusion operation. In this group, the fusion rate was high (83%), but many of these patients required upfront OCF and VBD because of their symptom pattern and craniocervical bony pathologic condition. For patients requiring odontoid resection, an endoscopic transoral/transnasal odontoidectomy is a viable treatment option with low morbidity.[19,20]

SURGICAL MANAGEMENT

As mentioned, there are several surgical techniques used in the treatment of CM. PFD is commonly acknowledged as the primary treatment for pediatric patients with CM1. There is still much debate about whether to perform duraplasty as part of the PFD because the evidence supports both methods as efficacious in treating symptoms of CM.[4,5] For patients with CCM, however, a broader set of procedures may be required; Brockmeyer[21] found that 56% of patients with complex CM required OCF and 22% required odontoid reduction. A detailed discussion of the surgical methods used and the evidence base behind them is beyond the scope of this article but we have chosen to highlight salient aspects of our techniques here.

PFDD: Suboccipital craniectomy, C1 laminectomy, duraplasty

- A horseshoe headrest is preferred for a standard PFDD. If the patient is undergoing OCF, then pin fixation is used.
- Neurophysiologic monitoring is used in all cases with CCM, especially in the setting of significant myelopathy, bulbar symptoms, or syringomyelia.
- The suboccipital muscle and fascia are opened with a "T-shaped" technique to allow for suspension of the musculature back to the nuchal line with tight fascial closure to aid in healing (**Fig. 3**).

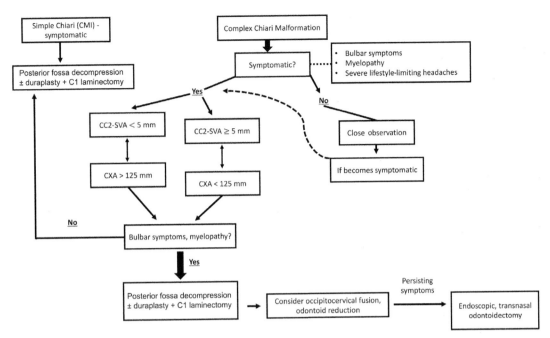

Fig. 2. Evidence-based treatment algorithm to manage CCMs in children.

- The craniectomy is performed with a perforating drill bit and completed with a craniotome. It is important to not remove more bone than is necessary to achieve decompression of the foramen magnum and suboccipital region. Particularly in the setting of a CCM with the potential for OCF, we limit the craniectomy to 3 × 3 cm in height and width.
- The dura is opened in a linear fashion, and the cerebellar tonsils are elevated and gently reduced from the bottom aspect until the fourth ventricular outlet can be visualized. This area is carefully explored to ensure there is no web or scar obstructing cerebrospinal fluid outflow.
- The subdural space is kept free of blood products to prevent postoperative nausea and vomiting. In addition, blood products may lead to arachnoiditis and subsequent scarring.
- The choice of dural substitute for expansile duraplasty can be synthetic dural substitute or pericranial autograft, with the final choice made by the surgeon. Recent evidence has suggested a similar complication profile for autograft and nonautologous graft[22] but with higher rates of pseudomeningocele formation and meningitis with nonautologous grafts.[22,23] In any scenario, achieving a watertight closure to prevent cerebrospinal fluid leak/fistula is the most important goal.

Occipitocervical Fusion and Odontoid Reduction

- For children requiring fusion for CCM, it is sufficient to incorporate only occiput-C2. Inclusion of C1 does not influence the fusion rate.[24]
- C2 screws can be placed within the pars interarticularis, in the pedicles, or crossing within the lamina. Whichever technique used, careful attention should be paid to vertebral artery anatomy and neural structures.
- After the instrumentation is placed, reduction of the odontoid can be achieved with distraction and extension of the instrumentation between the occiput and C2. Intraoperative three-dimensional scanning (O-arm, Medtronic, Inc., or AiRO, BrainLab, Inc.) can be used to verify adequate brainstem decompression.
- The most commonly used grafting option is rib autograft; however, compressed iliac crest allograft can also be used.[25] There are no differences in fusion rates between autograft and alternative graft materials.[26] The grafts are placed under tension and secured using multistranded titanium cables between the bony surfaces of the occiput and C2. Craniofacial screws are used to secure the rib against the occipital surface (see **Fig. 3**).
- The use of bone morphogenetic protein has been described.[27–30] Its use to promote

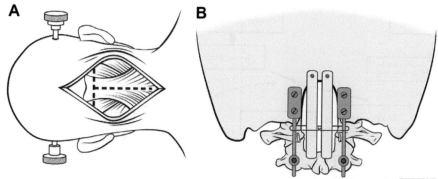

Fig. 3. PFDD and OCF. (*A*) T-shaped incision in the suboccipital fascia and musculature facilitating a watertight closure. (*B*) Odontoid reduction, OCF. Gray indicates the position of the OCF plates and rods; blue indicates the C2 pars screws; pink designates the occipital screws. (Figure reproduced with permission from Brockmeyer DL, Spader HS. Complex Chiari malformations in children: diagnosis and management. *Neurosurg Clin N Am.* 2015;26(4):555-560.)

arthrodesis at bone–bone interface points is at the discretion of the surgeon.

Transnasal Endoscopic Odontoid Resection

- These procedures should be performed with an experienced otolaryngologist with an endoscopic skillset. Tonsillectomy is sometimes performed to aid in the surgical exposure. Difficult airway management should be anticipated in any patient with CCM. A recent case series from Iyer and colleagues[19] reviews these concepts and presents outcomes from a combined neurosurgical-otolaryngologic approach.
- Surgical instruments can be passed either transorally or transnasally to access the pharyngeal mucosa, anterior ring of C1, and odontoid process. Care is taken during bony removal to avoid the carotid arteries laterally. The posterior longitudinal ligament is left intact. Intraoperative three-dimensional scanning (O-arm or AiRO) can be used to verify adequate odontoid resection.
- The pharyngeal mucosa is reapproximated by the otolaryngologist with interrupted absorbable sutures. Postoperative protocols are focused on graduated, early oral intake and mobilization.[19]

SUMMARY

Patients with CCM may be at risk for surgical failure if standard surgical techniques for treatment of CM are used; in some cases, reoperation and OCF with or without VBD may be required. We recommend a methodical approach to the management of these patients, with focus on clinical symptoms, most notably bulbar symptoms and myelopathy. Radiographic data including the C-C2SVA, CXA,

and pBC2 can be useful in guiding management. Specifically, patients with C-C2SVA of 5 mm or greater and CXA of less than 125° represent a more high-risk phenotype. Careful follow-up, monitoring of symptoms, and consideration of additional surgery in the setting of failure after PFDD in this high-risk cohort are necessary.

CLINICS CARE POINTS

- Patients with a "Complex Chiari" malformation may exhibit more severe symptoms caused by skull base and upper cervical anomalies due to direct brainstem compression and cervicomedullary crowding.

- The CXA, pBC2, and C-C2SVA are radiographic measurements that can be used as adjuncts when assessing children with CCMs.

- The current model emphasizes the presence of symptoms in surgical decision-making. If there are no symptoms present, then close observation with clinical and radiographic follow-up may be appropriate.

- For symptomatic children, evaluation of the degree of tonsillar herniation, as well as the pBC2, CXA, and C-C2SVA, is appropriate.

- In low-risk children, where the pBC2 is less than 9 mm, the C-C2SVA is less than 5 mm, and the CXA is greater than 125° with the absence of bulbar or myelopathic symptoms, the patient should undergo PFDD with C1 laminectomy.

- Patients with CCM may be at risk for surgical failure if standard surgical techniques for the treatment of CM are used; in some cases, re-operation and OCF with or without VBD may be required.

- Careful follow-up, monitoring of symptoms, and consideration of additional surgery in the setting of failure after PFDD in this high-risk cohort are necessary.
- Further large-scale studies are needed to determine evidence-based treatment algorithms for children with CCMs.

COPYRIGHT STATEMENT

I am a military Service member. This article was prepared as part of my official duties. Title 17, U.S.C., §105 provides that copyright protection under this title is not available for any work of the US Government. Title 17, U.S.C., §101 defines a US Government work as a work prepared by a military Service member or employee of the US Government as part of that person's official duties.

DISCLOSURE

The views expressed in this article are those of the author and do not necessarily reflect the official policy or position of the Department of the Navy, Department of Defense, nor the US Government.

REFERENCES

1. Caetano de Barros M, Farias W, Ataide L, et al. Basilar impression and Arnold-Chiari malformation. A study of 66 cases. J Neurol Neurosurg Psychiatry 1968;31(6):596–605.
2. Khalsa SSS, Geh N, Martin BA, et al. Morphometric and volumetric comparison of 102 children with symptomatic and asymptomatic Chiari malformation Type I. J Neurosurg Pediatr 2018;21(1):65–71.
3. Ho WSC, Brockmeyer DL. Complex Chiari malformation: using craniovertebral junction metrics to guide treatment. Childs Nerv Syst 2019;35(10):1847–51.
4. Akbari SHA, Yahanda AT, Ackerman LL, et al. Complications and outcomes of posterior fossa decompression with duraplasty versus without duraplasty for pediatric patients with Chiari malformation type I and syringomyelia: a study from the Park-Reeves Syringomyelia Research Consortium. J Neurosurg Pediatr 2022;30(1):39–51.
5. Lee A, Yarbrough CK, Greenberg JK, et al. Comparison of posterior fossa decompression with or without duraplasty in children with Type I Chiari malformation. Childs Nerv Syst 2014;30(8):1419–24.
6. Bollo RJ, Riva-Cambrin J, Brockmeyer MM, et al. Complex Chiari malformations in children: an analysis of preoperative risk factors for occipitocervical fusion. J Neurosurg Pediatr 2012;10(2):134–41.
7. Grabb PA, Mapstone TB, Oakes WJ. Ventral brain stem compression in pediatric and young adult patients with Chiari I malformations. Neurosurgery 1999;44(3):520–7. discussion 527-528.
8. Tubbs RS, Iskandar BJ, Bartolucci AA, et al. A critical analysis of the Chiari 1.5 malformation. J Neurosurg 2004;101(2 Suppl):179–83.
9. Nagashima C, Kubota S. Craniocervical abnormalities. Modern diagnosis and a comprehensive surgical approach. Neurosurg Rev 1983;6(4):187–97.
10. Smoker WR. Craniovertebral junction: normal anatomy, craniometry, and congenital anomalies. Radiographics 1994;14(2):255–77.
11. CreveCoeur TS, Yahanda AT, Maher CO, et al. Occipital-cervical fusion and ventral decompression in the surgical management of Chiari-1 malformation and syringomyelia: analysis of data from the Park-Reeves Syringomyelia Research Consortium. Neurosurgery 2021;88(2):332–41.
12. Ravindra VM, Iyer RR, Awad AW, et al. Defining the role of the condylar-C2 sagittal vertical alignment in Chiari malformation type I. J Neurosurg Pediatr 2020;26(4):439–44.
13. Ravindra VM, Iyer RR, Yahanda AT, et al. A multicenter validation of the condylar-C2 sagittal vertical alignment in Chiari malformation type I: a study using the Park-Reeves Syringomyelia Research Consortium. J Neurosurg Pediatr 2021;28(2):176–82.
14. Albert GW, Menezes AH, Hansen DR, et al. Chiari malformation Type I in children younger than age 6 years: presentation and surgical outcome. J Neurosurg Pediatr 2010;5(6):554–61.
15. Brockmeyer DL, Spader HS. Complex Chiari malformations in children: diagnosis and management. Neurosurg Clin N Am 2015;26(4):555–60.
16. Tubbs RS, Beckman J, Naftel RP, et al. Institutional experience with 500 cases of surgically treated pediatric Chiari malformation Type I. J Neurosurg Pediatr 2011;7(3):248–56.
17. Ono A, Suetsuna F, Ueyama K, et al. Surgical outcomes in adult patients with syringomyelia associated with Chiari malformation type I: the relationship between scoliosis and neurological findings. J Neurosurg Spine 2007;6(3):216–21.
18. Fenoy AJ, Menezes AH, Fenoy KA. Craniocervical junction fusions in patients with hindbrain herniation and syringohydromyelia. J Neurosurg Spine 2008;9(1):1–9.
19. Iyer RR, Grimmer JF, Brockmeyer DL. Endoscopic transnasal/transoral odontoid resection in children: results of a combined neurosurgical and otolaryngological protocolized, institutional approach. J Neurosurg Pediatr 2021;28(2):221–8.

20. Hankinson TC, Grunstein E, Gardner P, et al. Trans-nasal odontoid resection followed by posterior decompression and occipitocervical fusion in children with Chiari malformation Type I and ventral brainstem compression. J Neurosurg Pediatr 2010; 5(6):549–53.

21. Brockmeyer DL. The complex Chiari: issues and management strategies. Neurol Sci 2011;32(Suppl 3):S345–7.

22. Yahanda AT, Adelson PD, Akbari SHA, et al. Dural augmentation approaches and complication rates after posterior fossa decompression for Chiari I malformation and syringomyelia: a Park-Reeves Syringomyelia Research Consortium study. J Neurosurg Pediatr 2021;27(4):459–68.

23. Yahanda AT, Simon LE, Limbrick DD. Outcomes for various dural graft materials after posterior fossa decompression with duraplasty for Chiari malformation type I: a systematic review and meta-analysis. J Neurosurg 2021;135(5):1356–69.

24. Hankinson TC, Avellino AM, Harter D, et al. Equivalence of fusion rates after rigid internal fixation of the occiput to C-2 with or without C-1 instrumentation. J Neurosurg Pediatr 2010;5(4):380–4.

25. Iyer RR, Tuite GF, Meoded A, et al. A modified technique for occipitocervical fusion using compressed iliac crest allograft results in a high rate of fusion in the pediatric population. World Neurosurg 2017; 107:342–50.

26. Robinson LC, Anderson RCE, Brockmeyer DL, et al, Pediatric Craniocervical Society. Comparison of fusion rates based on graft material following occipitocervical and atlantoaxial arthrodesis in adults and children. Oper Neurosurg (Hagerstown) 2018;15(5): 530–7.

27. Fahim DK, Whitehead WE, Curry DJ, et al. Routine use of recombinant human bone morphogenetic protein-2 in posterior fusions of the pediatric spine: safety profile and efficacy in the early postoperative period. Neurosurgery 2010;67(5):1195–204. discussion 1204.

28. Lindley TE, Dahdaleh NS, Menezes AH, et al. Complications associated with recombinant human bone morphogenetic protein use in pediatric craniocervical arthrodesis. J Neurosurg Pediatr 2011;7(5): 468–74.

29. Simmonds MC, Brown JV, Heirs MK, et al. Safety and effectiveness of recombinant human bone morphogenetic protein-2 for spinal fusion: a meta-analysis of individual-participant data. Ann Intern Med 2013;158(12):877–89.

30. Mazur MD, Sivakumar W, Riva-Cambrin J, et al. Avoiding early complications and reoperation during occipitocervical fusion in pediatric patients. J Neurosurg Pediatr 2014;14(5):465–75.

Spine Deformity Associated with Chiari I Malformation and Syringomyelia

Somnath Das, MD[a,*], Lauren Stone, MD[b], Jakub Godzik, MD[a], Michael Kelly, MD[c]

KEYWORDS

- Chiari malformation • Syringomyelia • Scoliosis • Posterior fossa decompression

KEY POINTS

- It is not uncommon for patients to have the trio of Chiari Malformation 1, syringomyelia, and scoliosis.
- Diagnostic workup of these patients requires a careful attention to history, physical examination, and imaging.
- Should scoliosis be discovered in a patient with Chiari and syringomyelia, posterior fossa decompression may improve or stabilize scoliotic curves in about half of these patients. Emerging evidence indicated that younger age at time of posterior fossa decompression (PFD) and smaller pre-PFD curve may reduce likelihood of spinal fusion.
- Posterior fossa decompression likely stabilizes scoliosis by decompressing the syringomyelia, as opposed to relieving tonsillar herniation.
- The risk of new neurologic deficit after spina fusion is low but not negligible, particularly if performed before posterior fossa decompression.

BACKGROUND

Chiari I malformation (CM1) refers to descent of the cerebellar tonsils 5 mm or greater below the foramen magnum.[1] The most common presenting symptom for these patients is headache.[1,2] It is not uncommon for these patients to also present with abnormal spinal curvature[2]—it is estimated that approximately 20% of patients with CM1 have scoliosis.[3] The prevalence of scoliosis increases to between 30% and 70% when patients with CM1 have concurrent syringomyelia (CM1-S).[3,4] The pathophysiology correlating spinal deformity with CM1-S is not well understood, although there is some evidence proposing dysfunction of the anterior horn cells as a possible mechanism.[5] Managing CM1-associated deformity requires thoughtful workup and decision-making given few high-quality studies existing to guide clinical choices. In this article, we aim to summarize the current evidence in diagnosis and management of spinal deformity in patients with CM1-S.

INITIAL WORKUP AND DIAGNOSTIC STUDIES

History and physical examination are early clinical means to detect important, decision-altering elements for scoliosis with CM1. From an orthopedic standpoint, the first identified element is often the spinal deformity, noted by positive Adams forward bend or cosmetic complaints. A complete

[a] Department of Neurological Surgery, University of Alabama, 2000 6th Ave S, Birmingham, AL 35294, USA;
[b] Department of Orthopedic Surgery, University of California, San Diego, USA; [c] Department of Orthopedic Surgery, Rady Children's Hospital, San Diego, CA, USA
* Corresponding author.
E-mail address: sdas@uabmc.edu

Neurosurg Clin N Am 34 (2023) 151–157
https://doi.org/10.1016/j.nec.2022.08.011
1042-3680/23/© 2022 Elsevier Inc. All rights reserved.

neurological examination and focused history should be performed as part of the initial evaluation. Positive findings as postural headache, back pain, oropharyngeal dysfunction, and absence of or asymmetric abdominal reflexes should provoke suspicion of an underlying CM1 and be cause for MRI of the entire neural axis.[2,3] Early onset scoliosis (<10 years old) should undergo MRI scanning because 10% to 25% may have an underlying neural axis abnormality, and current evidence indicates that MRI is an appropriate screening tool in this population.[6–8] In adolescent idiopathic scoliosis (AIS), routine MRI screening for neural axis abnormalities is debated.[9,10] The prevalence of CM1 in patients presumed to have AIS is approximately 8%.[10]

Deformity surgeon's first images are typically standing scoliosis films. Scoliosis is defined by a coronal Cobb greater than 20° located anywhere within the spinal column. There are several characteristics that suggest, but do not unilaterally conclude, the presence of neuroaxis abnormality. The evidence for this, however, is limited. For example, hyperkyphosis (kyphosis > 40°, Lenke "+" sagittal plane modifier) has been suggested as a possible indicator of an underlying syrinx.[11,12] However, a recent retrospective study of patients with AIS treated with spinal fusion did not reveal association between degree of scoliosis and neural axis abnormalities.[13] The presence of a syrinx in another otherwise neurologically normal patient may also increase the likelihood of atypical curve features in patients with CM1.[14] For example, a left-thoracic curve has been previously described as a possible predictor neural axis abnormalities[15,16]; however, both prospective and retrospective studies have challenged this association.[17,18] Other atypical curves such as multiple thoracic curves merit further MRI screening.[3] If clinical suspicion exists then it is prudent to obtain an MRI study.

If a patient is discovered to have a CM1 and syrinx on MRI, further measurements are necessary in order to guide workup and treatment. By definition, CM1 is defined as 3 mm of tonsillar ectopia below the foramen magnum in children, and 5 mm in adults.[19] Some studies have reported that greater tonsillar herniation can predict if a patient will develop scoliosis[20,21]; however, this measurement does not seem to predict deformity severity.[21,22] A smaller clivo-axial angle (<125°) may also predict likelihood of deformity.[21] Should imaging not include the craniocervical junction, then the quality of the observed syrinx may also play a role in predicting a CM1-S. In a large multicenter study, those with scoliosis generally have longer and wider syrinxes and CM1. The presence of a holocord syrinx has been associated with the development of scoliosis.[22]

Guidelines for scoliosis screening in patients with CM1 are not defined. Given that most patients with CM1-S undergo MRI, it is reasonable to assume that some cases will be diagnosed via this imaging modality alone.[22,23] Practitioners may benefit from testing patients with the Adams forward bending test given its high sensitivity; however, this test may produce a false negative.[24] To date, no evidence exists whether either adolescents or patients aged younger than 10 years with CM1 or CM1-S should also be screened for concurrent scoliosis with X-rays. The theoretical concern of radiation exposure has been addressed by recent studies.[25] This question may be of benefit for future investigations. As with AIS, if there is suspicion then radiographs should be ordered. This can be limited to a posteroanterior upright spine radiograph to minimize radiation exposure.

TREATMENT
Bracing

Nonoperative treatment via bracing observation is a reasonable option in select patients with CM1 with scoliosis. Curves less than 20° may regress on their own or remain stable over time.[26] In general, bracing is appropriate for those patients with curve characteristics similar to AIS patients: skeletal immature patients with scoliosis measuring 20° to 40°.[3] Although bracing may slow progression of larger curves, regression of these curves is unlikely—especially if the patient is aged more than 10 years.[26–28]

Bracing may have a role to play in the management of patients with CM1-S who undergo the posterior fossa decompression (PFD). Sha and colleagues compared 22 patients with CM1-S who underwent decompression to 44 age and sex-matched AIS patients. The presenting curve magnitude between their 2 cohorts was not statistically significant (32.9° $\pm$ 6.3° vs 29.6° $\pm$ 6.4°; P = .052). Their comparison demonstrated the curve progression profile and likelihood of undergoing spinal fusion was similar in patients with CM1 who are braced following PFD to A1S.[29] Notably, these curves are smaller than the threshold for fusion noted in prior studies.[27,28]

Posterior Fossa Decompression

PFD plays a major role in the treatment of patients with CM1, particularly if there is concurrent syringomyelia. Chotai and colleagues studied the natural history of scoliosis in 43 patients with C1M. Approximately half their cohort had concurrent syringomyelia. In an average follow-up of 3 years, 13 patients (48%) underwent decompression alone, (15%) underwent spinal fusion, and 10 (37%) underwent both decompression and deformity correction. All but 1 patient who underwent surgical intervention (PFD, spinal fusion, or PFD + fusion) had a syrinx.[26] There is evidence that in select populations, PFD can halt scoliosis curve progression. In a review of 120 patients who underwent PFD, Hwang and colleagues[30] estimated that estimated that about one-third of scoliotic curves will improve in magnitude following PFD, and in an additional 20%, curves will not change within an average follow-up of 48 months. There was no association between preoperative curve magnitude and likelihood of progression; however, both groups had a magnitude less than 35° (34.13 ± 14.7° vs 35.0 ± 12.0°, $P = .82$).

Practitioners may choose to add duraplasty to their posterior fossa decompression. Few studies have examined the effect of duraplasty on scoliosis curve progression. In their 2017 meta-analysis of 1492 patients, Lu and colleagues[31] concluded that patients who undergo PFDD have greater clinical improvement compared with patients with PFD; however, outcomes on syrinx size and scoliosis progression were equivocal. Sadler and colleagues compared 346 patients who had undergone PFDD versus 51 PFD patients. In their study, patients who underwent duraplasty with PFD had significantly longer and wider syringes. Preoperative curve was similar between the 2 groups (29.9° for PFD vs 28.8° for duraplasty). Between the 2 groups, similar proportions of patients underwent subsequent fusion surgery (23% vs 19%, $P = .59$). PFD without duraplasty was associated with curve progression greater than 10° but there was no difference in likelihood of undergoing fusion. Age and larger preoperative curves were also associated with likelihood of spinal fusion. Although reduction of syrinx length and width was not correlated with curve progression in both cohorts, reduction of these dimensions was associated with a lower likelihood of fusion.[32]

The mechanism behind syrinx decompression and its relation to a patient's scoliotic progression is still being elucidated. It is thought that patients with CM1-S have impaired CSF flow dynamics.[33] Patients with CM1-S and scoliosis are more likely to have higher Cobb angles compared patients with CM1.[17] Posterior fossa decompression improves CSF dynamics and neurological symptoms by decreasing the velocity of cerebrospinal fluid within the syrinx.[34] The pathophysiology of whether CSF dynamics contributes to scoliosis

development is still under investigation; however, recent animal studies of kaolin-injected rabbits have shown a possible link between reduced spinal CSF velocity and development of scoliosis.[35] In addition, PFD may help restore innervation to the surrounding paraspinal muscles. In a study of 37 patients with CM1-S who underwent PFD followed by deformity correction, Sha and colleagues[36] demonstrated that decompression reduces levels of antiapoptotic markers and improves histological architecture muscle fiber biopsies taken from the uppermost instrumented vertebrae at fusion. Given that patients with CM1-S with scoliosis have wider and longer syrinxes, it is reasonable to assume that decompressing the syrinx—as opposed to relieving tonsillar herniation—is associated with scoliosis improvement following posterior fossa decompression.[4,32] These findings are further being explored in scoliotic patients with CM1 without syringomyelia. In their study of 32 patients (average age of 11 years) with CM1 and scoliosis (in which patients with CM1-S were excluded), O'Neill and colleagues[37] found that PFD was not associated with curve progression or likelihood of spinal fusion.

Spinal Deformity Surgery

High-quality evidence to guide surgical decision-making for Chiari 1-associated scoliosis is not extensive. To date, no definitive guidelines exist, although trends in expert decision-making can be culled from institutional experiences.

Current evidence suggests that the risk of perioperative complications, including intraoperative neuromonitoring (IOM) data changes and new neurological deficits, are higher in CM1-associated scoliosis surgeries versus AIS. Godzik and colleagues matched patients with AIS and patients with CM1-S by Cobb angle. There were no significant differences found for levels fused, operative time, or blood loss. They did report more neurologic complications in the CIM-S group (4 vs 0, 11%, $P = .04$). These numbers, however, are small, and greater preoperative kyphosis as well as posterior column osteotomies were associated with complications, both of which are independently associated with neurologic complications elsewhere. There is insufficient evidence to associate these 2 factors with Chiari-associated deformities.[38]

Tan and colleagues performed a matched cohort study comparing 21 patients with CIM-S and 120 patients with idiopathic syringomyelia (iSM). The authors reported no significant differences in levels fused, intraoperative

Table 1
Summary of evidence for posterior fossa decompression and Chiari I malformation-associated scoliosis

Author (* = CM1-S Only)	Study Type	* of CM1 Patients	Results
Hwaung et al, 2012	Systematic review	120	About one-half of scoliotic curves will improve or stabilize after PFD
Sha et al,[29] 2013	Case-control	22	Bracing after PFD attenuates curve progression equivalent to patients with AIS
Mackel et al,[27] 2016	Retrospective cohort	44	Patients presenting with curves >35° and at older than 10 years may be more likely to be fused after PFD
Chotai et al,[26] 2021	Natural history	43	Patients with syrinx were more likely to have Cobb >20°. Curves <20° were more likely to regress
Sha et al,[36] 2017*	Prospective case series	37	PFD decreases antiapoptotic activity and improves histological architecture in paraspinal muscle
Sadler et al,[32] 2021*	Retrospective multi-institutional	422	Patients who receive duraplasty are less likely to have curve progression compared with PFD alone
Luzzi et al,[34] 2021*	Prospective case series	14	PFD improves CSF flow dynamics by decreasing CSF within the syrinx

neuromonitoring changes, new neurologic deficits, primary curve correction (70.9% vs 69.5%), SRS-22 scores at 2 years, or global balance change. They conclude that posterior fusion is at least as effective for CM1-S and iSM.[39,40]

Radiographic outcomes are generally satisfactory in patients with CM1 treated with spine fusion reconstructions. Feng and colleagues studied 14 patients with CM1-S with 30 matched patients with AIS who underwent selective thoracolumbar fusion. They were able to achieve similar levels of curve correction both postoperatively and at 3-year follow-up without permanent neurological deficit; however, CM1-S generally required more fused vertebrae.[41] In a study comparing 63 patients with CM1 with left thoracic curves and 63 years of age and curve magnitude-matched patients with right thoracic curve, Jiang and colleagues[42] found that selective thoracic fusion seems to obtain effective outcomes in Chiari-associated curves, although leftward curves demonstrated less correction of the thoracolumbar/lumbar curve (56.9% vs 67.9%, $P = .023$) and more postoperative trunk shift.

The decision-making process behind treating CM1-S and scoliosis is still being actively investigated. It is generally well understood that decompression of the syrinx should likely take place before correction of underlying spinal deformity.[43] The aforementioned results by Godzik and colleagues[38] suggest a possible harm to these patients if the syrinx is not addressed first, and they suggest that scoliosis secondary to C1M should be treated as a succinct surgical entity compared with AIS. The results by Tan and colleagues did not find any neurological complications in their C1M-S and iSM cohorts who did not receive PFD before deformity correction. They report on CM1-S 21 patients who underwent one-stage posterior fusion surgery; more studies are needed to validate these findings across the expert spine community-namely in areas of discrepancy (neurological deficit) and long-term outcome (**Tables 1** and **2**).

Table 2
Summary of evidence for spinal correction surgery and Chiari I malformation-associated scoliosis

Author (* = CM1-S Only)	Study Type	* of CM1 Patients	Results
Mackel et al,[27] 2016	Retrospective multicenter	44	Patients presenting with curves >35° as well as those >10 years of age may require fusion after PFD
Godzik et al,[38] 2015*	Retrospective cohort	36	Although patients with CM1-S can have similar deformity correction, they may have higher neuromonitoring difficulties and neurological complications
Feng et al,[41] 2020*	Case control	14 (iSM + CM1)	Patients with syringomyelia-associated scoliosis can achieve similar deformity correction to AIS; however, additional levels may need to be fused
Jiang et al,[42] 2019	Retrospective multicohort	126	Patients with CM1 with both right and left thoracic curves can be managed with selective thoracic fusion. Right thoracic curves tend to have better correction
Tan et al,[40] 2020	Retrospective	22	One stage posterior fusion surgery achieved similar radiographic correction in patients with CM1-S and patients with AIS without significant neurologic deficits

SUMMARY

The management of patients with CM1-S with scoliosis involves complex decision-making with limited evidence. Idiopathic scoliosis patients who present at less than 10 years of age should be screened for underlying neural axis abnormalities with an MRI of the entire spine. Similarly, patients with AIS and neurological symptoms such as headaches, oropharyngeal dysfunction, absence of abdominal reflexes, weakness, or hyperreflexia should prompt the clinician to screen for an underlying neural axis abnormality. Early diagnosis and treatment of CM1 may result in resolution of scoliosis. Decompression of the syrinx improves CSF flow dynamics and denervation to the surrounding paraspinal muscles, which both possibly lead to attenuation of the scoliotic curve progression. The addition of duraplasty may reduce the likelihood of spinal fusion; however, more evidence is needed as to its effect on scoliotic curve progression. For patients who require spinal fusion, most evidence suggests that treating syringomyelia should precede deformity correction; however, future investigations may provide exceptions. Should the decision be made to fuse patients with CM1-S, it is possible to achieve reasonable correction in these patients, and surgeons should be aware of the potential for IOM-alerts and new neurological deficits.

ACKNOWLEDGMENTS

I would like to thank Dr. Jakub Godzik, Dr. Lauren Stone, and Dr. Michael Kelly for assistance with conception and writing this chapter.

DISCLOSURE

No pertinent conflicts of interest to disclose.

REFERENCES

1. Tubbs RS, Lyerly MJ, Loukas M, et al. The pediatric Chiari I malformation: a review. Child's Nervous Syst 2007;23(11):1239–50.

2. Pindrik J, Johnston JM Jr. Clinical presentation of Chiari I malformation and syringomyelia in children. Neurosurg Clin N Am 2015;26(4):509–14.

3. Kelly MP, Guillaume TJ, Lenke LG. Spinal deformity associated with chiari malformation. Neurosurg Clin N Am 2015;26(4):579–85.

4. Strahle JM, Taiwo R, Averill C, et al. Radiological and clinical associations with scoliosis outcomes after posterior fossa decompression in patients with Chiari malformation and syrinx from the Park-Reeves Syringomyelia Research Consortium. J Neurosurg Pediatr 2020;26(1):53–9.

5. Isu T, Iwasaki Y, Akino M, et al. Hydrosyringomyelia associated with a Chiari I malformation in children and adolescents. Neurosurgery 1990;26(4):591–6 [discussion: 596-7].

6. Zhang W, Sha S, Xu L, et al. The prevalence of intraspinal anomalies in infantile and juvenile patients with "presumed idiopathic" scoliosis: a MRI-based analysis of 504 patients. BMC Musculoskelet Disord 2016;17:189.

7. Gupta P, Lenke LG, Bridwell KH. Incidence of neural axis abnormalities in infantile and juvenile patients with spinal deformity. Is a magnetic resonance image screening necessary? Spine (Phila Pa 1976) 1998;23(2):206–10.

8. Dobbs MB, Lenke LG, Szymanski DA, et al. Prevalence of neural axis abnormalities in patients with infantile idiopathic scoliosis. J Bone Joint Surg Am 2002;84(12):2230–4.

9. Do T, Fras C, Burke S, et al. Clinical value of routine preoperative magnetic resonance imaging in adolescent idiopathic scoliosis. A prospective study of three hundred and twenty-seven patients. J Bone Joint Surg Am 2001;83(4):577–9.

10. Tully PA, Edwards BA, Mograby O, et al. Should all paediatric patients with presumed idiopathic scoliosis undergo MRI screening for neuro-axial disease? Child's Nervous Syst 2018;34(11):2173–8.

11. Whitaker C, Schoenecker PL, Lenke LG. Hyperkyphosis as an indicator of syringomyelia in idiopathic scoliosis: a case report. Spine (Phila Pa 1976) 2003; 28(1):E16–20.

12. Inoue M, Minami S, Nakata Y, et al. Preoperative MRI analysis of patients with idiopathic scoliosis: a prospective study. Spine (Phila Pa 1976) 2005;30(1): 108–14.

13. Swarup I, Derman P, Sheha E, et al. Relationship between thoracic kyphosis and neural axis abnormalities in patients with adolescent idiopathic scoliosis. J Child Orthop 2018;12(1):63–9.

14. Godzik J, Dardas A, Kelly MP, et al. Comparison of spinal deformity in children with Chiari I malformation with and without syringomyelia: matched cohort study. Eur Spine J 2016;25(2):619–26.

15. Spiegel DA, Flynn JM, Stasikelis PJ, et al. Scoliotic curve patterns in patients with Chiari I malformation and/or syringomyelia. Spine (Phila Pa 1976) 2003; 28(18):2139–46.

16. Wu L, Qiu Y, Wang B, et al. The left thoracic curve pattern: a strong predictor for neural axis abnormalities in patients with "idiopathic" scoliosis. Spine (Phila Pa 1976) 2010;35(2):182–5.

17. Strahle J, Smith BW, Martinez M, et al. The association between Chiari malformation Type I, spinal syrinx, and scoliosis. J Neurosurg Pediatr 2015;15(6): 607–11.

18. Fruergaard S, Ohrt-Nissen S, Dahl B, et al. Neural axis abnormalities in patients with adolescent idiopathic scoliosis: is routine magnetic resonance imaging indicated irrespective of curve severity? Neurospine 2019;16(2):339–46.

19. McClugage SG, Oakes WJ. The Chiari I malformation. J Neurosurg Pediatr 2019;24(3):217–26.

20. Godzik J, Kelly MP, Radmanesh A, et al. Relationship of syrinx size and tonsillar descent to spinal deformity in Chiari malformation Type I with associated syringomyelia. J Neurosurg Pediatr 2014; 13(4):368–74.

21. Luo M, Wu D, You X, et al. Are craniocervical angulations or syrinx risk factors for the initiation and progression of scoliosis in Chiari malformation type I? Neurosurg Rev 2021;44(4):2299–308.

22. Strahle JM, Taiwo R, Averill C, et al. Radiological and clinical predictors of scoliosis in patients with Chiari malformation type I and spinal cord syrinx from the Park-Reeves Syringomyelia Research Consortium. J Neurosurg Pediatr 2019;1–8. https://doi.org/10. 3171/2019.5.Peds18527.

23. Wright N. Imaging in scoliosis. Arch Dis Child 2000; 82(1):38.

24. Karachalios T, Sofianos J, Roidis N, et al. Ten-year follow-up evaluation of a school screening program for scoliosis. Is the forward-bending test an accurate diagnostic criterion for the screening of scoliosis? Spine (Phila Pa 1976) 1999;24(22):2318–24.

25. Oakley PA, Ehsani NN, Harrison DE. The scoliosis quandary: are radiation exposures from repeated x-rays harmful? Dose Response 2019;17(2). 1559325819852810.

26. Chotai S, Nadel JL, Holste KG, et al. Longitudinal scoliosis behavior in Chiari malformation with and without syringomyelia. J Neurosurg Pediatr 2021; 28(5):585–91.

27. Mackel CE, Cahill PJ, Roguski M, et al. Factors associated with spinal fusion after posterior fossa decompression in pediatric patients with Chiari I malformation and scoliosis. J Neurosurg Pediatr 2016;25(6):737–43.

28. Brockmeyer D, Gollogly S, Smith JT. Scoliosis associated with Chiari 1 malformations: the effect of suboccipital decompression on scoliosis curve progression: a preliminary study. Spine (Phila Pa 1976) 2003;28(22):2505–9.

29. Sha S, Zhu Z, Sun X, et al. Effectiveness of brace treatment of chiari malformation–associated scoliosis after posterior fossa decompression: a comparison with idiopathic scoliosis. Spine 2013;38(5):299–305.

30. Hwang SW, Samdani AF, Jea A, et al. Outcomes of Chiari I-associated scoliosis after intervention: a meta-analysis of the pediatric literature. Childs Nerv Syst 2012;28(8):1213–9.

31. Lu VM, Phan K, Crowley SP, et al. The addition of duraplasty to posterior fossa decompression in the surgical treatment of pediatric Chiari malformation Type I: a systematic review and meta-analysis of surgical and performance outcomes. J Neurosurg Pediatr 2017;20(5):439–49.

32. Sadler B, Skidmore A, Gewirtz J, et al. Extradural decompression versus duraplasty in Chiari malformation type I with syrinx: outcomes on scoliosis from the Park-Reeves Syringomyelia Research Consortium. J Neurosurg Pediatr 2021;1–9. https://doi.org/10.3171/2020.12.Peds20552.

33. Oldfield EH, Muraszko K, Shawker TH, et al. Pathophysiology of syringomyelia associated with Chiari I malformation of the cerebellar tonsils. Implications for diagnosis and treatment. J Neurosurg 1994;80(1):3–15.

34. Luzzi S, Giotta Lucifero A, Elsawaf Y, et al. Pulsatile cerebrospinal fluid dynamics in Chiari I malformation syringomyelia: Predictive value in posterior fossa decompression and insights into the syringogenesis. J Craniovertebr Junction Spine 2021;12(1):15–25.

35. Zhao Z, Li T, Bi N, et al. Continuous Hypodynamic Change of Cerebrospinal Fluid Flow as A Potential Factor Working for Experimental Scoliotic Formation. Scientific Rep 2020;10(1):6821.

36. Sha S, Li Y, Qiu Y, et al. Posterior fossa decompression in Chiari I improves denervation of the paraspinal muscles. J Neurol Neurosurg Psychiatr 2017;88(5):438.

37. O'Neill NP, Miller PE, Hresko MT, et al. Scoliosis with Chiari I malformation without associated syringomyelia. Spine Deform 2021;9(4):1105–13.

38. Godzik J, Holekamp TF, Limbrick DD, et al. Risks and outcomes of spinal deformity surgery in Chiari malformation, Type 1, with syringomyelia versus adolescent idiopathic scoliosis. Spine J 2015;15(9):2002–8.

39. Zhang Y, Lin G, Zhang J, et al. Radiographic evaluation of posterior selective thoracolumbar or lumbar fusion for moderate Lenke 5C curves. Arch Orthop Trauma Surg 2017;137(1):1–8.

40. Tan H, Lin Y, Rong T, et al. Surgical Scoliosis Correction in Chiari-I Malformation with Syringomyelia Versus Idiopathic Syringomyelia. J Bone Joint Surg Am 2020;102(16):1405–15.

41. Feng F, Shen H, Chen X, et al. Selective thoracolumbar/lumbar fusion for Syringomyelia-associated scoliosis: a case-control study with Lenke 5C adolescent idiopathic scoliosis. BMC Musculoskelet Disord 2020;21(1):749.

42. Jiang L, Qiu Y, Xu L, et al. Selective thoracic fusion for adolescent thoracic scoliosis secondary to Chiari I malformation: a comparison between the left and the right curves. Eur Spine J 2019;28(3):590–8.

43. Akhtar OH, Rowe DE. Syringomyelia-associated scoliosis with and without the Chiari I malformation. J Am Acad Orthop Surg 2008;16(7):407–17.

Role of Chiari Decompression in Managing Spinal Deformity Associated with Chiari I Malformation and Syringomyelia

Silky Chotai, MD[a], Diane Jewon Aum, MD[b], Jennifer Mae Strahle, MD[b],*

KEYWORDS

- Chiari malformation • Scoliosis • Syringomyelia • Outcomes • Posterior fossa decompression

KEY POINTS

- Posterior fossa decompression is a durable management option for pediatric patients with CM-I, syringomyelia, and scoliosis.
- There exists significant variability in scoliosis outcomes following PFD for CM-I and syringomyelia.
- Early decompression, younger age, smaller curve at the time of PFD, and greater reduction in syrinx after PFD are associated with improved outcomes.

INTRODUCTION

Chiari Malformation-I (CM-I) is defined as cerebellar tonsil position 5 mm or more below the foramen magnum.[1–3] CM-I is often associated with syringomyelia with baseline rates of 21% in an imaging population of Chiari and up to 70% in those undergoing surgical decompression of CM-1.[1,4–6] Several theories have been proposed to explain the relationship between CM-I and syringomyelia including small posterior fossa, hindbrain dysgenesis, craniocervical junction abnormalities and altered CSF hydrodynamics.[7–17] Scoliosis is a common spinal deformity observed in the pediatric neurosurgical population. Idiopathic scoliosis is the most common type of scoliosis in the pediatric population. Scoliosis associated with neurologic conditions has frequency been grouped together under the term neuromuscular scoliosis, however there is significant variability within this category. Chiari-syrinx- associated scoliosis is usually included under this category, but is different from scoliosis associated with spinal dysraphism, cerebral palsy and other neuromuscular disorders.[6,10] Scoliosis is present in up to 20% of patients with CM-I and over 80% of patients with CM-I and syringomyelia.[1 2,18–21] Although the association between CM-I and scoliosis remains unclear, the association between syringomyelia and scoliosis is well-reported.[4,7–9,12,13,15,16]

Posterior fossa decompression (PFD) for CM-I is considered the standard management strategy for symptomatic CM-I.[3,6,22,23,24–29] After PFD, about a 50-100% reduction in syringomyelia associated with CM-I has been reported in the literature.[17,23,24,25,27,28,30–32] Some studies have demonstrated the value of PFD in stabilizing

[a] Department of Neurosurgery, Vanderbilt University Medical Center, 1161 21st Avenue South #D3300, Nashville, TN, 37232, USA; [b] Department of Neurosurgery, Washington University School of Medicine, One Children's Place, Suite 4S20, Saint Louis, MO 63110-1077, USA

* Corresponding author. Saint Louis Children's Hospital, One Children's Place, Suite 4S20, Saint Louis, MO 63110-1077.

E-mail address: strahlej@wustl.edu

Neurosurg Clin N Am 34 (2023) 159–166
https://doi.org/10.1016/j.nec.2022.09.007
1042-3680/22/© 2022 Elsevier Inc. All rights reserved.

scoliosis.[2,9,18,20,33–37] The reported improvement or stabilization of scoliosis after PDF is variable with about 18% to 70% of patients needing spinal fusion after PFD.[19,20,36–39] Therefore, the role of PFD in the management of all scoliosis associated with CM-I with and without syringomyelia remains a matter of debate.

The goal of this article is to 1) summarize theories defining the association of scoliosis and CM-I with and without syringomyelia, 2) discuss the role of PFD in the management of CM-I-associated scoliosis, and 3) discuss short-term and long-term outcomes for this cohort of patients.

SCOLIOSIS AND CM-I WITH AND WITHOUT SYRINGOMYELIA

The most accepted proposed theory for the development of syrinx in the setting of CM-I is that the reduction in CSF spaces in the posterior fossa, surrounding foramen magnum and upper cervical spinal canal alter CSF dynamics resulting in syringomyelia.[5,13,15,16,30,31] There are several theories on how low tonsil position results in syrinx formation and the exact mechanism is not fully known at this time. One theory, describes that the restriction in pathways for CSF produces a water-hammer effect where the arterial pulses from the arteries including those associated with the choroid plexus, which normally would transmit CSF freely down the foramen magnum, are now retained in the brain, resulting in an abnormal craniospinal pressure gradient. Furthermore, the low-lying cerebellar tonsils might obstruct the fourth ventricular outlet foramina and create a one-way valve further impeding CSF movement into the spinal subarachnoid space and rerouting it instead into the central canal. With each cardiac cycle, systole forces CSF out of the cranium, and the progressive fluid accumulation within the central canal results in the formation of a syrinx. Finally, the spinal subarachnoid pressure may be increased and transmit fluid along Virchow-robin spaces into the spinal cord with CSF accumulating within the central canal.[40,41] The syrinx in turn can cause asymmetrical injury to the cells in the anterior horn of the spinal cord. This may result in denervation to and weakness of paraspinal muscles contributing to the development of scoliosis.[42,43]

In patients with CM-I and scoliosis without syringomyelia, there are speculations that compression of the cervicomedullary junction by the low-lying cerebellar tonsils may cause direct upper cervical spinal cord injury resulting in interference with postural tonic reflexes and scoliosis development.[8] However, studies have demonstrated that CM-I is not independently associated with scoliosis and therefore scoliosis may be a coincidental finding in patients with CM-I without syrinx.[20] [35] [20,37,44]

Posterior Fossa Decompression

When CM-I is associated with syringomyelia the decision to proceed with posterior fossa decompression is not controversial. The techniques for PFD include bone decompression only, extradural lysis of sclerotic tissue and removal of the outer layer of the dura, intradural extra-arachnoid durotomy with expansile duraplasty; intra-arachnoid lysis of scarring and adhesions, coagulation of herniated tonsil, partial tonsillectomy, opening of foramen magendie and obex plugging.[4,14,19,22,24–28,32,45–47] Recent studies have demonstrated that extradural techniques are as effective as intradural techniques for a select group of patients.[2,30,31,47] For patients with syringomyelia, there are speculations that PFD with duraplasty might be needed.[2] In a retrospective study of 85 patients undergoing PFD with duraplasty, the authors noted that the maximal syrinx reduction can be expected within 3 months after PFD for patients with CM-I and syrinx, and the coagulation of tonsil was associated with early syrinx regression.[46] Another study of 380 patients with CM-I and syrinx, from Park-Reeves Syringomyelia registry, demonstrated that PFD with duraplasty and younger age at the time of surgery were associated with greater syrinx resolution.[48] These studies suggest that duraplasty and intradural techniques might be considered in patients with CM-I and syrinx. However, larger cohort prospective studies are needed to provide any definite recommendations on need for intradural techniques for PFD, particularly in young patients, where the risks of dural opening may be greater related to the persistence of the occipital sinus.

Given that CM-I-associated syringomyelia is closely tied to the development of scoliosis, the effect of syrinx on scoliosis progression may be alleviated by PFD. The majority of studies evaluating scoliosis outcomes after PFD are small and based on single centers with varied findings.[2,17–19,33,35–37,29] [2,17–19,33,35-37,49] Analysis of patients enrolled in the 42 center multicenter consortium, Park-Reeves Syringomyelia Research consortium, has allowed for evaluation of a larger cohort of patients. Through a combined prospective/retrospective study, 397 patients, were evaluated, including 346 (87%) who underwent PFD with duraplasty and 51 (13%) who underwent PFD without duraplasty.[36] After adjusting for age, sex, preoperative curve magnitude, length, and width of the syrinx, extradural decompression

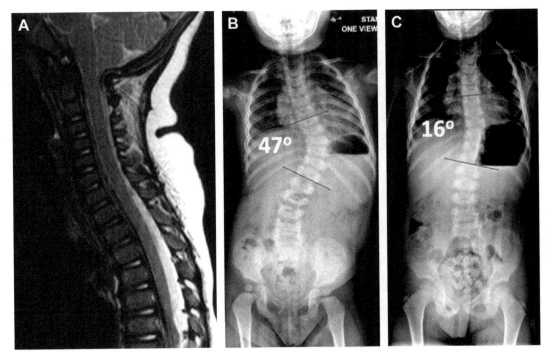

Fig. 1. Figure 1 depicts a patient with CM-I with scoliosis and no syrinx, who demonstrated spontaneous improvement in scoliosis after conservative management with (a) initial T2-weighted MRI brain and cervical spine, (b) initial AP x-ray demonstrating scoliosis (47 degrees), and (c) follow-up AP x-ray at 3 years demonstrating improvement of scoliosis curve (16 degrees). The patient was casted from ages 4 months to 3 years old, after which she was switched to a back brace.

was associated with curve progression > 10 degrees compared to PFD with duraplasty. The rates of spinal fusion, however, were similar between the groups. Greater syrinx reduction after PFD was associated with a decreased need for fusion surgery. While this study favored PFD with duraplasty for CM-I with syrinx and scoliosis, further data on the comparison of PFD techniques for this cohort of patients is needed.

Outcomes

CM-I with scoliosis and no syrinx
Numerous studies have reported outcomes following PFD in patients with CM-I-associated scoliosis with and without syringomyelia.[2,18–20,33–35,38,39,49–53] Although there exist some variations in outcomes for patients with CM-I with scoliosis and no syrinx,[2] most patients may not require any surgical treatment with respect to their CM-I. In a retrospective review of 32 patients with CM-I and scoliosis with no syrinx, O'Neill NP and colleagues[35] reported that CM-I without syringomyelia has minimal effect on scoliosis progression. In their study, the scoliosis curvature stabilized in the non-surgical population at an average progression of 1.0°. **Fig. 1** depicts a patient with CM-I with scoliosis and no syrinx, who demonstrated spontaneous improvement in scoliosis after conservative management with (a)

initial T2-weighted MRI brain and cervical spine, (b) initial AP x-ray demonstrating scoliosis (47 degrees), and (c) follow-up AP x-ray at 3 years demonstrating improvement of scoliosis curve (16 degrees). The patient was casted from ages 4 months to 3 years old, after which she was switched to a brace.

CM-I with scoliosis and syrinx
There is significant variability in curve progression in patients with CM-I with syrinx and scoliosis.[2,19,34,37] Of the 21 patients with CM-I associated scoliosis with syringomyelia who underwent PFD with duraplasty, Brockmeyer D and colleagues[33] demonstrated that 13 (62%) had curve improvement or stabilization and 8 patients (38%) had curve progression. They noted that older children (<12 years) or those with an advanced curve at the time of presentation had fewer chances of curve improvement. Similar results have been demonstrated by several authors, suggesting that early PFD when patients are younger and have smaller curves might be associated with scoliosis curve stabilization.[39 37 18,39] Other factors associated with progression in curve magnitude after surgery include older age at the time of decompression, the degree of the initial scoliotic curve, the curve location, and syrinx

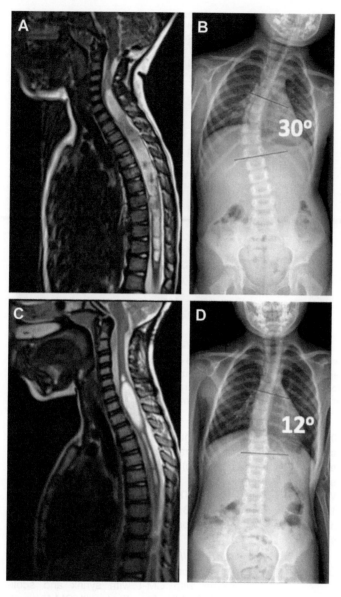

Fig. 2. **Figure 2** depicts a patient with CM-I with scoliosis and syrinx, who demonstrated improvement of scoliosis and syrinx after bone and duraplasty decompression: (a) preoperative MRI brain and spine, (b) preoperative AP x-ray demonstrating scoliosis (30 degrees), (c) postoperative MRI at 2-year follow-up with improvement in syrinx and (d) postoperative AP x-ray demonstrating improvement of scoliosis curve (12 degrees). This patient was braced starting 1 year after surgery, which was discontinued at 2-year follow-up.

reduction after surgery. In a retrospective series of 79 patients with CM-I, syrinx, and scoliosis, Krieger MD and colleagues[34] reported that CM-I decompression alone was adequate for mild scoliosis with a curve magnitude less than 20°. The patients with a curve magnitude greater than 20° required bracing and/or fusion surgery 70% of the time in addition to the PFD. Antonello FJ and colleagues[38] demonstrated that each increase in the degree of preoperative curve magnitude was associated with an 11% increase in the likelihood of scoliotic curve progression. **Fig. 2** depicts a patient with CM-I with scoliosis and syrinx, who demonstrated improvement of scoliosis and syrinx after bone and duraplasty decompression: (a) preoperative MRI brain and spine, (b) preoperative AP

x-ray demonstrating scoliosis (30 degrees), (c) postoperative MRI at 2-year follow-up with improvement in syrinx and (d) postoperative AP x-ray demonstrating improvement of scoliosis curve (12 degrees). This patient was braced starting 1 year after surgery, which was discontinued at 2-year follow-up. **Fig. 3** depicts a patient with CM-I with scoliosis and syrinx, who demonstrated progression of scoliosis after bone-only decompression: (a) preoperative T2-weighted MRI brain and spine, (b) preoperative AP x-ray demonstrating scoliosis (26 degrees), (c) postoperative MRI at 5-year follow-up demonstrating decrease in syrinx and (d) postoperative AP x-ray demonstrating progression of scoliosis curve (35 degrees). This patient was braced starting 1-month after surgery

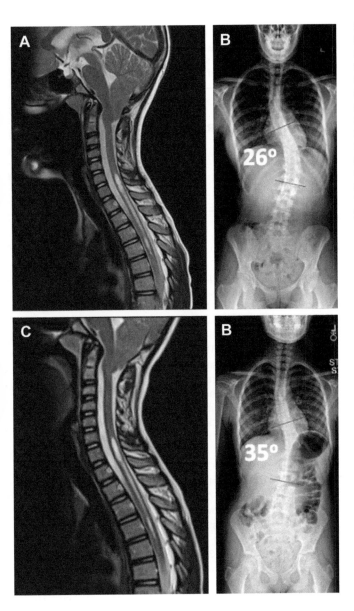

Fig. 3. **Figure 3** depicts a patient with CM-I with scoliosis and syrinx, who demonstrated progression of scoliosis after bone-only decompression: (a) preoperative T2-weighted MRI brain and spine, (b) preoperative AP x-ray demonstrating scoliosis (26 degrees), (c) postoperative MRI at 5-year follow-up demonstrating decrease in syrinx and (d) postoperative AP x-ray demonstrating progression of scoliosis curve (35 degrees). This patient was braced starting 1-month after surgery and continues to wear a back brace at night 4 years following surgery.

and continues to wear a back brace during nighttime at 4 years following surgery.

Natural History of Chiari-syrinx associated scoliosis prior to surgical decompression Few studies have reported the presurgical natural behavior of scoliosis in patients with CM-I and syrinx.[2,49] In our review of 43 patients with CM-I and scoliosis with and without syrinx, followed for a mean of 3.13 ± 2.04 years *before* surgery, 27 patients (63%) ultimately underwent either PFD or scoliosis correction surgery. We noted that the rate change in curve magnitude was statistically similar before (0.054° ± 0.79°) and after (0.042° ± 0.33°) surgery (p = 0.45) for patients who underwent PFD surgery only.[2] Therefore there may be factors involved in scoliosis progression in the setting of CM-1 and

syrinx outside of syrinx size alone that have yet to be determined. A retrospective study of 309 patients with or without scoliosis and with CM-I and syrinx, from Park-Reeves registry, demonstrated that scoliosis was associated with wider syrinxes, longer syrinxes, syrinxes with their rostral extent located in the cervical spine, and holocord syrinxes.[20] Notably, there was no association with tonsil position and scoliosis in this cohort.

Long-term outcomes for patients with CM-I and scoliosis with and without syrinx

Only a handful of studies have reported long-term outcomes for patients with CM-I and scoliosis with and without syrinx.[49,54] Ravindra and colleagues[49] reported long-term outcomes for 28 patients who underwent PFD for CM-I-associated scoliosis. The authors noted that the durability of PFD on curve stability was poor. After a mean of 88.3 ± 15.4 months after PFD, 30% of patients had late curve progression. The authors noted that a lower clival-axial angle, pBC2 > 9 mm, and higher initial Cobb angle were associated with the need for fusion surgery. After adjusting for pertinent variables, lower clival-axial angle was independently associated with a need for delayed fusion surgery. In a retrospective review of 65 patients with CM-I, syrinx, and scoliosis, Verhoftse B and colleagues[54] reported that 58% of patients underwent decompression before 10 years of diagnosis. At a mean follow-up of 6.9 years (range 2.0–20.4), syrinx size reduced in about 70% of patients after PFD, scoliosis improved in 40%, and stabilized in 26%, and progressed in 34% of cases. The authors noted that the greater curve improvement within the first-year post-decompression and smaller curves at presentation decreased the risk of spinal fusion.

SUMMARY

Posterior fossa decompression is a durable surgical management option for pediatric patients with CM-I, syringomyelia, and scoliosis. There exists significant variability in scoliosis outcomes following PFD for CM-I and syringomyelia. Early decompression, younger age, smaller curve at the time of PFD, and greater reduction in syrinx size after PFD are associated with curve stabilization after posterior fossa decompression.

CLINICS CARE POINTS

- From the available evidence at this point in time, it is unlikely that there exists a direct relationship between tonsil position and scoliosis in the absence of a syrinx. Therefore, surgical management of a Chiari malformation in the absence of syrinx should be based on Chiari symptoms and not the presence of scoliosis alone.

- There is significant variability in curve progression in patients with CM-I associated syringomyelia and scoliosis.

- Older age at the time of PFD and larger curve magnitude are associated with the need for surgical correction of scoliosis after PFD.

- The risk of delayed surgical correction of scoliosis is not well-reported. Lower clival-axial angle is associated with the need for later surgical correction of scoliosis

- Further multicenter studies are needed to evaluate the natural history of CM-I with syrinx and scoliosis and long-term scoliosis outcomes after surgery.

DISCLOSURE

None.

REFERENCES

1. Strahle J, Muraszko KM, Kapurch J, et al. Chiari malformation Type I and syrinx in children undergoing magnetic resonance imaging. J Neurosurg Pediatr 2011;8(2):205–13.
2. Chotai S, Nadel JL, Holste KG, et al. Longitudinal scoliosis behavior in Chiari malformation with and without syringomyelia. J Neurosurg Pediatr 2021; 28(5):585–91.
3. Ladner TR, Westrick AC, Wellons JC 3rd, et al. Health-related quality of life in pediatric Chiari Type I malformation: the Chiari Health Index for Pediatrics. J Neurosurg Pediatr 2016;17(1):76–85.
4. Shane Tubbs R, McGirt Matthew J, Jerry Oakes W. Surgical experience in 130 pediatric patients with Chiari I malformations. J Neurosurg 2003;99(2): 291–6.
5. Wu YW, Chin CT, Chan KM, et al. Pediatric Chiari I malformations: do clinical and radiologic features correlate? Neurology 1999;53(6):1271–6.
6. Krieger MD, McComb JG, Levy ML. Toward a simpler surgical management of Chiari I malformation in a pediatric population. Pediatr Neurosurg 1999;30(3):113–21.
7. Baisden J. Controversies in Chiari I malformations. Surg Neurol Int 2012;3(Suppl 3):S232–7.
8. Batzdorf U, McArthur DL, Bentson JR. Surgical treatment of Chiari malformation with and without syringomyelia: experience with 177 adult patients. J Neurosurg 2013;118(2):232–42.
9. Haroun RI, Guarnieri M, Meadow JJ, et al. Current opinions for the treatment of syringomyelia and chiari malformations: survey of the Pediatric Section of the American Association of Neurological Surgeons. Pediatr Neurosurg 2000;33(6):311–7.
10. Heiss JD, Suffredini G, Smith R, et al. Pathophysiology of persistent syringomyelia after decompressive craniocervical surgery. Clinical article. J Neurosurg Spine 2010;13(6):729–42.
11. Isu T, Sasaki H, Takamura H, et al. Foramen magnum decompression with removal of the outer layer of the dura as treatment for syringomyelia occurring with Chiari I malformation. Neurosurgery 1993;33(5): 844–9 [discussion: 849-850].

12. Lee HS, Lee SH, Kim ES, et al. Surgical results of arachnoid-preserving posterior fossa decompression for Chiari I malformation with associated syringomyelia. J Clin Neurosci 2012;19(4):557–60.

13. Massimi L, Caldarelli M, Frassanito P, et al. Natural history of Chiari type I malformation in children. Neurol Sci 2011;32(Suppl 3):S275–7.

14. Munshi I, Frim D, Stine-Reyes R, et al. Effects of posterior fossa decompression with and without duraplasty on Chiari malformation-associated hydromyelia. Neurosurgery 2000;46(6):1384–9 [discussion: 1389-1390].

15. Sekula RF Jr, Arnone GD, Crocker C, et al. The pathogenesis of Chiari I malformation and syringomyelia. Neurol Res 2011;33(3):232–9.

16. Williams B. The distending force in the production of communicating syringomyelia. Lancet 1970; 2(7662):41–2.

17. Genitori L, Peretta P, Nurisso C, et al. Chiari type I anomalies in children and adolescents: minimally invasive management in a series of 53 cases. Child's Nervous Syst 2000;16(10–11):707–18.

18. Eule JM, Erickson MA, O'Brien MF, et al. Chiari I malformation associated with syringomyelia and scoliosis: a twenty-year review of surgical and nonsurgical treatment in a pediatric population. Spine (Phila Pa 1976) 2002;27(13):1451–5.

19. Hwang SW, Samdani AF, Jea A, et al. Outcomes of Chiari I-associated scoliosis after intervention: a meta-analysis of the pediatric literature. Childs Nerv Syst 2012;28(8):1213–9.

20. Strahle JM, Taiwo R, Averill C, et al. Radiological and clinical predictors of scoliosis in patients with Chiari malformation type I and spinal cord syrinx from the Park-Reeves Syringomyelia Research Consortium. J Neurosurg Pediatr 2019;24(5):1–8.

21. Szuflita NS, Phan TN, Boulter JH, et al. Nonoperative management of enlarging syringomyelia in clinically stable patients after decompression of Chiari malformation type I. J Neurosurg Pediatr 2021;28(1):1–6.

22. Chotai S, Kshettry VR, Lamki T, et al. Surgical outcomes using wide suboccipital decompression for adult Chiari I malformation with and without syringomyelia. Clin Neurol Neurosurg 2014;120:129–35.

23. Chotai S, Medhkour A. Surgical outcomes after posterior fossa decompression with and without duraplasty in Chiari malformation-I. Clin Neurol Neurosurg 2014;125:182–8.

24. Limonadi FM, Selden NR. Dura-splitting decompression of the craniocervical junction: reduced operative time, hospital stay, and cost with equivalent early outcome. J Neurosurg 2004;101(2 Suppl): 184–8.

25. Litvack ZN, Lindsay RA, Selden NR. Dura splitting decompression for Chiari I malformation in pediatric patients: clinical outcomes, healthcare costs and resource utilization. Neurosurgery 2013;72(6): 922–9.

26. Shane Tubbs R, Beckman J, Naftel RP, et al. Institutional experience with 500 cases of surgically treated pediatric Chiari malformation Type I. J Neurosurg Pediatr 2011;7(3):248–56.

27. Yilmaz A, Kanat A, Musluman AM, et al. When is duraplasty required in the surgical treatment of Chiari malformation type I based on tonsillar descending grading scale? World Neurosurg 2011;75(2): 307–13.

28. Yundt KD, Park TS, Tantuwaya VS, et al. Posterior fossa decompression without duraplasty in infants and young children for treatment of Chiari malformation and achondroplasia. Pediatr Neurosurg 1996; 25(5):221–6.

29. Attenello FJ, McGirt MJ, Gathinji M, et al. Outcome of Chiari-associated syringomyelia after hindbrain decompression in children: analysis of 49 consecutive cases. Neurosurgery 2008;62(6):1307–13 [discussion: 1313].

30. Caldarelli M, Novegno F, Vassimi L, et al. The role of limited posterior fossa craniectomy in the surgical treatment of Chiari malformation Type I: experience with a pediatric series. J Neurosurg 2007;106(3 Suppl):187–95.

31. Chauvet D, Carpentier A, George B. Dura splitting decompression in Chiari type 1 malformation: clinical experience and radiological findings. Neurosurg Rev 2009;32(4):465–70.

32. Durham SR, Fjeld-Olenec K. Comparison of posterior fossa decompression with and without duraplasty for the surgical treatment of Chiari malformation Type I in pediatric patients: a meta-analysis. J Neurosurg Pediatr 2008;2(1):42–9.

33. Brockmeyer D, Gollogly S, Smith JT. Scoliosis associated with Chiari 1 malformations: the effect of suboccipital decompression on scoliosis curve progression: a preliminary study. Spine (Phila Pa 1976) 2003;28(22):2505–9.

34. Krieger MD, Falkinstein Y, Bowen IE, et al. Scoliosis and Chiari malformation Type I in children. J Neurosurg Pediatr 2011;7(1):25–9.

35. O'Neill NP, Miller PE, Hresko MT, et al. Scoliosis with Chiari I malformation without associated syringomyelia. Spine Deform 2021;9(4):1105–13.

36. Sadler B, Skidmore A, Gewirtz J, et al. Extradural decompression versus duraplasty in Chiari malformation type I with syrinx: outcomes on scoliosis from the Park-Reeves Syringomyelia Research Consortium. J Neurosurg Pediatr 2021;28(2):1–9.

37. Strahle JM, Taiwo R, Averill C, et al. Radiological and clinical associations with scoliosis outcomes after posterior fossa decompression in patients with Chiari malformation and syrinx from the Park-Reeves Syringomyelia Research Consortium. J Neurosurg Pediatr 2020;26(1):53–9.

38. Attenello FJ, McGirt MJ, Atiba A, et al. Suboccipital decompression for Chiari malformation-associated scoliosis: risk factors and time course of deformity progression. J Neurosurg Pediatr 2008;1(6):456–60.

39. Mackel CE, Cahill PJ, Roguski M, et al. Factors associated with spinal fusion after posterior fossa decompression in pediatric patients with Chiari I malformation and scoliosis. J Neurosurg Pediatr 2016;25(6):737–43.

40. Oldfield EH, Muraszko K, Shawker TH, et al. Pathophysiology of syringomyelia associated with Chiari I malformation of the cerebellar tonsils. Implications for diagnosis and treatment. J Neurosurg 1994; 80(1):3–15.

41. Heiss JD, Jarvis K, Smith RK, et al. Origin of syrinx fluid in syringomyelia: a physiological study. Neurosurgery 2019;84(2):457–68.

42. Sha S, Li Y, Qiu Y, et al. Posterior fossa decompression in Chiari I improves denervation of the paraspinal muscles. J Neurol Neurosurg Psychiatry 2017; 88(5):438–44.

43. Zhao Z, Li T, Bi N, et al. Continuous hypodynamic change of cerebrospinal fluid flow as a potential factor working for experimental scoliotic formation. Sci Rep 2020;10(1):6821.

44. Strahle J, Smith BW, Martinez M, et al. The association between Chiari malformation Type I, spinal syrinx, and scoliosis. J Neurosurg Pediatr 2015;15(6): 607–11.

45. Akbari SHA, Yahanda AT, Ackerman LL, et al. Complications and outcomes of posterior fossa decompression with duraplasty versus without duraplasty for pediatric patients with Chiari malformation type I and syringomyelia: a study from the Park-Reeves Syringomyelia Research Consortium. J Neurosurg Pediatr 2022;30(1):1–13.

46. Chotai S, Chan EW, Ladner TR, et al. Timing of syrinx reduction and stabilization after posterior fossa decompression for pediatric Chiari malformation type I. J Neurosurg Pediatr 2020;26(2):193–9.

47. Yahanda AT, Adelson PD, Akbari SHA, et al. Dural augmentation approaches and complication rates after posterior fossa decompression for Chiari I malformation and syringomyelia: a Park-Reeves Syringomyelia Research Consortium study. J Neurosurg Pediatr 2021;27(4):459–68.

48. Hale AT, Adelson PD, Albert GW, et al. Factors associated with syrinx size in pediatric patients treated for Chiari malformation type I and syringomyelia: a study from the Park-Reeves Syringomyelia Research Consortium. J Neurosurg Pediatr 2020;1–11.

49. Ravindra VM, Onwuzulike K, Heller RS, et al. Chiari-related scoliosis: a single-center experience with long-term radiographic follow-up and relationship to deformity correction. J Neurosurg Pediatr 2018; 21(2):185–9.

50. Luo M, Wu D, You X, et al. Are craniocervical angulations or syrinx risk factors for the initiation and progression of scoliosis in Chiari malformation type I? Neurosurg Rev 2021;44(4):2299–308.

51. Zhu Z, Wu T, Zhou S, et al. Prediction of Curve Progression After Posterior Fossa Decompression in Pediatric Patients With Scoliosis Secondary to Chiari Malformation. Spine Deform 2013;1(1):25–32.

52. Sha S, Zhu Z, Sun X, et al. Effectiveness of brace treatment of Chiari malformation-associated scoliosis after posterior fossa decompression: a comparison with idiopathic scoliosis. Spine (Phila Pa 1976) 2013;38(5):E299–305.

53. Chotai S, Basem J, Gannon S, et al. Effect of Posterior Fossa Decompression for Chiari Malformation-I on Scoliosis. Pediatr Neurosurg 2018;53(2):108–15.

54. Verhofste BP, Davis EA, Miller PE, et al. Chiari I malformations with syringomyelia: long-term results of neurosurgical decompression. Spine Deform 2020; 8(2):233–43.

Assessing Clinical Outcome Measures in Chiari I Malformation

Nishit Mummareddy, MD[a,1], Akshay Bhamidipati, MS[b,1],
Chevis N. Shannon, DrPH, MBA, MPH, MERC[c,*]

KEYWORDS

- Chiari I malformation • Clinical outcomes • Outcome measures • Clinical assessment tools • Adult
- Pediatrics

KEY POINTS

- Presentation and management of Chiari I malformation patients varies widely.
- Clinical outcome measures tools help standardize assessment of post-management outcomes.
- Generic and disease-specific instruments have been studied, each with its own pros and cons.

INTRODUCTION

Chiari I malformation (CM1) is a common diagnosis with a prevalence estimated between 0.5% and 3.6%.[1–4] However, the natural history of CM1 is not well established and symptom onset is often insidious. As such, patients can have a wide variety of presentations from completely asymptomatic individuals to patients who suffer from debilitating diseases.[5–7] Indications for treatment and techniques for decompression are variable and debated.[8,9] With varying degrees of severity and heterogeneity in the management for CM1 patients, assessing clinical outcomes is often difficult and is currently an active area of research. Historically, outcomes were assessed using several general disability outcomes scales however, several Chiari-specific scales have been developed and are now preferred in assessing outcomes.[10–15] Therefore, the purpose of this article is to consider, evaluate, and compare the clinical outcomes measurement tools that are used to assess patients with CM1.

ADULTS

Chiari is often a congenital and/or pediatric diagnosis, however, many children are not evaluated and diagnosed until their teen or early adult lives (20s to 30s). Because of this, adults may present with different signs and symptoms, or may be referred for evaluation based on incidental findings. In addition, most adults can articulate their pain severity, location, and frequency, better than children, making the use of non-disease specific outcome measures more reliable.

General Outcome Measures

- The visual analog scale (VAS) is a two-item questionnaire and scores pain on a scale of 0 to 10.[16]
- The Neck Disability scale (NDI) is a 10-item questionnaire developed to assess severity of functional disability in patients reporting neck pain.[17]
- The headache disability index (HDI) is a 25-item patient-reported tool used in patients

[a] Department of Neurological Surgery, Vanderbilt University Medical Center, Nashville, TN 37232, USA;
[b] School of Medicine, Vanderbilt University, Nashville, TN 37232, USA; [c] Department of Neurosurgery, University of Alabama at Birmingham, Birmingham, AL 35294, USA
[1] Present address: Medical Center North, 1161 21st Avenue South, Room/Suite T-4224F, Nashville, TN 37232, USA.
* Corresponding author. 1008 FOT, 510 20th Street South, Birmingham, AL 35294.
E-mail address: cnshannon@uabmc.edu

Neurosurg Clin N Am 34 (2023) 167–174
https://doi.org/10.1016/j.nec.2022.08.010
1042-3680/23/© 2022 Elsevier Inc. All rights reserved.

reporting disability and pain due to severe and chronic headaches.[18]

- The SF-12 is a health-related quality-of-life questionnaire consisting of 12 questions that measure eight health domains to assess physical and mental health.[19]
- The Zung Self-Rating Depression Scale is a 20-item patient-reported survey quantifying a depressed state by rating the four common characteristics of depression: the pervasive effect, the physiologic equivalents, other disturbances, and psychomotor activities.[12]
- EQ-5D is a standardized patient-reported measure of health-related quality of life developed to assess health status in terms of five dimensions of health including mobility, self-care, usual activities, pain/discomfort and anxiety/depression.[20]

Previous studies have assessed the effectiveness of using general outcome measures for evaluating physical (pain frequency and severity) and psychosocial wellbeing in adults with Chiari.[21,22] Godil and colleagues conducted a study in 2013 to assess the validity of multiple nondisease specific outcomes measures in adult CM1 patients including, a VAS for neck pain and headaches (VAS-Neck and VAS-Head), Neck Disability Index (NDI), Headache Disability Index (HDI), Zung Self-Rating Depression Scale (Zung), Euro-Qol-5D [EQ-5D], and SF-12 Physical and Mental Component Scales (SF-12 PCS and SF-12 MCS).[21] They found the NDI most effectively measured pain, whereas the SF-12 Physical Component Scale and the EQ-5D were effective in measuring general health-related quality of life. However, a major limitation of this study is the outcome of interest, meaningful improvement, defined by the authors for this study as "level of improvement in general health after suboccipital decompression". The authors note that no gold standard exists to clearly assess this type of outcome in adult patients treated for CM1. In addition, this 50-patient study had 1-year postoperative pain, disability, and QoL assessments conducted via phone interviews by an independent investigator not involved with clinical care. This type of assessment could create the opportunity for interviewer bias and recall bias on the part of the patient. A study conducted by Almotairi, and colleagues[22] evaluated CM1 patients 3-month post-surgery using the EQ-5D and the Hospital Anxiety and Depression Scale. This study showed a significant difference in health-related quality of life, as measured by the EQ-5D. However, only 13 patients were followed in this study, so results should be taken with caution.

Chiari Symptom Profile

Developed in 2013, the Chiari Symptom Profile (CSP) is a 57-item patient-reported self-reported questionnaire evaluating physical, functional, social, and psychological domains primarily in adults. Each question is answered using a Likert system with 0 representing "Never" and 4 representing "All the time." Scores for CSP range from 0 to 228 with 0 representing no disability.[15] Mueller and Oro' found this tool to be reliable and valid in the patient cohort evaluated. Although the CSP is extremely comprehensive, disease-specific, and shows promise, there has been no validation study done comparing normative patients and no external validation from other institutions (**Table 1**).

Chicago Chiari Outcome Scale

The Chicago Chiari Outcome Scale (CCOS) was developed in 2012 to evaluate postoperative changes in Chiari patients. The CCOS encompasses four domains:

- Pain symptoms: headaches, neck pain, and dysesthetic pain in arms
- Non-pain symptoms: dysphagia, vertigo, weakness, and syrinx.
- Functionality: assessed the patient's ability to perform daily responsibilities.
- Complications: wound infection, meningitis, and cerebrospinal fluid leak.

Each domain is scored from 1 to 4 with 4 signifying a better outcome. An overall score is calculated by summing the individual domains with a score of 16 representing "Excellent Outcome" and a score of 4 representing "Incapacitated Outcome".[11]

Aliaga and colleagues developed and validated the CCOS using data captured from a chart review of 146 adult and pediatric patients previously undergoing first-time treatment for CM1. In addition to having a CCOS score each of the patients were also stratified as having improved/unchanged/worse postoperatively based on the quality-of-life change for the patients. Five blinded raters were used, and the results showed good reliability without significant variance between the raters.[11] Authors found that the CCOS assigned higher scores to those who were noted as "improved" postoperatively, and proportionately lower scores to those who were "unchanged or worse". Limitations of this validation study included (1) the retrospective chart review without patient confirmation, (2) data were only captured at one moment in time, versus multiple postoperative clinic visits, and (3) the

Table 1
Strengths and limitations of outcome measures

Outcome Measure	Population	Strengths	Limitations
Generic Outcome Measures			
VAS	Adult	Externally validated Quick Patient reported	Generic Cannot be compared between individuals
NDI	Adult	Externally validated Effectively measures pain Patient reported	Generic Specific to neck pain and cervical radiculopathy
HDI	Adult	Externally validated Evaluates functional and emotional impact on QoL Patient reported	Generic Limited to headache specific QoL measures
SF-12	Adult	Externally validated Patient reported Effectively measures QoL Validated to track changes over time	Generic
ZDS	Adult	Externally validated Patient reported	Generic Primarily evaluates mood
EQ-5D	Adult	Externally validated Effectively measures QoL Quantitative comparisons	Generic
PedsQL	Pediatric	Externally validated Patient reported	Generic
PROMIS	Pediatric	Externally validated Patient reported	Generic Time intensive
HUI3	Both	Externally validated Patient reported Effectively measures QoL	Generic
Chiari Specific Outcome Measures			
CCOS	Both	Externally validated Most used Time efficient	Certain domains can be difficult to interpret Not patient reported Clusters at higher scores
CSP	Adult	Patient-reported Rigorous internal validation	Needs external validation Time requirement
CHIP	Pediatric	Patient-reported Rigorous internal validation	Needs external validation Time requirement
SI	Pediatric	Includes clinical and imaging characteristics Externally validated	QoL metrics susceptible to recall bias Weak association with surgical outcomes Limited patient input

subjective labeling of 'improved, unchanged, or worse' was used as the standard outcome measure creating bias and potentially reducing the reliability of these results.

PEDIATRICS
Pediatric Quality of Life Inventory

The Pediatric Quality of Life Inventory (PedsQL) is a self-reported (by patient or parent) quality of life inventory with 23 questions assessing physical, social, emotional, and school functioning. Using a Likert scale, the PedsQL is scored on a scale from 0 "never" to 4 "almost always".[23] PedsQL has been used extensively to assess pediatric neurosurgery outcomes in posterior fossa brain tumor, myelomeningocele, and vascular malformation patients.[24–27] In fact, Hansen and colleagues reported that the PedsQL was one of the most frequently used inventories in pediatric neurosurgery.[26] Through our review we were able to only identify one study that investigated this tool's use in a Chiari-1 patient population. In a study analyzing 87 pediatric patients with CM1 undergoing decompression, Raygani and colleagues reported that individuals who had severe disability as measured by the PedsQL had improvement in their scores postoperatively.[28] However, inconsistent results that were not were seen at different time points and across respondents (patient vs parents). In addition, this study was retrospective in nature, and due to the lack of data available for each patient, including lack of preoperative baseline data missing for 47 patients, the authors aggregated the data for analysis. Due to the limitations of this study, it is unclear if the conclusions the authors drew were appropriate. Currently, there is an ongoing multi-center study by investigators in the UK using PedsQL to measure children's health-related quality of life (HRQoL) in patients with CM1 and we look forward to those results.[29] The widespread use of the PedsQL is likely due to its simplicity, quick administration (less than 5 min), high reliability as well as it being translated to many different languages. The biggest limitation of this tool is due to it being a generic measure. Especially in younger patients or patients with multiple comorbidities, it is difficult to identify the exact causes for lower quality of life.

The Patient-Reported Outcomes Measurement Information Systems

PROMIS is a web-based publicly available health outcomes system created by the National Institutes of Health (NIH), to measure patient-reported health status for physical, mental, and social well-being. This tool has been used to measure health symptoms and health-related quality of life domains such as pain, fatigue, depression, and physical function, often reported in patients with a variety of chronic disease diagnoses. Multiple studies have evaluated the use of PROMIS in populations such as adult seen in dermatology and optometry clinics, adults presenting in the emergency department, adults in the orthopedic trauma ICU, as well as patients seen in the juvenile arthritis clinic, in pediatrics with hip disease, and in home health

patients.[30–36] Most studies felt that the general measurement tool was adequate for capturing factors impacting the health of their patients and easily adaptable in the settings used. However, several noted that when compared with disease-specific instruments PROMIS was less effective and difficult to interpret making the utility less impactful. Only one study we found used PROMIS to investigate Chiari outcomes. Savchuck and colleagues used the mobility, cognition, peer relation, anxiety, fatigue, pain, and sleep domains of PROMIS to create a preference score ranging from 0 to 1 with 1 representing perfect health. This pilot study included 20 pediatric patients who underwent posterior fossa decompression for Chiari 1 malformation. The results showed moderate improvement in quality of life as measured with the most improvement seen in anxiety and pain.[37] As mentioned this was a pilot study of only 20 patients and as not been replicated in a larger sample size, therefore results of this study remain in question.

Health Utilities Index Mark 3

Health Utilities Index Mark 3 (HUI3) is a general health rating scale that measures health-related quality of life. The HUI3 score is based on 8 attributes: vision, hearing, speech, ambulation, dexterity, emotion, cognition, and pain. Each attribute is scored on a scale from 1 to 5/6 (depending on the attribute) with 1 indicating the best possible health state in each domain.[38] HUI3 has been extensively validated in the general pediatric population, and in children diagnosed with cancer, acute illness, and pulmonary illnesses and found to be both reliable and generalizable.[26,39,40] In addition, HUI3 has been evaluated in children with cerebral palsy, and found to be effective in measuring psychometric properties, but does not include dimensions and factors directly impacting this patient group and therefore was unable to adequately assess the quality of life in the cerebral palsy population.[41]

A study by Ladner and colleagues used the HUI3 to compare and validate a disease-specific quality of life instrument. In their study, they found the HUI3 domains of vision, speech, cognition, and pain were able to show a difference between the CM-I population and their control group, with Chiari patients having lower scores. However, as the purpose of the Ladner study was not to validate HUI3 in the pediatric Chiari population, no information can be gleaned regarding the effectiveness of this instruction to properly measure the quality of life in this patient group.

No other studies have used HUI3 to evaluate post-surgical outcomes in pediatric patients undergoing treatment for CM1. Therefore, we are unable to determine whether the HUI3 is an effective outcome measure in this patient population.

Chicago Chiari Outcome Scale

Yarbrough and colleagues conducted a study to externally validated the CCOS using retrospective data from 215 pediatric patients previously undergoing first-time treatment for CM-1.[42] Similar to the original study, they reported a good reliability among the raters. This study found that the CCOS was consistent in scoring postoperative outcomes when compared with general physician assessment. However, very poor reliability for the functionality component was reported, affecting the overall score's reliability. The authors stated that although this was a strong step forward in identifying a disease-specific tool, it did not remove the subjectivity from clinical assessment, and the ambiguous scoring scale was not adequate in clearly stratifying patients by severity of symptoms, postoperative improvement, and complications.[42] Unlike the other tools discussed in this article, the CCOS is not patient reported. Instead, it is designed for a reviewer to assess outcome metrics via chart review. which opens the instrument to interrater variability, and subjectivity and bias in interpretation.

Chiari Health Index for Pediatrics

The Chiari Health Index for Pediatrics (CHIP) is a 45-item patient-reported questionnaire that evaluates the health-related quality of life (HRQL) in pediatric patients, 5 years and older, with Chiari 1 malformation. It is comprised of 4 components making up 2 domains. The physical domain includes pain severity (5 questions), pain frequency (5 questions), nonpain symptoms (11 questions), and the Psychosocial domain includes all psychosocial/cognitive questions (24 questions). Question scales range from "No pain or Never", with a score of 0, to "Severe or Almost Always", with a score of 1. Each domain gets a score between 0 and 1 with higher numbers representing the higher quality of life.[13]

Ladner and colleagues validate the CHIP in several stages. First, the scores from each component were compared between patients with Chiari 1 malformation and healthy controls. Results showed that for each individual domain the Chiari patient group scored lower than the healthy controls, noting the lower quality of life. Second, scores on the CHIP questionnaire were compared between symptomatic and asymptomatic Chiari patients with the symptomatic patients scoring significantly lower compared with asymptomatic patients. Lastly, the individual domains of the CHIP questionnaire were compared with scores from the validated HUI3 revealing a good correlation.[13]

A follow-up study was conducted by Sellyn and colleagues evaluating the effectiveness of the CHIP to measure short-term quality of life changes. The study included 63 patients who underwent initial treatment for their Chiari 1 malformation, were seen in the same clinic for follow-up, and had at least 1 postoperative CHIP survey completed. The CHIP was compared with surgical success and noted as improvements in clinical and/or radiographic symptoms. The results showed an increase in overall scores from baseline to postoperative evaluation. The CHIP scores were also significantly correlated with changes in symptomatology, especially the resolution of syrinx.[43]

The limitations of CHIP continue to be the single-center evaluation of this quality-of-life instrument and the inconsistency of survey responders between pre- and postoperative survey completion. The CHIP was recently used as the quality-of-life instrument in a 35-center PCORI-funded study. That study, currently in data analysis and write-up phase, looked at the quality of life, measured by the CHIP, intervention type, and long-term follow-up.

Chiari Severity Index

The Chiari Severity Index (CSI) was developed in 2015 by Greenberg and colleagues using both imaging and clinical parameters to predict postoperative outcomes. In a sample of 158 pediatric patients, clinical parameters such as headache type as well as myelopathic symptoms along with imaging characteristics such as syrinx size were recorded. In addition, patients were asked to complete a two-question survey to evaluate their quality-of-life improvement after surgery. By performing sequential sequestration for both clinical and imaging parameters followed by integrating the two, a three-tiered severity index was created. Grade 1 included patients with "classic-Chiari" or "poorly localized" headaches. A majority of the Grade 1 patients (32/46) had either no syrinx or <6 mm of syrinx. In this severity group, 83% improved postoperatively. Grade 2 included patients with either frontotemporal headaches, no headaches, or myelopathic symptoms along with no syrinx or <6 mm of syrinx. In this severity group, 66% improved postoperatively. Grade 3 included patients with either frontotemporal headaches, no headaches, or myelopathic symptoms along with >6 mm of syrinx. In this severity group, 45% improved postoperatively.[14]

Several studies have investigated the role of CSI in predicting treatment outcomes. Pisapia and colleagues studied 189 pediatric patients who were treated with posterior fossa decompression, of which 176 had data to formulate a CSI grade. Their results did not reveal a clear association between CSI grade and postoperative outcomes irrespective of extradural decompression or intradural decompression. They note that this may have been due to how postoperative outcomes were measured.[44]

Grangeon and colleagues evaluated 49 adult patients to study headache resolution postoperatively after decompression surgery. In their cohort, 38 patients had CSI grades, and they reported 82.6% favorable outcomes for CSI Grade 1 patients, 62.5% for CSI Grade 2 patients, and 42.8% for CSI grade 3 patients. However, statistically significance was not met.[45] Feghali and colleagues also studied an adult Chiari I patient population and found a similar decreasing percentage of favorable postoperative outcomes with increasing CSI grade. They too also reported this association was not statistically significant.[46] They postulate this may be due to differences in adult versus pediatric outcomes postoperatively.

DISCUSSION

For this article, we identified general and disease-specific outcome measures that have been used in both the CM1 adult and pediatric populations. There are pros and cons to incorporating any of these tools into routine clinical care.

When considering general outcome measures, we cannot deny the simplicity of using these instruments across all patients seen in a single clinic. These tools are easily adapted into clinical practice, often shorter surveys with broad questions related to health that do not necessarily require significant recall, thereby reducing recall bias. In addition, most are self-reported reducing subjectivity bias. In adults, these general outcome measures, like the VAS, EQ-5D, and the HDI, may be more impactful as adults are, most often, able to articulate symptoms such as pain frequency and pain severity better than children, making interpretability clearer. As with adult-specific outcome measure, pediatric measures, such as the PedsQL, is again an easily adopted, simply understood, survey with Likert scale questions. Parents completing this survey can do so while waiting to be seen and clinic staff can administer quickly, as it is generalizable to most patient groups. PROMIS has similar positive factors and has been found to be extremely comprehensive with broad questions that can apply to most patient populations (both adult and pediatric). Several of the general measures, HUI3, SF-12, PROMIS, also do a respectable job of identifying psychosocial factors such as depression and anxiety, which can often impact treatment success. For this reason, some sections or domains of these tools could be considered for standard use in the clinic setting.

However, in most of the studies we looked at the general outcome measure did not do a sufficient job of identifying factors that specifically impact patients with chronic diagnoses such as Chiari. The questions asked are broad and do not often address the chronic nature of the symptoms seen by these patients. In addition, the questions do not provide the detail, such as limb numbness and weakness, headache location, pain severity, gait and balance, often seen in this patient population and needed in clinical decision-making.

Over the last 6 to 10 years we have seen multiple disease-specific instruments validated in both populations and there seems to be a trend toward using these tools over general outcome measures.[42] The CSI, the CCOS, the CSP, and the CHIP have all been validated in recent years.

CCOS was the first to be developed in 2012, and has been used the most for Chiari outcomes research.[47–49] CCOS was initially validated using a patient population of both adult and pediatric patients; thus, subsequent studies have used CCOS in both populations and have been externally validated.[11,42] Furthermore, the simplicity of the CCOS allows it to be time-efficient as only five questions need to be answered. Despite these strengths, the CCOS does have several limitations including the retrospective nature of the scale and the scoring interpretability. The CSI has also been validated. externally validated and has been used in multiple previously published studies. Although several of the studies found clinical significance, they were unable to achieve statistical significance. In addition, this scale is a preoperative scoring scale looking at predicting postoperative outcomes. The CSP and CHIP were created with rigorous validation methods. Both surveys were tested to ensure a comprehensive, appropriate, and efficient group of questions were used to measure Chiari-I specific outcomes. The CHIP has been shown to be valid when looking at short-term outcomes in pediatric Chiari patients previously undergoing surgical intervention. However, this study was conducted by the original validation team. At this time neither the CSP nor the CHIP has been externally validated (see **Table 1**). The CHIP has recently been included in a 35-center prospective funded study. That study is currently in data analysis and writeup.

All the disease-specific outcome measures discussed provide comprehensive questions that are specific to the factors, symptoms, and psychosocial characteristics of this patient population. This information is impactful and necessary for treatment decision-making and long-term management. There are still several important areas that still need to be explored and studied. The CSP and the CHIP need to be externally validated in their current validated populations and validation or modification and validation needs to occur in other Chiari patient populations. The scoring scale and interpretability of the CCOS needs to be addressed to properly differentiate between patient symptoms, complications, and postoperative improvement.

SUMMARY

This article highlights the variety of general and disease-specific outcome measures used in both the pediatric and adult CM1 patient populations. Although general measures can be associated with clinical outcomes and quality of life, that association is not often found to be statistically significant, and they do not often have the capabilities to assess and measure factors that directly impact the Chiari patient population. However, limitations exist when considering the disease-specific outcome measures, as these tools most often have not been rigorously evaluated externally from the initial validation or have been externally validated but results cannot be replicated. Identifying an outcomes measurement tool for both adults and patients will contribute to the clinical tools available to providers for decision-making and management.

DISCLOSURE

None.

REFERENCES

1. Meadows J, Kraut M, Guarnieri M, et al. Asymptomatic Chiari Type I malformations identified on magnetic resonance imaging. J Neurosurg 2000;92(6):920–6.
2. Strahle J, Muraszko Karin M, Joseph K, et al. Chiari malformation Type I and syrinx in children undergoing magnetic resonance imaging. J Neurosurg Pediatrics 2011;8(2):205–13.
3. Aitken Leslie A, Lindan Camilla E, Stephen S, et al. Chiari Type I Malformation in a Pediatric Population. Pediatr Neurol 2009;40(6):449–54.
4. Vernooij Meike W, Arfan IM, Tanghe Hervé L, et al. Incidental Findings on Brain MRI in the General Population. N Engl J Med 2007;357(18):1821–8.
5. Bezuidenhout Abraham F, Chang Y-M, Heilman Carl B, et al. Headache in Chiari Malformation. Neuroimaging Clin N Am 2019;29(2):243–53.
6. Almotairi F. Andersson Mats., Andersson Olof., et al. Swallowing Dysfunction in Adult Patients with Chiari I Malformation. J Neurol Surg B Skull Base 2018; 79(06):606–13.

7. McClugage Samuel G, Jerry OW. The Chiari I malformation. J Neurosurg Pediatr 2019;24(3):217–26.
8. Alden TD, Ojemann JG, Park TS. Surgical treatment of Chiari I malformation: indications and approaches. Neurosurg Focus 2001;11(1):E2.
9. Jörg Klekamp. Surgical Treatment of Chiari I Malformation—Analysis of Intraoperative Findings, Complications, and Outcome for 371 Foramen Magnum Decompressions. Neurosurgery 2012;71(2):365–80.
10. Yarbrough Chester K, Greenberg Jacob K, Park TS. Clinical Outcome Measures in Chiari I Malformation. Neurosurg Clin N Am 2015;26(4):533–41.
11. Aliaga L, Hekman Katherine E, Reza Y, et al. A Novel Scoring System for Assessing Chiari Malformation Type I Treatment Outcomes. Neurosurgery 2012; 70(3):656–65.
12. ZUNG WW. A Self-Rating Depression Scale. Arch Gen Psychiat 1965;12(1):63–70.
13. Ladner Travis R, Westrick Ashly C, Wellons John C, et al. Health-related quality of life in pediatric Chiari Type I malformation: the Chiari Health Index for Pediatrics. J Neurosurg Pediatr 2016;17(1):76–85.
14. Greenberg Jacob K, Yarbrough Chester K, Radmanesh Alireza, et al. The Chiari Severity Index: A Preoperative Grading System for Chiari Malformation Type 1. Neurosurgery 2015;76(3):279–85.
15. Mueller Diane M. Oro' John J. The Chiari Symptom Profile. J Neurosci Nurs 2013;45(4):205–10.
16. Gallagher EJ, Liebman M, Bijur Polly E. Prospective validation of clinically important changes in pain severity measured on a visual analog scale. Ann Emerg Med 2001;38(6):633–8.
17. Vernon H, Mior S. The Neck Disability Index: a study of reliability and validity. J Manipulative Physiol Ther 1991;14(7):409–15.
18. Jacobson Gary P, Ramadan Nabih M, Norris Lisa, et al. Headache Disability Inventory (HDI): Short-term Test-Retest Reliability and Spouse Perceptions. Headache J Head Face Pain 1995;35(9):534–9.
19. Ware JE, Kosinski M, Keller susan D. A 12-Item Short-Form Health Survey: Construction of Scales and Preliminary Tests of Reliability and Validity. Med Care 1996;34(3):220–33.
20. Group The EuroQol. EuroQol - a new facility for the measurement of health-related quality of life. Health Policy 1990;16(3):199–208.
21. Godil Saniya S, Parker Scott L, Zuckerman Scott L, et al. Accurately Measuring Outcomes After Surgery for Adult Chiari I Malformation: Determining the Most Valid and Responsive Instruments. Neurosurgery 2013;72(5):820–7.
22. Almotairi Fawaz S. Hellström Per., Skoglund Thomas., et al. Chiari I malformation—neuropsychological functions and quality of life. Acta Neurochir 2020;162(7):1575–82.
23. Varni James W, Seid M, Kurtin Paul S. PedsQL™ 4.0: Reliability and Validity of the Pediatric Quality

of Life Inventory™ Version 4.0 Generic Core Scales in Healthy and Patient Populations. Med Care 2001; 39(8):800–12.

24. Nishit M, Dewan MC, Huang A, et al. Intrauterine closure of myelomeningocele is associated with superior long-term quality of life than postnatal closure: a single-center study. J Neurosurg Pediatr 2019; 24(2):115–9.

25. Kulkarni Abhaya V, Piscione J, Shams I, et al. Long-term quality of life in children treated for posterior fossa brain tumors. J Neurosurg Pediatr 2013; 12(3):235–40.

26. Hansen D, Vedantam A, Valentina B, et al. Health-related quality of life outcomes and level of evidence in pediatric neurosurgery. J Neurosurg Pediatr 2016; 18(4):480–6.

27. Goethe E, LoPresti Melissa A, Zhao Michelle, et al. Quality of Life in Pediatric Neurosurgery: Comparing Parent and Patient Perceptions. World Neurosurg 2020;134:e306–10.

28. Shawyon B, Zieles K, Jea A. PedsQL for prediction of postoperative patient-reported outcomes following Chiari decompression surgery. J Neurosurg Pediatr 2020;25(3):268–73.

29. Piper Rory J, Afshari Fardad T, Soon Wai C, et al. UK Chiari 1 Study: protocol for a prospective, observational, multicentre study. Bmj Open 2021;11(4):e043712.

30. Esaa F, James P, Alice P, et al. The utility of PROMIS domain measures in dermatologic care. Arch Dermatol Res 2021;313(1):17–24.

31. Rebecca T, Wang CM, Murray E, et al. PROMIS Computer Adaptive Tests and Their Correlation With Disease Activity in Juvenile Idiopathic Arthritis. Jcr J Clin Rheumatol 2019. https://doi.org/10.1097/rhu.0000000000001171. Publish Ahead of Print(4):131–5.

32. Snavely Joseph E, Weiner Joseph A, Johnson Daniel J, et al. Preoperative PROMIS Scores Predict Postoperative Outcomes in Lumbar Spine Surgery Patients. Spine 2021;46(17):1139–46.

33. O'Hara Nathan N, Richards John T, Archie O, et al. Is PROMIS the new standard for patient-reported outcomes measures in orthopaedic trauma research? Inj 2020;51:S43–50.

34. Porter Randall S, Holt K, Ramchandran Rajeev S. Implementation of PROMIS® in an Optometry Clinic. Patient Relat Outcome Meas 2021;12:307–12.

35. Kurt K, Stump Timothy E, Jacob K, et al. Diagnostic operating characteristics of PROMIS scales in screening for depression. J Psychosom Res 2021; 147:110532.

36. Donato Giuseppe L, Perry Daniel C, Abdullah B, et al. PROMIS Paediatric Mobility tool is correlated with accelerometer-measured physical activity in children with hip diseases. Bone Jt J 2021;103-B(2):405–10.

37. Savchuk S, Jin MC, Choi S, et al. Incorporating patient-centered quality-of-life measures for outcome assessment after Chiari malformation type I decompression in a pediatric population: a pilot study. J Neurosurg Pediatr 2022;29(2):200–7.

38. Horsman J, Furlong W, Feeny D, et al. The Health Utilities Index (HUI): concepts, measurement properties and applications. Health Qual Life Out 2003; 1(1):54.

39. Chen P, Melissa Hudson M, Li M, et al. Health utilities in pediatric cancer patients and survivors: a systematic review and meta-analysis for clinical implementation. Qual Life Res 2022;31(2):343–74.

40. Cunha F, Almeida-Santos L, Teixeira-Pinto A, et al. Health-related quality of life of pediatric intensive care survivors. J Pediatr 2011;88(1):25–32.

41. Mpundu-Kaambwa C, Chen G, Elisabeth H, et al. A review of preference-based measures for the assessment of quality of life in children and adolescents with cerebral palsy. Qual Life Res 2018;27(7): 1781–99.

42. Yarbrough Chester K, Greenberg Jacob K, Smyth Matthew D, et al. External validation of the Chicago Chiari Outcome Scale: Clinical article. J Neurosurg Pediatr 2014;13(6):679–84.

43. Sellyn Georgina E, Tang AR, Zhao S, et al. Effectiveness of the Chiari Health Index for Pediatrics instrument in measuring postoperative health-related quality of life in pediatric patients with Chiari malformation type I. J Neurosurg Pediatr 2021;27(2):139–44.

44. Pisapia Jared M, Merkow Maxwell B, Danielle B, et al. External validity of the chiari severity index and outcomes among pediatric chiari I patients treated with intra- or extra-Dural decompression. Child's Nerv Syst 2017;33(2):313–20.

45. Lou G, Laurent P, Gilard Vianney, et al. Predictive Factors of Headache Resolution After Chiari Type 1 Malformation Surgery. World Neurosurg 2018;110: e60–6.

46. James F, Xie Y, Chen Y, et al. External validation of current prediction systems of improvement after decompression surgery in Chiari malformation type I patients: can we do better? J Neurosurg 2020; 134(5):1466–71.

47. Lorenzo G, Mahmoud M, Daniel Roy T, et al. Long-term outcome of surgical treatment of Chiari malformation without syringomyelia. J Neurosurg Sci 2020;64(4). https://doi.org/10.23736/s0390-5616.17.04063-2.

48. Michael Lumintang L, Vivas-Buitrago T, Domingo Ricardo A, et al. Prognostic significance of C1–C2 facet malalignment after surgical decompression in adult Chiari malformation type I: a pilot study based on the Chicago Chiari Outcome Scale. J Neurosurg Spine 2021;34(2):171–7.

49. Gilmer Holly S, Xi M, Young Sonja H. Surgical Decompression for Chiari Malformation Type I: An Age-Based Outcomes Study Based on the Chicago Chiari Outcome Scale. World Neurosurg 2017;107: 285–90.

Idiopathic Intracranial Hypertension and Vascular Anomalies in Chiari I Malformation

David C. Lauzier, BS[a],*, Sarah N. Chiang, BS[a],
Arindam R. Chatterjee, MD[a,b,c], Joshua W. Osbun, MD[a,b,c]

KEYWORDS

- Chiari I • Dural venous stenosis • Idiopathic intracranial hypertension

KEY POINTS

- Idiopathic intracranial hypertension and Chiari I malformation may share common pathophysiologic mechanisms.
- There is a high rate of dural venous sinus stenosis in both patient groups.
- Understanding these mechanisms may improve treatment provided to these patients.

INTRODUCTION

Idiopathic intracranial hypertension (IIH), sometimes referred to as pseudotumor cerebri, is a disorder of elevated intracranial pressure (ICP) that causes headaches, papilledema, vision changes, and pulsatile tinnitus.[1,2] In severe cases, it can progress to irreversible optic nerve damage and blindness.[3] IIH most commonly presents in women of child-bearing age with elevated body mass index (BMI).[4] Prior study has firmly established elevated BMI, female sex, and the presence of certain steroid hormones as factors contributing to the development of IIH.[5,6] BMI elevations cause IIH by increasing intra-abdominal pressure and central venous pressure (CVP), leading to decreased cerebrospinal fluid (CSF) reabsorption.[7] Female sex hormones act through adipocyte conversion of androstenedione into estrone, which stimulates CSF production.[8] In both cases, the pressure gradients necessary for normal CSF flow and drainage are disrupted.

Recent studies of IIH have emphasized the role cerebral venous anomalies play in its pathogenesis and progression, with some suggesting that IIH in this setting should be classified as "vascular intracranial hypertension," rather than truly idiopathic.[9–11] Specifically, venous sinus stenosis has garnered considerable attention in relation to IIH. In patients who fail to demonstrate improvement following conservative and pharmacologic treatment for IIH, targeting venous sinus stenosis with venous sinus stenting (VSS) provides an alternative to traditional treatment procedures such as optic nerve sheath fenestration (ONSF) or CSF shunting.[12,13] Despite clinical success in treating IIH by targeting venous sinus stenosis, it remains unclear if the development of stenosis is an inciting event for the development of intracranial hypertension or if it is a consequence of sustained compression of the venous sinuses from elevated ICP.[9]

Chiari I malformation is another disease closely associated with abnormal intracranial fluid dynamics and pressures.[14,15] Causes of Chiari I

[a] Department of Neurological Surgery, Washington University School of Medicine; [b] Mallinckrodt Institute of Radiology, Washington University School of Medicine; [c] Department of Neurology, Washington University School of Medicine
* Corresponding author. 510 S. Kingshighway Boulevard.
E-mail address: dlauzier@wustl.edu

Neurosurg Clin N Am 34 (2023) 175–183
https://doi.org/10.1016/j.nec.2022.09.008
1042-3680/23/© 2022 Elsevier Inc. All rights reserved.

malformation include genetic diseases, pathologic conditions of the basal skull, and conditions causing caudal traction of the brainstem.[16] It has been observed that a subset of patients present with both IIH and Chiari I malformation.[17] Therefore, some investigators have proposed common underlying mechanisms between IIH and Chiari I malformation, because both involve impaired intracranial compliance and present in similar patient populations.[18,19] Furthermore, there may be an elevated prevalence of venous sinus stenosis and venous disease in patients with Chiari I malformation.[20,21]

With recent work identifying the possible interplay of intracranial hypertension, cerebral venous anomalies, and Chiari I malformation, it is imperative to pause and review the literature to guide future preclinical and clinical studies in this area. This article summarizes the mechanisms connecting these conditions and reviews their diagnostic and treatment strategies.

Mechanisms

Venous sinus stenosis and idiopathic intracranial hypertension

Causes of venous hypertension are multifactorial and include elevated BMI, heart failure, and pulmonary hypertension. Elevated CVP results in increased ICP by increasing cerebral venous pressure and decreasing venous outflow.[22] Alongside these extracranial causes, a growing body of evidence has suggested that venous sinus stenosis is a major cause of elevated cerebral venous pressure.[23] Following the report of a single patient with IIH that resolved after stenting of the transverse sinus, Farb and colleagues[24] identified venous sinus stenosis in 93% of patients with IIH and only 7% of controls using magnetic resonance venography, suggesting that IIH and venous anomalies are intimately related.[24,25] Subsequent reports have confirmed that venous sinus stenosis is nearly always present in patients with IIH but rarely observed in controls without IIH.[23,26] Although the involvement of venous outflow in the pathogenesis of IIH was initially posited in the late nineteenth century, the findings of Farb and colleagues[24] were the first to provide evidence of venous sinus stenosis in this pathologic condition.[27]

Venous sinus stenosis contributes to elevated ICP by interfering with CSF drainage. For proper CSF drainage from the subarachnoid spaces to the venous system, a pressure gradient of approximately 3 to 5 mm Hg is required.[28,29] Elevated cerebral venous pressure secondary to venous sinus stenosis impairs CSF drainage due to disruption of this gradient, subsequently increasing ICP.[10] Significant flow impairments may develop with angiographic stenosis of only 30% to 35%.[30] In a large series by Riggeal and colleagues[23] examining patients with IIH and transverse sinus stenosis, the median degree of stenosis was 56%, but severity of stenosis was not correlated with clinical course. It is theorized that once stenosis reaches a certain threshold, the transstenosis pressure gradient is severe enough to resist additional external compression, leading to coexistence of high ICP and venous pressure.[31] At this point, compensatory mechanisms and collateral pathways develop to mollify the progression of venous pressures by allowing CSF absorption at higher pressure thresholds.[32] Signs of increased collateralization including dilation of the occipital emissary vein are frequently observed in patients with stenosis-associated IIH and sparingly in those without.[32]

Venous sinus stenosis is broadly categorized as either extrinsic or intrinsic. Because of the collapsibility of dural venous sinuses, high ICP compresses these structures and leads to extrinsic stenosis.[27] The transverse sinuses in particular are vulnerable to collapse in the setting of ICP elevation.[12] Extrinsic stenosis is associated with an angiographic appearance of long segment stenosis with obtuse margins.[13] Intrinsic stenosis occurs due to local filling defects secondary to fixed intravenous structures that hinder venous blood flow including arachnoid granulations, fenestrations, and chronic thrombus.[27] Intrinsic stenosis is associated with an angiographic appearance of short segment stenosis with acute margins.[13] Extrinsic stenosis typically improves with reductions in ICP, whereas intrinsic stenosis does not.[27] Following the development of stenosis, venous pressures increase proximal to the occlusion[30,33]; this creates a positive feedback loop, where additional increases in ICP can worsen extrinsic compression and stenosis.[33] Removal of CSF interrupts this process, with some studies reporting temporary resolution of venous sinus stenosis following CSF diversion via shunting.[34,35] Stenting of the venous sinuses provides another method to disrupt the positive feedback loop. However, underlying causes of ICP elevations may be extracranial, and in these cases, stenting does not address the cause of the increased ICP.

Venous sinus stenosis and idiopathic intracranial hypertension in relation to Chiari I malformation

A relationship between IIH and Chiari I malformation was proposed nearly concurrently with the first reports of an association between IIH and venous sinus stenosis. Bejjani and colleagues[36,37] first proposed a relationship between IIH and Chiari I in 2003 following their publication of a series that described 6 patients with Chiari I malformation that failed to improve following posterior fossa decompression but improved with ventriculoperitoneal shunting, repeated lumbar puncture, or pharmacologic treatment with acetazolamide. In light of these findings, the investigators suggested that IIH and certain forms of Chiari I malformation are variants of the same disease process. In their model, tonsillar ectopia characteristic of Chiari I malformation develops in cases in which craniocephalic disproportion is present, which allows for ICP to drive the cerebellar tonsils caudally. In their hypothesis, ectopy of the cerebellar tonsils is a consequence of ICP elevations.

The initial observation by Bejjani and colleagues of patients with IIH and tonsillar ectopy unresponsive to posterior fossa decompression but responsive to CSF diversion has been reported in several series, with this process now named "Chiari pseudotumor syndrome."[38–40] The inverse has also been reported, where patients with concomitant IIH and tonsillar ectopia fail to improve after treatment with CSF shunting, but respond well to posterior fossa decompression.[19] Recent estimates suggest tonsillar ectopy fulfilling criteria for Chiari I malformation is present in 10% to 24% of patients with clinically confirmed IIH.[19,41] It remains unclear if some patients with Chiari I malformation carry a secondary diagnosis of IIH, or if patients with IIH develop secondary tonsillar ectopia that is mislabeled as Chiari I malformation.

Given the prevalence of venous sinus stenosis in patients with IIH and the frequent copresentation of IIH and Chiari I malformation, Saindane and colleagues[20] examined the prevalence of transverse sinus stenosis (VSS) in patients with Chiari I malformation. The investigators found that 33% of patients with Chiari I malformation had unilateral or bilateral VSS, a significantly higher rate than in control subjects. Furthermore, these investigators conducted a multivariable analysis that demonstrated that presence of VSS was an independent predictor of Chiari I malformation, accounting for age, sex, and BMI. Patients with both Chiari I and VSS were also found to have a greater degree of pituitary flattening, perhaps reflecting the severity or chronicity of ICP elevations. In another study, Fric and Eide[18] found that elevated ICP was a predictor of tonsillar ectopia, but smaller posterior cranial fossa volume was not. In a study of venous anomalies in patients with craniosynostosis, Copeland and colleagues[21] found that patients with dural venous sinus stenosis were more likely to have Chiari I malformation and elevated ICP. However, this study population may not be reflective of the general spectrum of comorbidities in patients with IIH, tonsillar ectopy, or venous sinus stenosis.

Absence of a unifying mechanism

Separate analyses have found that elevated ICP is significantly associated with tonsillar ectopia diagnostic of Chiari I malformation, and that VSS is present at an elevated rate in patients with Chiari I malformation and IIH.[18,20] Despite these findings, the underlying mechanism for these processes remains unclear (**Fig. 1**.). In some cases, peripheral factors like elevated BMI may lead to IIH secondary to increased CVP, thereby increasing ICP, causing extrinsic stenosis, and ultimately forcing the cerebellar tonsils to herniate inferiorly through the foramen magnum.[19] In other cases, intrinsic stenosis could cause cerebral venous pressure elevations, increasing ICP, and causing both extrinsic stenosis and tonsillar herniation. A predisposition for Chiari I malformation may even be the inciting event, where patients with Chiari I malformation have inherently abnormal CSF dynamics that lead to elevated ICP and subsequent stenosis. In each of these models, the positive feedback loops described in patients with IIH explains the progressive worsening of affected patients.[33] Given the absence of a clear mechanism unifying these processes, these varying hypotheses underscore the need for preclinical and translational study into the relationship of IIH, venous sinus stenosis, and Chiari I malformation.

Clinical application

Although there is ambiguity surrounding the underlying relationships between IIH, Chiari I malformation, and venous sinus stenosis, the presentation, diagnosis, and treatment of these conditions is well-defined and reviewed in this section. Of greatest relevance to our previous discussion are patients presenting with "Chiari pseudotumor syndrome."[42]

Presentation and Diagnosis

Idiopathic intracranial hypertension

IIH is characterized by ICP elevations that produce a constellation of potentially devastating symptoms. The most common of these is a pulsatile, retro-orbital headache that is positional and exacerbated by certain eye movements.[43,44] This headache is often accompanied by nausea, diplopia, pulsatile "whooshing" tinnitus, ataxia, dizziness, and loss of vision related to papilledema.[27,45] In IIH that is not medically or surgically addressed, loss of vision may become permanent due to irreversible damage to afferent visual pathways in the optic nerve.[46] Therefore, prompt recognition and

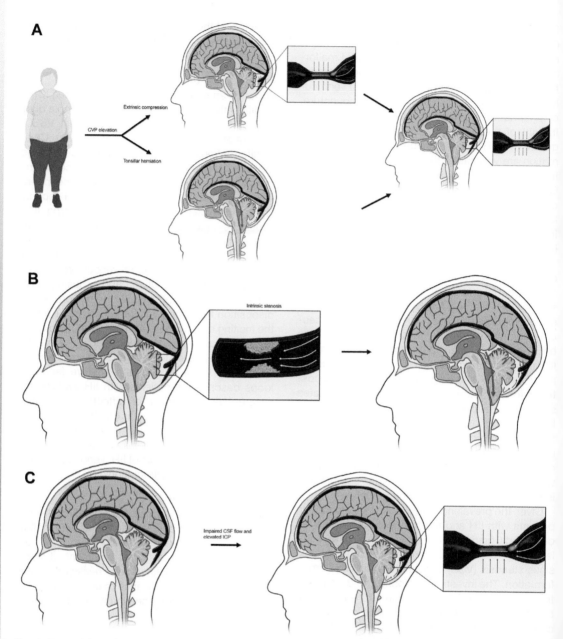

Fig. 1. Potential mechanisms explaining the relationship and copresentation of IIH, Chiari I malformation, and dural venous stenosis. (*A*) A sequence of events in which peripheral factors lead to ICP elevations, which then causes extrinsic compression on the venous sinuses that generates stenosis as well as caudal displacement of the cerebellar tonsils. (*B*) A sequence of events in which local filling defects secondary to accumulation of arachnoid granulations and chronic thrombus lead to intrinsic stenosis, which then causes increased cerebral venous pressure, impairs CSF flow, and causes ICP elevations that lead to caudal displacement of the cerebellar tonsils. (*C*) A sequence of events in which aberrant CSF flow associated with a Chiari I malformation leads to ICP elevations, extrinsic compression on the venous sinuses, and caudal displacement of the cerebellar tonsils.

diagnosis of IIH is necessary to avoid these long-term complications.[47]

Diagnosis of IIH is made according to the Dandy criteria, which are as follows: signs and symptoms of ICP (papilledema, vomiting, visual changes, headache, nausea), an absence of localizing signs,

increased CSF pressure on lumbar puncture without abnormal CSF electrolytes or cytology (typically defined as >25 cm H_2O), and no identifiable cause for increased ICP.[48] For proper diagnosis of IIH, all the aforementioned criteria must be met. When ruling out a mass causing increased

ICP, MRI or computed tomography (CT) may also demonstrate an empty sella.[5] For patients who fail to experience symptomatic improvement after conservative medical treatment, a vascular cause of IIH may be suspected. In these cases, stenting is often considered. In preparation for stenting, an angiographic workup is first conducted to exclude other vascular causes of increased ICP. This workup may also identify the presence of an abnormal cerebral venous pressure gradient, suggesting the patient will benefit from stenting.[12,49,50] The current gold standard for diagnosing venous sinus stenosis and associated pressure gradients is cerebral venography with manometry.

Chiari I malformation

Patients with Chiari I malformation may be asymptomatic or may present with symptoms including headache, neck pain, altered sensation, vertigo, and loss of coordination.[51] Similar to IIH, the most common symptom of Chiari I malformation is a headache.[16] However, this headache differs from that in IIH because it is described as being in the occipital or upper cervical region.[52] Classically, patients have a "tussive" headache brought on by coughing, laughing, straining, or other actions that induce a Valsalva maneuver. Patients with associated syringomyelia may complain of numbness over the back and shoulders in a "cape-like" distribution. In more severe cases, autonomic dysfunction may be present, caused by brainstem compression.[53] Finally, an association between postural orthostatic tachycardia syndrome and Chiari I malformation has been described.[54] However, orthostatic intolerance may not be directly attributable to brainstem compression, and a causal relationship has yet to be established.[55]

When Chiari I malformation is suspected based on presenting symptoms or prior history, diagnostic steps are straightforward, with MRI being the most widely used imaging modality for diagnosis.[16] Owing to the association of syringomyelia with Chiari I, the cervical spine should also be included in imaging sequences. In situations in which MRI is not possible, CT or CT myelography may be reasonable. Diagnosis of Chiari I requires herniation of the cerebellar tonsils at least 3 to 5 mm inferior to the basion-opisthion line through the foramen magnum.[56]

Management

Idiopathic intracranial hypertension

Patients presenting with IIH are first managed conservatively, and management is largely directed toward preventing vision loss. When patients with IIH have elevated BMIs, weight loss can reduce CVP.[57] In cases in which weight loss is unattainable through lifestyle changes, bariatric surgery has demonstrated success in reducing IIH for certain patients.[58] When symptoms do not resolve with conservative approaches, pharmacologic treatment with acetazolamide is often pursued to minimize CSF secretion by the choroid plexus by inhibiting carbonic anhydrase.[50] However, there is conflicting evidence regarding the efficacy of acetazolamide, with a recent systematic review concluding that there was insufficient evidence to recommend or reject the efficacy of this therapy in patients with IIH.[59,60] Moreover, many patients are unable to tolerate escalating doses of acetazolamide secondary to side effects of dizziness, lightheadedness, nausea, and increased urination, and are therefore unable to achieve a therapeutic effect. Other medications sometimes used in patients with IIH include loop diuretics and somatostatin analogues, although the efficacy of these is less well characterized.[61,62]

In many patients suffering from IIH, both conservative and pharmacologic treatment may not be adequate to improve symptoms.[5] Procedural interventions available include ONSF, CSF diversion, or VSS. Lumbar puncture is commonly used as a bridging therapy before pursuing more permanent interventions. ONSF is preferred in cases in which visual symptoms are predominant, because it shows little efficacy in improving headache and other symptoms.[63] However, ONSF frequently requires a second surgery and over one-third of patients require later CSF diversion to achieve symptomatic resolution.[64] In headache-predominant patients, CSF diversion is typically selected despite nearly 80% of patients redeveloping headache in long-term follow-up.[65] Therefore, treatment goals should be aimed at reducing ICP rather than long-term headache control, because headache is likely multifactorial. For patients who fail the aforementioned conventional treatments, VSS has emerged as an option to increase CSF drainage at arachnoid granulations by restoring the necessary pressure gradient for this process.[66] Symptoms improve in up to 94% of patients following VSS.[5,67] Because the pulsatile tinnitus commonly associated with IIH may be partially attributable to venous sinus stenosis and the accelerated, turbulent blood flow it causes, this symptom of IIH may also be amenable to VSS.[68–70] Indeed, studies suggest that 93% to 100% of patients with IIH and pulsatile tinnitus experience a resolution of tinnitus after VSS,[69,71,72] whereas patients with IIH and nonpulsatile tinnitus are less likely to report improvement after stenting.[68] Despite the ability of VSS to address many symptoms of vascular IIH, severe complications including subdural hematoma, in-stent thrombosis, and subarachnoid hemorrhage are known to occur.[73] Venous stenting continues to be an area of interest, with an active trial currently examining the performance of the first stent designed specifically for use in dural venous sinuses.[74]

Chiari I Malformation

Treatment goals in symptomatic Chiari I malformation are to relieve compression at the cervicomedullary junction, restore normal CSF circulation, and minimize syrinx size.[75] The overwhelming majority of surgeries performed to treat Chiari I malformation involve a suboccipital craniectomy at the level of the C1 posterior arch, with or without associated duroplasty.[16,76] Other treatments including tonsillar resection are sparingly performed due to associated complications.[76]

Copresenting Idiopathic Intracranial Hypertension and Chiari I Malformation

Connecting Chiari I and IIH clinically is the Chiari pseudotumor syndrome, in which patients with apparent Chiari I malformation do not respond to Chiari decompression but demonstrate clinical improvement following CSF diversion.[40,42] The reverse process was described by Aiken and colleagues[19] in one patient with tonsillar ectopia greater than 5 mm who required surgical decompression after CSF diversion failed to improve her symptoms.[77] However, this second case seems to be considerably less common than Chiari pseudotumor syndrome. In the context of these findings, workup for IIH in patients with Chiari I malformation may be warranted to anticipate possible treatment failures. Although increased attention has been provided toward venous anomalies in the context of IIH and Chiari I malformation, minimal evidence currently supports targeting venous anomalies to resolve both, with a single case report currently describing sustained improvements in a patient with Chiari I malformation and IIH after VSS.[17] More clinical and translational research is needed to understand the potential relationships between Chiari I, IIH, and venous abnormalities.

SUMMARY

Mounting clinical evidence has identified a relationship between IIH, venous anomalies, and Chiari I malformation, but a precise mechanism explaining the high prevalence of these conditions in tandem with one another continues to elude investigators. There is a clear need for preclinical and translational studies to elucidate the causal

mechanisms of these pathologic conditions in relation to each other. Sustained investigation of the treatment of venous anomalies in IIH may also yield benefits for patients with Chiari I malformation.

CLINICS CARE POINTS

- Patients with Chiari I malformation present with IIH and stenosis of the venous sinuses at an elevated rate.
- Mechanisms explaining the relationship between IIH, Chiari I, and venous anomalies remain elusive.
- Some patients with Chiari I malformation and IIH will fail to respond to posterior fossa decompression and require CSF diversion.
- Further study of VSS may provide superior treatment options for patients with these conditions.

DISCLOSURE

J.W.Osbun is a consultant for Microvention and Medtronic.

REFERENCES

1. Thanki S, Guerrero W, Mokin M. Treatment of Pseudotumor Cerebri (Sinus Stenosis). Neurosurg Clin N Am 2022;33(2):207–14.
2. Mallery RM, Friedman DI, Liu GT. Headache and the pseudotumor cerebri syndrome. Curr Pain Headache Rep 2014;18(9):446.
3. Corbett JJ, Savino PJ, Thompson HS, et al. Visual loss in pseudotumor cerebri. Follow-up of 57 patients from five to 41 years and a profile of 14 patients with permanent severe visual loss. Arch Neurol 1982;39(8):461–74.
4. Friedman DI. The pseudotumor cerebri syndrome. Neurol Clin 2014;32(2):363–96.
5. Toscano S, Lo Fermo S, Reggio E, et al. An update on idiopathic intracranial hypertension in adults: a look at pathophysiology, diagnostic approach and management. J Neurol 2021;268(9):3249–68.
6. Biousse V, Bruce BB, Newman NJ. Update on the pathophysiology and management of idiopathic intracranial hypertension. J Neurol Neurosurg Psychiatry 2012;83(5):488–94.
7. Bloomfield GL, Ridings PC, Blocher CR, et al. A proposed relationship between increased intraabdominal, intrathoracic, and intracranial pressure. Crit Care Med 1997;25(3):496–503.

8. O'Reilly MW, Westgate CS, Hornby C, et al. A unique androgen excess signature in idiopathic intracranial hypertension is linked to cerebrospinal fluid dynamics. JCI Insight 2019;4(6). https://doi.org/10.1172/jci.insight.125348.

9. De Simone R, Ranieri A, Sansone M, et al. Dural sinus collapsibility, idiopathic intracranial hypertension, and the pathogenesis of chronic migraine. Neurol Sci 2019;40(Suppl 1):59–70.

10. Fargen KM. Idiopathic intracranial hypertension is not idiopathic: proposal for a new nomenclature and patient classification. J Neurointerv Surg 2020; 12(2):110–4.

11. Iencean SM, Ciurea AV. Intracranial hypertension: classification and patterns of evolution. J Med Life 2008;1(2):101–7.

12. Levitt MR, Hlubek RJ, Moon K, et al. Incidence and predictors of dural venous sinus pressure gradient in idiopathic intracranial hypertension and non-idiopathic intracranial hypertension headache patients: results from 164 cerebral venograms. J Neurosurg 2017;126(2):347–53.

13. Patsalides A, Oliveira C, Wilcox J, et al. Venous sinus stenting lowers the intracranial pressure in patients with idiopathic intracranial hypertension. J Neurointerv Surg 2019;11(2):175–8.

14. Langridge B, Phillips E, Choi D. Chiari Malformation Type 1: A Systematic Review of Natural History and Conservative Management. World Neurosurg 2017; 104:213–9.

15. Jayamanne C, Fernando L, Mettananda S. Chiari malformation type 1 presenting as unilateral progressive foot drop: a case report and review of literature. BMC Pediatr 2018;18(1):34.

16. Kular S, Cascella M. Chiari I malformation. Stat-Pearls; 2022.

17. Chung CY, John S, Luciano MG, et al. Reduction in Syrinx Size and Severity After Venous Sinus Stenting in a Patient With Pseudotumor Cerebri and Chiari Malformation: Technical Case Report. Oper Neurosurg (Hagerstown) 2016;12(2):E197–201.

18. Fric R, Eide PK. Comparative observational study on the clinical presentation, intracranial volume measurements, and intracranial pressure scores in patients with either Chiari malformation Type I or idiopathic intracranial hypertension. J Neurosurg 2017;126(4):1312–22.

19. Aiken AH, Hoots JA, Saindane AM, et al. Incidence of cerebellar tonsillar ectopia in idiopathic intracranial hypertension: a mimic of the Chiari I malformation. AJNR Am J Neuroradiol 2012;33(10):1901–6.

20. Saindane AM, Bruce BB, Desai NK, et al. Transverse sinus stenosis in adult patients with Chiari malformation type I. AJR Am J Roentgenol 2014;203(4): 890–6.

21. Copeland AE, Hoffman CE, Tsitouras V, et al. Clinical Significance of Venous Anomalies in Syndromic

Craniosynostosis. Plast Reconstr Surg Glob Open 2018;6(1):e1613.

22. Maissen G, Narula G, Strassle C, et al. Functional relationship of arterial blood pressure, central venous pressure and intracranial pressure in the early phase after subarachnoid hemorrhage. Technol Health Care 2021. https://doi.org/10.3233/THC-212956.

23. Riggeal BD, Bruce BB, Saindane AM, et al. Clinical course of idiopathic intracranial hypertension with transverse sinus stenosis. Neurology 2013;80(3): 289–95.

24. Farb RI, Vanek I, Scott JN, et al. Idiopathic intracranial hypertension: the prevalence and morphology of sinovenous stenosis. Neurology 2003;60(9): 1418–24.

25. Higgins JN, Owler BK, Cousins C, et al. Venous sinus stenting for refractory benign intracranial hypertension. Lancet 2002;359(9302):228–30.

26. Higgins JN, Gillard JH, Owler BK, et al. MR venography in idiopathic intracranial hypertension: unappreciated and misunderstood. J Neurol Neurosurg Psychiatry 2004;75(4):621–5.

27. Dinkin M, Oliveira C. Men Are from Mars, Idiopathic Intracranial Hypertension Is from Venous: The Role of Venous Sinus Stenosis and Stenting in Idiopathic Intracranial Hypertension. Semin Neurol 2019;39(6): 692–703.

28. Pollay M. The function and structure of the cerebrospinal fluid outflow system. Cerebrospinal Fluid Res 2010;7:9.

29. Welch K, Friedman V. The cerebrospinal fluid valves. Brain Sep 1960;83:454–69.

30. West JL, Greeneway GP, Garner RM, et al. Correlation between angiographic stenosis and physiologic venous sinus outflow obstruction in idiopathic intracranial hypertension. J Neurointerv Surg 2019; 11(1):90–4.

31. Coffman SA, Singh J, Wolfe S, et al. Unexpected occlusion of the contralateral transverse sinus after stenting for idiopathic intracranial hypertension. Interv Neuroradiol 2018;24(6):718–21.

32. Hedjoudje A, Piveteau A, Gonzalez-Campo C, et al. The Occipital Emissary Vein: A Possible Marker for Pseudotumor Cerebri. AJNR Am J Neuroradiol 2019;40(6):973–8.

33. Fargen KM. A unifying theory explaining venous sinus stenosis and recurrent stenosis following venous sinus stenting in patients with idiopathic intracranial hypertension. J Neurointerv Surg 2021; 13(7):587–92.

34. Buell TJ, Raper DMS, Pomeraniec IJ, et al. Transient resolution of venous sinus stenosis after high-volume lumbar puncture in a patient with idiopathic intracranial hypertension. J Neurosurg 2018;129(1):153–6.

35. Onder H, Gocmen R, Gursoy-Ozdemir Y. Reversible transverse sinus collapse in a patient with idiopathic

intracranial hypertension. J Neurointerv Surg 2016; 8(4):e16.

36. Bejjani GK. Association of the Adult Chiari Malformation and Idiopathic Intracranial Hypertension: more than a coincidence. Med Hypotheses 2003;60(6): 859–63.

37. Bejjani GK, Cockerham KP, Rothfus WE, et al. Treatment of failed Adult Chiari Malformation decompression with CSF drainage: observations in six patients. Acta Neurochir (Wien) 2003;145(2):107–16. discussion 116.

38. Kurschel S, Maier R, Gellner V, et al. Chiari I malformation and intra-cranial hypertension:a case-based review. Childs Nerv Syst 2007;23(8):901–5.

39. Sinclair N, Assaad N, Johnston I. Pseudotumour cerebri occurring in association with the Chiari malformation. J Clin Neurosci 2002;9(1):99–101.

40. Fagan LH, Ferguson S, Yassari R, et al. The Chiari pseudotumor cerebri syndrome: symptom recurrence after decompressive surgery for Chiari malformation type I. Pediatr Neurosurg 2006;42(1):14–9.

41. Banik R, Lin D, Miller NR. Prevalence of Chiari I malformation and cerebellar ectopia in patients with pseudotumor cerebri. J Neurol Sci 2006;247(1):71–5.

42. Alnemari A, Mansour TR, Gregory S, et al. Chiari I malformation with underlying pseudotumor cerebri: Poor symptom relief following posterior decompression surgery. Int J Surg Case Rep 2017;38:136–41.

43. Ahlskog JE, O'Neill BP. Pseudotumor cerebri. Ann Intern Med 1982;97(2):249–56.

44. Giuseffi V, Wall M, Siegel PZ, et al. Symptoms and disease associations in idiopathic intracranial hypertension (pseudotumor cerebri): a case-control study. Neurology 1991;41:239–44, 2 (Pt 1).

45. Round R, Keane JR. The minor symptoms of increased intracranial pressure: 101 patients with benign intracranial hypertension. Neurology 1988; 38(9):1461–4.

46. Wall M, Johnson CA, Cello KE, et al. Visual Field Outcomes for the Idiopathic Intracranial Hypertension Treatment Trial (IIHTT). Invest Ophthalmol Vis Sci 2016;57(3):805–12.

47. Best J, Silvestri G, Burton B, et al. The Incidence of Blindness Due to Idiopathic Intracranial Hypertension in the UK. Open Ophthalmol J 2013;7:26–9.

48. Dandy WE. Intracranial Pressure without Brain Tumor: Diagnosis and Treatment. Ann Surg 1937; 106(4):492–513.

49. Liu KC, Starke RM, Durst CR, et al. Venous sinus stenting for reduction of intracranial pressure in IIH: a prospective pilot study. J Neurosurg 2017; 127(5):1126–33.

50. Committee NIIHSGW, Wall M, McDermott MP, et al. Effect of acetazolamide on visual function in patients with idiopathic intracranial hypertension and mild visual loss: the idiopathic intracranial hypertension treatment trial. JAMA 2014;311(16):1641–51.

51. Aitken LA, Lindan CE, Sidney S, et al. Chiari type I malformation in a pediatric population. Pediatr Neurol 2009;40(6):449–54.

52. Tubbs RS, Beckman J, Naftel RP, et al. Institutional experience with 500 cases of surgically treated pediatric Chiari malformation Type I. J Neurosurg Pediatr 2011;7(3):248–56.

53. Selmi F, Davies KG, Weeks RD. Type I Chiari deformity presenting with profound sinus bradycardia: case report and literature review. Br J Neurosurg 1995;9(4):543–5.

54. Gourishankar A, Belton MD, Hashmi SS, et al. Demographic and clinical features of pediatric patients with orthostatic intolerance and an abnormal head-up tilt table test: A retrospective descriptive study. Pediatr Neonatol 2020;61(1):68–74.

55. Garland EM, Robertson D. Chiari I malformation as a cause of orthostatic intolerance symptoms: a media myth? Am J Med 2001;111(7):546–52.

56. Lawrence BJ, Urbizu A, Allen PA, et al. Cerebellar tonsil ectopia measurement in type I Chiari malformation patients show poor inter-operator reliability. Fluids Barriers CNS 2018;15(1):33.

57. Sinclair AJ, Burdon MA, Nightingale PG, et al. Low energy diet and intracranial pressure in women with idiopathic intracranial hypertension: prospective cohort study. BMJ 2010;341:c2701.

58. Manfield JH, Yu KK, Efthimiou E, et al. Bariatric Surgery or Non-surgical Weight Loss for Idiopathic Intracranial Hypertension? A Systematic Review and Comparison of Meta-analyses. Obes Surg 2017;27(2):513–21.

59. Ball AK, Howman A, Wheatley K, et al. A randomised controlled trial of treatment for idiopathic intracranial hypertension. J Neurol 2011;258(5):874–81.

60. Piper RJ, Kalyvas AV, Young AM, et al. Interventions for idiopathic intracranial hypertension. Cochrane Database Syst Rev 2015;8:CD003434.

61. McCarthy KD, Reed DJ. The effect of acetazolamide and furosemide on cerebrospinal fluid production and choroid plexus carbonic anhydrase activity. J Pharmacol Exp Ther 1974;189(1): 194–201.

62. Panagopoulos GN, Deftereos SN, Tagaris GA, et al. Octreotide: a therapeutic option for idiopathic intracranial hypertension. Neurol Neurophysiol Neurosci 2007;1.

63. Alsuhaibani AH, Carter KD, Nerad JA, et al. Effect of optic nerve sheath fenestration on papilledema of the operated and the contralateral nonoperated eyes in idiopathic intracranial hypertension. Ophthalmology 2011;118(2):412–4.

64. Satti SR, Leishangthem L, Chaudry MI. Meta-Analysis of CSF Diversion Procedures and Dural Venous Sinus Stenting in the Setting of Medically Refractory Idiopathic Intracranial Hypertension. AJNR Am J Neuroradiol 2015;36(10):1899–904.

65. Sinclair AJ, Kuruvath S, Sen D, et al. Is cerebrospinal fluid shunting in idiopathic intracranial hypertension worthwhile? A 10-year review. Cephalalgia 2011;31(16):1627–33.

66. Albuquerque FC, Dashti SR, Hu YC, et al. Intracranial venous sinus stenting for benign intracranial hypertension: clinical indications, technique, and preliminary results. World Neurosurg 2011;75(5–6): 648–52. ; discussion 592-5.

67. Teleb MS, Cziep ME, Issa M, et al. Stenting and angioplasty for idiopathic intracranial hypertension: a case series with clinical, angiographic, ophthalmological, complication, and pressure reporting. J Neuroimaging 2015;25(1):72–80.

68. Funnell JP, Craven CL, Thompson SD, et al. Pulsatile versus non-pulsatile tinnitus in idiopathic intracranial hypertension. Acta Neurochir (Wien) 2018;160(10): 2025–9.

69. Hui FK, Abruzzo T, Ansari SA. Endovascular Interventions for Idiopathic Intracranial Hypertension and Venous Tinnitus: New Horizons. Neuroimaging Clin N Am 2016;26(2):289–99.

70. Zhao P, Jiang C, Lv H, et al. Why does unilateral pulsatile tinnitus occur in patients with idiopathic intracranial hypertension? Neuroradiology 2021;63(2): 209–16.

71. Puffer RC, Mustafa W, Lanzino G. Venous sinus stenting for idiopathic intracranial hypertension: a review of the literature. J Neurointerv Surg 2013; 5(5):483–6.

72. Yang IH, Pereira VM, Lenck S, et al. Endovascular treatment of debilitating tinnitus secondary to cerebral venous sinus abnormalities: a literature review and technical illustration. J Neurointerv Surg 2019; 11(8):841–6.

73. Townsend RK, Jost A, Amans MR, et al. Major complications of dural venous sinus stenting for idiopathic intracranial hypertension: case series and management considerations. J Neurointerv Surg 2022;14(1). https://doi.org/10.1136/neurintsurg-2021-017361.

74. Fargen KM, Kittel C, Amans MR, et al. A national survey of venous sinus stenting practices for idiopathic intracranial hypertension. J Neurointerv Surg 2022. https://doi.org/10.1136/neurintsurg-2022-018832.

75. Zhao JL, Li MH, Wang CL, et al. A Systematic Review of Chiari I Malformation: Techniques and Outcomes. World Neurosurg 2016;88:7–14.

76. Arnautovic A, Splavski B, Boop FA, et al. Pediatric and adult Chiari malformation Type I surgical series 1965-2013: a review of demographics, operative treatment, and outcomes. J Neurosurg Pediatr 2015;15(2):161–77.

77. Vaphiades MS, Eggenberger ER, Miller NR, et al. Resolution of papilledema after neurosurgical decompression for primary Chiari I malformation. Am J Ophthalmol 2002;133(5):673–8.

Cerebrospinal Fluid Leaks, Spontaneous Intracranial Hypotension, and Chiari I Malformation

Rahul Kumar, MD, PhD[a], Jeremy K. Cutsforth-Gregory, MD[b],
Waleed Brinjikji, MD[a,c],*

KEYWORDS

- Spontaneous intracranial hypotension • CSF leak • CSF-Venous fistula • Brain sag
- Chiari malformation

KEY POINTS

- SIH occurs because of cerebrospinal fluid (CSF) leakage across the spinal dural membrane leading to characteristic postural headache and brain sag on cranial imaging.
- Spinal imaging can provide further evidence of CSF leakage while advanced modalities can be used to localize the site of CSF egress.
- A tiered consensus approach for managing spontaneous intracranial hypotension (SIH) patients uses multidisciplinary expertise and progresses through conservative treatment, percutaneous therapies, and surgical interventions.
- Differentiating SIH from other headache causes, such as Chiari malformation I, which can share certain imaging features but are managed differently, is imperative.

INTRODUCTION

Spontaneous intracranial hypotension (SIH) results from transdural egress of cerebrospinal fluid (CSF) in the spine. In contrast to secondary intracranial hypotension caused by iatrogenic dural defects (ie, after lumbar puncture or craniospinal surgery), SIH usually results from one of 3 patterns of spinal CSF leakage: (1) spinal dural rent with associated disc osteophyte, (2) spinal nerve root sleeve diverticulum tear, or (3) CSF-venous fistula. The most common symptom of SIH is headache worsened by upright posture and/or Valsalva maneuver, likely due to decreased buoyant force of intracranial contents leading to brain sagging and traction on pain-sensitive intracranial dura.

Although inclusion of "hypotension" in SIH implies decreased CSF pressure as a *sine non qua* for diagnosis, most patients do not have decreased CSF pressures, and thus radiographic findings consistent with intracranial hypotension have emerged as an important diagnostic marker. Although cranial imaging can be used to suggest a diagnosis of SIH, spinal imaging is necessary to localize CSF leakage and provide a target for definitive intervention. Furthermore, diagnosis of SIH via cranial imaging requires careful distinction from other disease processes, such as Chiari malformations, with some shared radiographic findings but, critically, distinct management approaches.

A multidisciplinary and tiered management paradigm has emerged for SIH. With an increasing reliance on precise localization of CSF leak or fistula with dynamic spinal imaging, technical nuances with many of these approaches may

[a] Department of Neurosurgery, Mayo Clinic, 200 1st Street Southwest, Rochester, MN 55905, USA;
[b] Department of Neurology, Mayo Clinic, 200 1st Street Southwest, Rochester, MN 55905, USA;
[c] Department of Radiology, Mayo Clinic, 200 1st Street Southwest, Rochester, MN 55905, USA
* Corresponding author. 200 1st Street Southwest, Rochester, MN, 55905.
E-mail address: brinjikji.waleed@mayo.edu

Neurosurg Clin N Am 34 (2023) 185–192
https://doi.org/10.1016/j.nec.2022.08.012
1042-3680/23/© 2022 Elsevier Inc. All rights reserved.

Abbreviations	
CM-1	Chiari malformation type I
CVF	CSF-venous fistula
SIH	spontaneous intracranial hypotension
SLEC	spinal longitudinal extradural CSF

influence diagnostic yield. Furthermore, advances in endovascular treatment of CSF-venous fistulas may eliminate the need for invasive spinal surgery in a subset of patients with SIH. Although diagnosis and management of SIH can be nuanced, continued technical and experiential advances will hopefully provide definitive cure for a greater number of patients with this debilitating condition.

EPIDEMIOLOGY AND CLINICAL FEATURES

Annual incidence of SIH across all age groups has been estimated at 4 to 5 per 100,000 based on small community-based studies.[1,2] A higher incidence is becoming apparent, however, as a result of greater practitioner awareness and improved diagnostic criteria.[3–7] Mean patient age is estimated at 45 years with a wide range (childhood to late adulthood) and female predominance (3:2).[8,9]

Orthostatic headache, with intensification in the upright position and improvement with recumbency, is by far the most common symptom in SIH, reported in 98.5% of patients in a meta-analysis of published cases.[10] The orthostatic pattern may be lost over time, with concurrent alterations in CSF fluid dynamics pressures.[5,11] Nonorthostatic headache patterns, including Valsalva-induced, exertional, nonpositional, thunderclap, and even reverse orthostatic, may also occur.[12–14] As such, the differential diagnosis of SIH is broad and includes migraine and other common causes of headache, leading to significant rates of misdiagnosis and diagnostic delay.[6,15,16]

Headache is rarely the only symptom of SIH, and in some patients, it is not present at all. SIH is often accompanied by a constellation of vestibulocochlear symptoms. Dizziness or vertigo occurs in up to half of patients, whereas hearing abnormalities, including both hypoacusis and hyperacusis as well as pulsatile tinnitus, occur in up to one-third.[10] Such symptoms may be attributable to altered pressure gradients across the vestibulocochlear apparatus.[17–20] Given decreased buoyant force conferred by CSF, brain sagging and cranial nerve traction can lead to cranial neuropathies manifesting as facial numbness, diplopia, or dysgeusia.[21–24]

Brain sag may also play a key role in the development of more sinister intracranial pathologic conditions encountered in the setting of SIH. Subdural fluid collections may develop in SIH secondary to traction imposed on the cerebral convexities due to brain sag, leading to hygroma or frank hematoma formation.[25–28] Superficial siderosis may represent a delayed manifestation of recurrent cycles of subclinical bleeding of stretched bridging veins (in the head) or hemorrhage at focal dural defects (in the spine) in patients with SIH.[29–32] Rare instances of cerebral venous sinus thrombosis and coma have been also been identified among patients with SIH.[33–35] The identification and treatment of the underlying spinal CSF leak is fundamental to preventing recurrence of all these sequelae.

PATHOPHYSIOLOGY

CSF leakage across the spinal dura is the cause of SIH. Given that the normal CSF pressure gradient (relative to atmospheric pressure) transitions from negative to positive in the upper cervical region when upright, CSF leakage and associated orthostatic symptoms develop with CSF egress at levels caudal to this equilibrium point.[36] CSF leakage at the level of the skull base has not been associated with SIH except for single report in a young child.[37,38]

Spinal CSF leaks underlying SIH have been classified into 3 types (**Table 1**).[9] Type 1 leaks are identified in approximately 25% of SIH cases and are defined by vertical tears in the spinal dura with Type 1a representing ventral defects (96%) and type 1b representing postero-lateral defects (4%).[9] Type 2 leaks are associated with spinal nerve root diverticula, with type 2a representing simple diverticula (91%) and type 2b corresponding to complex diverticula or dural ectasia (9%). Type 3 leaks consist of CSF-venous fistula (CVF). Although CVF were first described in 2014 and reported to account for approximately 3% of SIH in a 2016 observational series, CVF comprise approximately 50% of SIH cases in our tertiary referral practice.[9,39]

Intrinsic dural deficiency secondary to connective tissue disease has been postulated as an

Table 1
Classification of cerebrospinal fluid leak types in spontaneous intracranial hypotension

	Type 1	Type 2	Type 3
Relative incidence	25%	40%	5%[a]
Pathogenesis	Vertical spinal dural tears	Spinal nerve root diverticula	CSF-venous fistula
Subtypes	1A (ventral) 1B (posterolateral)	2A (simple) 2B (complex)	—
SLEC	Common	Occasional	Rare
Key diagnostic studies	Hyperdynamic CT myelogram		Digital subtraction myelogram
Definitive treatment	Microsurgical exploration and dural repair		Transvenous embolization Microsurgical ligation

[a] Up to one-third of cases may be "indeterminate." In our practice, type 3 CSF leaks accounted for nearly half of cases.

underlying predisposition for SIH in some patients. An increased incidence of dural ectasia, meningeal diverticula, and SIH has been reported in patients with Marfan syndrome (*FBN1* mutation).[40,41] SIH has also been reported in patients with Ehlers-Danlos type II (*COL5A1/2* mutations), Klippel-Trenaunay syndrome (*PIK3CA* mutation), and autosomal dominant polycystic kidney disease (*PKD1/2* mutation).[42–44] Fibrillopathies not meeting major diagnostic criteria but with physical examination findings suggestive of connective tissue disease may occur in up to one-fourth of SIH patients.[40,45,46] Familial incidence of SIH has also been reported.[47]

In type 3 CSF leaks, unidirectional loss of CSF into the venous system through CVF occurs. Abnormal fistulous connection between the spinal subarachnoid space and paraspinal venous system leads to CSF loss without collection in the epidural space, which occurs characteristically in type 1 and 2 CSF leaks. Approximately 80% of fistulous connections originate from nerve root sleeve diverticulum.[48] Although drainage most commonly occurs into a segmental spinal vein, the internal and epidural venous plexuses may also communicate with CVF leading to characteristics imaging findings for each pattern. Although the underlying cause of CVF formation is poorly understood, rupture of proliferated or protruding spinal arachnoid granulations into paraspinal venous complex may result in CVF.[48–50]

DIAGNOSIS

Careful and systematic diagnostic evaluation of patients suspected to have SIH is critical. Given the sensitivity of less than 50% for low opening

pressure (<6 cm CSF), cranial and spinal imaging abnormalities are central to SIH diagnosis, including in the International Classification of Headache Disorders (ICHD-3).[3–5,51] Although cranial imaging only provides indirect evidence of CSF volume depletion in SIH, brain MRI is commonly performed in the initial workup of headache and is the preferred starting point in patients with suspected SIH. Spinal imaging can provide additional information suggestive of causative pathologic condition and directly localize the site of CSF leak to identify a target for treatment. The diagnostic evaluation of SIH generally starts with noninvasive brain and spine MRI, followed by invasive spinal imaging modalities, such as myelography, which can guide downstream therapeutic interventions.[52]

Abnormal findings on brain MRI in SIH can be attributed to intracranial CSF loss, with the Monro-Kellie doctrine dictating a compensatory increase in blood compartment (brain tissue does not expand to fill the space left by lost CSF). Both gadolinium-enhanced and noncontrasted brain MRI can be used in the diagnosis of SIH.[53] Characteristic features include pachymeningeal enhancement/hyperintensity, subdural fluid collections, venous sinus engorgement, pituitary hyperemia, and brain sag.[54] A recent meta-analysis showed pooled estimates for these findings ranging from 20% to 75%. As such, no single imaging finding on brain MRI detects all cases of SIH, and normal findings are reported in approximately 20% of patients.[8] Additionally, interobserver reliability in discerning imaging findings can vary significantly.[4]

Radionuclide cisternography can also be used in the initial diagnostic workup of SIH and can

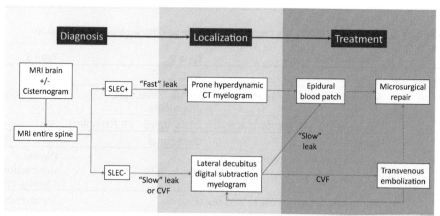

Fig. 1. Management workflow for suspected spontaneous intracranial hypotension. SLEC, spinal longitudinal extradural CSF; CVF, CSF-venous fistula.

provide both direct and indirect evidence of CSF leak.[55] Indirect makers of CSF leak include limited tracer activity at the cerebral convexities coupled with early radiotracer identification in the kidneys/bladder suggestive of rapid systemic uptake via the epidural venous plexus.[56,57] Direct signs of CSF leak include radiotracer accumulation outside of the subarachnoid space but poor spatial resolution can limit precise anatomic localization of CSF leak with cisternography. As such, up to a third of patients undergoing cisternography may fail to exhibit direct signs of CSF leak sufficient for guiding therapeutic intervention.[58]

A wide spectrum of spinal imaging has been used in the diagnostic workup of SIH.[51] Spine MRI can provide evidence of an extradural CSF collection, suggesting the presence of a Type 1 or rarely 2 CSF leak but noninvasive MRI is generally unable to provide precise anatomic localization of CSF leak.[8] More effective myelographic techniques are more invasive and include digital subtraction myelography (DSM), CT myelography, and MR myelography (intrathecal gadolinium is off label).[8,59] In patients with spinal longitudinal extradural CSF (SLEC) identified on MRI of spine suggesting fast CSF leak, our practice is to perform prone hyperdynamic CT myelogram. In patients without SLEC suggesting slow CSF leak or CSF-venous fistula, we favor performing lateral decubitus DSM, particularly in patients with Bern SIH score greater than two.[60]

TREATMENT

A tiered consensus approach for managing SIH patients progresses through conservative treatment, percutaneous therapies, and surgical interventions (**Fig. 1**). The treatment of SIH, much like

its diagnosis, is a multidisciplinary endeavor involving neurology, neuroradiology, and neurosurgery. Definitive management usually hinges on precise anatomic localization of the site of spinal CSF leak, which provides a direct therapeutic target. Conservative management strategies, including bed rest, hydration, theophylline, nonsteroidal anti-inflammatory medications, sodium intake, and caffeine, can be pursued while attempts are made to delineate a therapeutic target.[61–65] Ultimately, conservative management often only plays a temporizing role with less than 10% of patients exhibiting durable response.[66]

Epidural blood patching with autologous blood or fibrin is generally the next step in management on failure of conservative strategies. In nontargeted approaches, approximately 10 to 20 mL of autologous blood is injected into the epidural space. Although some patients may benefit from additional epidural blood patching procedures after initial failure, successive attempts are curative in diminishing subsets of patients.[67,68] In instances of failed site-directed epidural blood patches or those with multiple possible leak sites, large volume procedures using 40 to 70 mL of autologous blood can be used.[69] Response rates vary widely for epidural patching with response rates ranging from 30% to 90% and are confounded by inconsistent patient selection.[66–68,70,71]

DISTINGUISHING CHIARI MALFORMATION AND SPONTANEOUS INTRACRANIAL HYPOTENSION

Although both SIH and Chiari 1 malformation (CM-1) can cause headache, multiple distinguishing features should be noted to prevent inadvertent misdiagnosis (**Table 2**). Both SIH and CM-1 can

Table 2
Differentiating features of spontaneous intracranial hypotension (SIH) and Chiari 1 malformation (CM-1)

	SIH	CM-1
Epidemiology	Children to adults Middle-aged women	Children to adults Symptomatic in early middle age
Pathophysiology	Spontaneous loss of CSF across spinal dura	Congenital crowding of posterior fossa
Presentation	Orthostatic and/or Valsalva headache Vestibulocochlear syndromes Frontotemporal dementia	Occipital-cervical headache aggravated by Valsalva Lower cranial nerve dysfunction Upper cervical cord syndromes Hydrocephalus
Imaging features	Brain sag Pachymeningeal enhancement Subdural fluid collections Cerebral sinus venous engorgement Rare syrinx	Cerebellar tonsillar descent below foramen magnum "Peg-like"/pointed tonsillar morphology Preservation of prepontine cistern Majority with syrinx
Treatment	Percutaneous epidural blood patch Microsurgical repair of spinal dural defect Transvenous embolization of CVF	Suboccipital craniectomy ± expansion duraplasty

be characterized by cerebellar tonsillar ectopia, defined as tonsillar protrusion below the foramen magnum, and headache. CM-1 occurs because of congenitally small posterior fossa and is managed with surgical decompression.[72,73] Given the clinical and radiographic overlap between these 2 conditions, SIH can be misdiagnosed as CM-1 and result in misguided posterior fossa decompression.[6,58,74] Prior reports have described tonsillar descent in SIH as "acquired" or "pseudo" Chiari malformation but such descriptors are confusing and misleading.[36,75,76] "Chiari malformation" should be reserved for cases of congenital structural anomaly, with the cerebellar tonsils instead described as "low-lying" or "ectopic" in patients with SIH. Understanding the underlying pathophysiology of SIH and CM-1 allows recognition of distinct clinical and imaging features and thus facilitates accurate diagnosis.

Headache is a common presenting symptoms in both CM-1 and SIH. In SIH, headache is commonly orthostatic and diffuse compared with CM-1, where headache often localizes to the occipital or upper cervical region and is aggravated by Valsalva or other maneuvers that increase intracranial pressure.[8,77,78] Both conditions can occur across the gamut of age but CM-1 is often diagnosed in early childhood, whereas SIH is more commonly diagnosed in middle age.[8]

Downward herniation of cerebellar tonsils through the foramen magnum is universally identified in patients with CM-1 because of hindbrain crowding. In SIH, CSF loss results in brain sagging, which is characterized by caudal shift of the midbrain relative to the tentorium, downsloping of the third ventricular floor, and flattening of the ventral pons.[79] Morphometric assessments of these characteristics have been incorporated into scoring systems using measurements of the mamillopontine distance (pathologic 6.5 mm or less), prepontine cistern (pathologic 5 mm or less), and suprasellar cistern (pathologic 4 mm or less).[4] Although syringohydromyelia is commonly associated with CM-1 despite a wide range of reported incidence ranging from 25% to 75%, only rare association with SIH have been noted.[80–85] Furthermore, pachymeningeal enhancement and subdural fluid collections are characteristics of SIH but not of CM-1.

DISCLOSURE

No pertinent disclosures related to this study.
Acknowledgment

REFERENCES

1. Schievink WI, Maya MM, Moser F, et al. Frequency of spontaneous intracranial hypotension in the emergency department. J Headache Pain 2007;8(6):325–8.

2. Schievink WI, Maya MM, Moser FG, et al. Incidence of spontaneous intracranial hypotension in a community: Beverly Hills, California, 2006-2020. Cephalalgia 2022;42(4–5):312–6.

3. Headache Classification Committee of the International Headache Society (IHS) The International Classification of Headache Disorders, 3rd edition. Cephalalgia 2018;38(1):1–211.

4. Dobrocky T, Grunder L, Breiding PS, et al. Assessing Spinal Cerebrospinal Fluid Leaks in Spontaneous Intracranial Hypotension With a Scoring System Based on Brain Magnetic Resonance Imaging Findings. JAMA Neurol 2019;76(5):580–7.

5. Kranz PG, Tanpitukpongse TP, Choudhury KR, et al. How common is normal cerebrospinal fluid pressure in spontaneous intracranial hypotension? Cephalalgia 2016;36(13):1209–17.

6. Schievink WI. Misdiagnosis of spontaneous intracranial hypotension. Arch Neurol 2003;60(12):1713–8.

7. Schievink WI, Maya MM, Louy C, et al. Diagnostic criteria for spontaneous spinal CSF leaks and intracranial hypotension. AJNR Am J Neuroradiol 2008; 29(5):853–6.

8. D'Antona L, Jaime Merchan MA, Vassiliou A, et al. Clinical Presentation, Investigation Findings, and Treatment Outcomes of Spontaneous Intracranial Hypotension Syndrome: A Systematic Review and Meta-analysis. JAMA Neurol 2021;78(3):329–37.

9. Schievink WI, Maya MM, Jean-Pierre S, et al. A classification system of spontaneous spinal CSF leaks. Neurology 2016;87(7):673–9.

10. Schievink WI. Spontaneous Intracranial Hypotension. N Engl J Med 2021;385(23):2173–8.

11. Hani L, Fung C, Jesse CM, et al. Insights into the natural history of spontaneous intracranial hypotension from infusion testing. Neurology 2020;95(3):e247–55.

12. Mokri B, Aksamit AJ, Atkinson JL. Paradoxical postural headaches in cerebrospinal fluid leaks. Cephalalgia 2004;24(10):883–7.

13. Chang T, Rodrigo C, Samarakoon L. Spontaneous intracranial hypotension presenting as thunderclap headache: a case report. BMC Res Notes 2015;8:108.

14. Mokri B, Posner JB. Spontaneous intracranial hypotension: the broadening clinical and imaging spectrum of CSF leaks. Neurology 2000;55(12):1771–2.

15. Bond KM, Benson JC, Cutsforth-Gregory JK, et al. Spontaneous Intracranial Hypotension: Atypical Radiologic Appearances, Imaging Mimickers, and Clinical Look-Alikes. AJNR Am J Neuroradiol 2020; 41(8):1339–47.

16. Kim YJ, Cho HY, Seo DW, et al. Misdiagnosis of Spontaneous Intracranial Hypotension as a Risk Factor for Subdural Hematoma. Headache 2017; 57(10):1593–600.

17. Fontaine N, Charpiot A, Debry C, et al. A case of spontaneous intracranial hypotension: from Meniere-like syndrome to cerebral involvement. Eur Ann Otorhinolaryngol Head Neck Dis 2012;129(3):153–6.

18. Schon F, Karunakaran A, Shanmuganathan S, et al. Orthostatic hearing loss: audiovestibular manifestations of spontaneous intracranial hypotension. Pract Neurol 2021;21:61–5.

19. Ferrante E, Olgiati E, Sangalli V, et al. Early pain relief from orthostatic headache and hearing changes in spontaneous intracranial hypotension after epidural blood patch. Acta Neurol Belg 2016; 116(4):503–8.

20. Sakano H, Jafari A, Allehaiby W, et al. Spontaneous Intracranial Hypotension May Be an Under-recognized Cause of Endolymphatic Hydrops. Otol Neurotol 2020;41(7):e860–3.

21. Sajjadi A, Chang I, Djalilian M, et al. Facial Nerve Paralysis Due to Spontaneous Intracranial Hypotension. Ear Nose Throat J 2021;100(3):NP137–8.

22. Cipriani D, Rodriguez B, Hani L, et al. Postural changes in optic nerve and optic nerve sheath diameters in postural orthostatic tachycardia syndrome and spontaneous intracranial hypotension: A cohort study. PLoS One 2019;14(10):e0223484.

23. Fichtner J, Ulrich CT, Fung C, et al. Sonography of the optic nerve sheath diameter before and after microsurgical closure of a dural CSF fistula in patients with spontaneous intracranial hypotension - a consecutive cohort study. Cephalalgia 2019;39(2):306–15.

24. Mokri B, Piepgras DG, Miller GM. Syndrome of orthostatic headaches and diffuse pachymeningeal gadolinium enhancement. Mayo Clin Proc 1997; 72(5):400–13.

25. Beck J, Gralla J, Fung C, et al. Spinal cerebrospinal fluid leak as the cause of chronic subdural hematomas in nongeriatric patients. J Neurosurg 2014; 121(6):1380–7.

26. Schievink WI, Maya MM, Moser FG, et al. Spectrum of subdural fluid collections in spontaneous intracranial hypotension. J Neurosurg 2005;103(4):608–13.

27. Takahashi K, Mima T, Akiba Y. Chronic Subdural Hematoma Associated with Spontaneous Intracranial Hypotension: Therapeutic Strategies and Outcomes of 55 Cases. Neurol Med Chir (Tokyo) 2016;56(2):69–76.

28. Kim JH, Roh H, Yoon WK, et al. Clinical Features of Patients With Spontaneous Intracranial Hypotension Complicated With Bilateral Subdural Fluid Collections. Headache 2019;59(5):775–86.

29. Schievink WI, Maya M, Moser F, et al. Long-term Risks of Persistent Ventral Spinal CSF Leaks in SIH: Superficial Siderosis and Bibrachial Amyotrophy. Neurology 2021;97(19):e1964–70.

30. Kumar N, McKeon A, Rabinstein AA, et al. Superficial siderosis and csf hypovolemia: the defect (dural) in the link. Neurology 2007;69(9):925–6.

31. Schievink WI, Maya MM, Nuno M. Chronic cerebellar hemorrhage in spontaneous intracranial hypotension: association with ventral spinal cerebrospinal fluid leaks: clinical article. J Neurosurg Spine 2011; 15(4):433–40.

32. Webb AJ, Flossmann E, Armstrong RJ. Superficial siderosis following spontaneous intracranial hypotension. Pract Neurol 2015;15(5):382–4.

33. Oien M, Cutsforth-Gregory JK, Garza I, et al. Prevalence of cerebral vein thrombosis among patients with spontaneous intracranial hypotension. Interv Neuroradiol 2021. https://doi.org/10.1177/15910199211065912. 15910199211065912.

34. Takai K, Niimura M, Hongo H, et al. Disturbed Consciousness and Coma: Diagnosis and Management of Intracranial Hypotension Caused by a Spinal Cerebrospinal Fluid Leak. World Neurosurg 2019;121: e700–11.

35. Schievink WI, Maya MM, Moser FG, et al. A serious complication of spontaneous intracranial hypotension. Neurology 2018;90(19):e1638–45.

36. Kranz PG, Gray L, Amrhein TJ. Spontaneous Intracranial Hypotension: 10 Myths and Misperceptions. Headache 2018;58(7):948–59.

37. Schievink WI, Schwartz MS, Maya MM, et al. Lack of causal association between spontaneous intracranial hypotension and cranial cerebrospinal fluid leaks. J Neurosurg 2012;116(4):749–54.

38. Schievink WI, Michael LM 2nd, Maya M, et al. Spontaneous Intracranial Hypotension Due to Skull-Base Cerebrospinal Fluid Leak. Ann Neurol 2021;90(3): 514–6.

39. Schievink WI, Moser FG, Maya MM. CSF-venous fistula in spontaneous intracranial hypotension. Neurology 2014;83(5):472–3.

40. Mokri B, Maher CO, Sencakova D. Spontaneous CSF leaks: underlying disorder of connective tissue. Neurology 2002;58(5):814–6.

41. Fattori R, Nienaber CA, Descovich B, et al. Importance of dural ectasia in phenotypic assessment of Marfan's syndrome. Lancet 1999;354(9182):910–3.

42. Schievink WI, Gordon OK, Tourje J. Connective tissue disorders with spontaneous spinal cerebrospinal fluid leaks and intracranial hypotension: a prospective study. Neurosurgery 2004;54(1):65–70 [discussion: 70–1].

43. Madhavan AA, Kim DK, Carr CM, et al. Association Between Klippel-Trenaunay Syndrome and Spontaneous Intracranial Hypotension: A Report of 4 Patients. World Neurosurg 2020;138:398–403.

44. Schievink WI, Torres VE. Spinal meningeal diverticula in autosomal dominant polycystic kidney disease. Lancet 1997;349(9060):1223–4.

45. Schrijver I, Schievink WI, Godfrey M, et al. Spontaneous spinal cerebrospinal fluid leaks and minor skeletal features of Marfan syndrome: a microfibrillopathy. J Neurosurg 2002;96(3):483–9.

46. Liu FC, Fuh JL, Wang YF, et al. Connective tissue disorders in patients with spontaneous intracranial hypotension. Cephalalgia 2011;31(6):691–5.

47. Larrosa D, Vazquez JL, Mateo I, et al. [Familial spontaneous intracranial hypotension]. Neurologia 2009; 24(7):485–7.

48. Kranz PG, Amrhein TJ, Gray L. CSF Venous Fistulas in Spontaneous Intracranial Hypotension: Imaging Characteristics on Dynamic and CT Myelography. AJR Am J Roentgenol 2017;209(6):1360–6.

49. Kranz PG, Gray L, Malinzak MD, et al. CSF-Venous Fistulas: Anatomy and Diagnostic Imaging. AJR Am J Roentgenol 2021;217(6):1418–29.

50. Kido DK, Gomez DG, Pavese AM Jr, et al. Human spinal arachnoid villi and granulations. Neuroradiology 1976;11(5):221–8.

51. Farb RI, Nicholson PJ, Peng PW, et al. Spontaneous Intracranial Hypotension: A Systematic Imaging Approach for CSF Leak Localization and Management Based on MRI and Digital Subtraction Myelography. AJNR Am J Neuroradiol 2019;40(4):745–53.

52. Dobrocky T, Nicholson P, Hani L, et al. Spontaneous intracranial hypotension: searching for the CSF leak. Lancet Neurol 2022;21(4):369–80.

53. Tosaka M, Sato N, Fujimaki H, et al. Diffuse pachymeningeal hyperintensity and subdural effusion/hematoma detected by fluid-attenuated inversion recovery MR imaging in patients with spontaneous intracranial hypotension. AJNR Am J Neuroradiol 2008;29(6):1164–70.

54. Schievink WI. Spontaneous spinal cerebrospinal fluid leaks and intracranial hypotension. JAMA 2006;295(19):2286–96.

55. Moriyama E, Ogawa T, Nishida A, et al. Quantitative analysis of radioisotope cisternography in the diagnosis of intracranial hypotension. J Neurosurg 2004;101(3):421–6.

56. Sehgal AK, Sethi RS, Raghavan S, et al. Radionuclide cisternography: A prudent investigation in diagnosing spontaneous intracranial hypotension. Indian J Nucl Med 2013;28(1):42–4.

57. Ishihara S, Otani N, Shima K. Spontaneous intracranial hypotension (SIH): the early appearance of urinary bladder activity in RI cisternography is a pathognomonic sign of SIH? Acta Neurochir Suppl 2003;86:587–9.

58. Schievink WI, Meyer FB, Atkinson JL, et al. Spontaneous spinal cerebrospinal fluid leaks and intracranial hypotension. J Neurosurg 1996;84(4):598–605.

59. Chazen JL, Talbott JF, Lantos JE, et al. MR myelography for identification of spinal CSF leak in spontaneous intracranial hypotension. AJNR Am J Neuroradiol 2014;35(10):2007–12.

60. Kim DK, Carr CM, Benson JC, et al. Diagnostic Yield of Lateral Decubitus Digital Subtraction Myelogram Stratified by Brain MRI Findings. Neurology 2021; 96(9):e1312–8.

61. Turek G, Rogala A, Zabek M, et al. Bed regime as a lifesaving factor in spontaneous intracranial hypotension. Neurol Neurochir Pol 2021;55(4):407–9.

62. Tyagi A. Management of spontaneous intracranial hypotension. Pract Neurol 2016;16(2):87–8.

63. Williams EC, Buchbinder BR, Ahmed S, et al. Spontaneous intracranial hypotension: presentation, diagnosis, and treatment. Anesthesiology 2014; 121(6):1327–33.

64. Camann WR, Murray RS, Mushlin PS, et al. Effects of oral caffeine on postdural puncture headache. A double-blind, placebo-controlled trial. Anesth Analg 1990;70(2):181–4.

65. Arshed S, Enakuaa S, Nai Q, et al. A rare case of orthostatic headache due to spontaneous intracranial hypotension. Clin Case Rep 2016;4(2):192–4.

66. Wu JW, Hseu SS, Fuh JL, et al. Factors predicting response to the first epidural blood patch in spontaneous intracranial hypotension. Brain 2017;140(2): 344–52.

67. Sencakova D, Mokri B, McClelland RL. The efficacy of epidural blood patch in spontaneous CSF leaks. Neurology 2001;57(10):1921–3.

68. Berroir S, Loisel B, Ducros A, et al. Early epidural blood patch in spontaneous intracranial hypotension. Neurology 2004;63(10):1950–1.

69. Griauzde J, Gemmete JJ, Chaudhary N, et al. Large-volume blood patch to multiple sites in the epidural space through a single-catheter access site for treatment of spontaneous intracranial hypotension. AJNR Am J Neuroradiol 2014;35(9):1841–6.

70. He FF, Li L, Liu MJ, et al. Targeted Epidural Blood Patch Treatment for Refractory Spontaneous Intracranial Hypotension in China. J Neurol Surg B Skull Base 2018;79(3):217–23.

71. Pagani-Estevez GL, Cutsforth-Gregory JK, Morris JM, et al. Procedural predictors of epidural blood patch efficacy in spontaneous intracranial hypotension. Reg Anesth Pain Med 2019;44:212–20.

72. Stovner LJ, Bergan U, Nilsen G, et al. Posterior cranial fossa dimensions in the Chiari I malformation: relation to pathogenesis and clinical presentation. Neuroradiology 1993;35(2):113–8.

73. McClugage SG, Oakes WJ. The Chiari I malformation. J Neurosurg Pediatr 2019;24(3):217–26.

74. Kingston W, Hoxworth J, Halker-Singh R. Spontaneous intracranial hypotension diagnosed as Chiari I malformation. Neurology 2017;88(13):1294.

75. Haider AS, Sulhan S, Watson IT, et al. Spontaneous Intracranial Hypotension Presenting as a "Pseudo-Chiari 1. Cureus 2017;9(2):e1034.

76. Onal H, Ersen A, Gemici H, et al. Acquired Chiari I Malformation Secondary to Spontaneous Intracranial Hypotension Syndrome and Persistent Hypoglycemia: A Case Report. J Clin Res Pediatr Endocrinol 2018;10(4):391–4.

77. Thunstedt DC, Schmutzer M, Fabritius MP, et al. Headache characteristics and postoperative course in Chiari I malformation. Cephalalgia 2022;42(9): 879–87.

78. Taylor FR, Larkins MV. Headache and Chiari I malformation: clinical presentation, diagnosis, and controversies in management. Curr Pain Headache Rep 2002;6(4):331–7.

79. Houk JL, Amrhein TJ, Gray L, et al. Differentiation of Chiari malformation type 1 and spontaneous intracranial hypotension using objective measurements of midbrain sagging. J Neurosurg 2021;1–8.

80. Milhorat TH, Chou MW, Trinidad EM, et al. Chiari I malformation redefined: clinical and radiographic findings for 364 symptomatic patients. Neurosurgery 1999;44(5):1005–17.

81. Speer MC, Enterline DS, Mehltretter L, et al. Review Article: Chiari Type I Malformation with or Without Syringomyelia: Prevalence and Genetics. J Genet Couns 2003;12(4):297–311.

82. Strahle J, Muraszko KM, Kapurch J, et al. Chiari malformation Type I and syrinx in children undergoing magnetic resonance imaging. J Neurosurg Pediatr 2011;8(2):205–13.

83. Gad KA, Yousem DM. Syringohydromyelia in Patients with Chiari I Malformation: A Retrospective Analysis. AJNR Am J Neuroradiol 2017;38(9): 1833–8.

84. Kranz PG, Viola RJ, Gray L. Resolution of syringohydromyelia with targeted CT-guided epidural blood patching. J Neurosurg 2011;115(3):641–4.

85. Sharma P, Sharma A, Chacko AG. Syringomyelia in spontaneous intracranial hypotension. Case report. J Neurosurg 2001;95(5):905–8.

Printed and bound by CPI Group (UK) Ltd, Croydon, CR0 4YY

08/05/2025

01864715-0018